Urban Health

Urban Health

EDITED BY
SANDRO GALEA, CATHERINE K. ETTMAN,
AND DAVID VLAHOV

OXFORD
UNIVERSITY PRESS

OXFORD
UNIVERSITY PRESS

Oxford University Press is a department of the University of Oxford. It furthers
the University's objective of excellence in research, scholarship, and education
by publishing worldwide. Oxford is a registered trade mark of Oxford University
Press in the UK and certain other countries.

Published in the United States of America by Oxford University Press
198 Madison Avenue, New York, NY 10016, United States of America.

Library of Congress Cataloging-in-Publication Data
Names: Galea, Sandro, editor. | Ettman, Catherine K., editor. |
Vlahov, David, editor.
Title: Urban health / edited by Sandro Galea, Catherine K. Ettman,
David Vlahov.
Other titles: Urban health (Galea)
Description: Oxford ; New York : Oxford University Press, [2019] |
Includes bibliographical references and index.
Identifiers: LCCN 2018046822 | ISBN 9780190915858 (hardcover : alk. paper) |
ISBN 9780190915841 (pbk. : alk. paper)
Subjects: | MESH: Urban Health
Classification: LCC RA566.7 | NLM WA 380 | DDC 362.1/042—dc23
LC record available at https://lccn.loc.gov/2018046822

3 5 7 9 8 6 4 2

Paperback printed by Sheridan Books, Inc., United States of America
Hardback printed by Bridgeport National Bindery, Inc., United States of America

CONTENTS

ACKNOWLEDGMENTS

We are indebted to the editorial guidance of Chad Zimmerman at Oxford, who continues to support our work with unfailing good humor, optimism, and incisive thinking. We would like to acknowledge all our colleagues who have participated in International Society for Urban Health meetings over the years and who contributed to the Journal of Urban Health; they have much sharpened our thinking about the field. As always, we thank our families for their support as we took on this book amidst many other ongoing projects.

CONTRIBUTORS

Yazan A. Al-Ajlouni
School of Medicine, New York
  University, New York, NY

Amélia Augusta de Lima Friche
School of Medicine, Federal University
  of Minas Gerais, Belo Horizonte,
  Brazil

Sanjay Basu
School of Medicine, Stanford University,
  Palo Alto, CA

Renée Boynton-Jarrett
School of Medicine, Boston University,
  Boston, MA

Ben Brisbois
School of Health Sciences, University of
  Northern British Columbia, Prince
  George, Canada

Kathleen A. Cagney
Population Research Center, University
  of Chicago, Chicago, IL

Waleska Teixeira Caiaffa
School of Medicine, Federal University of
  Minas Gerais, and
Observatory for Urban Health,
  Belo Horizonte, Brazil

Brian C. Castrucci
de Beaumont Foundation, Bethesda, MD

Basile Chaix
INSERM, Sorbonne Université, Institut
  Pierre Louis d'Epidémiologie et de
  Santé Publique, Paris, France

Wen Chen
School of Public Health, Sun Yat-Sen
  University, Guangzhou, China

Sally Chew
Vital Strategies, New York, NY

Chris M. Coombe
School of Public Health, University
  of Michigan, Ann Arbor, MI

Jason Corburn
College of Environmental Design,
  School of Public Health, University
  of California Berkeley, Berkeley, CA

Elizabeth A. Corcoran
de Beaumont Foundation,
  Bethesda, MD

Mike Davies
Bartlett School of Environment,
  Energy and Resources, University
  College London,
  London, UK

Carlos Dora
Mailman School of Public Health,
    Columbia University, New York,
    NY, and
World Health Organization, Geneva,
    Switzerland

Dustin T. Duncan
School of Medicine, New York
    University, New York, NY

Alexa K. Eisenberg
School of Public Health, University of
    Michigan, Ann Arbor, MI

Catherine K. Ettman
School of Public Health, Boston
    University, Boston, MA, and
School of Public Health, Brown
    University, Providence, RI

Alex Ezeh
Dornsife School of Public Health, Drexel
    University, Philadelphia, PA, and
School of Public Health, University
    of Witwatersrand, Johannesburg,
    South Africa

Eric Fong
The Chinese University of Hong Kong,
    Shatin, Hong Kong

Nicholas Freudenberg
Graduate School of Public Health and
    Health Policy, City University of
    New York, New York, NY

Sandro Galea
School of Public Health, Boston
    University, Boston, MA

Joseph S. Griffin
School of Public Health, University of
    California Berkeley, Berkeley, CA

Oliver Gruebner
Humboldt-Universität zu Berlin, Berlin,
    Germany, and
University of Zurich, Zurich, Switzerland

Guia Guffanti
McLean Hospital, Belmont, MA

Michael K. Gusmano
School of Public Health, Rutgers,
    the State University of New Jersey,
    Piscataway Township, NJ

Brian J. Hall
University of Macau, Taipa, Macau, and
Bloomberg School of Public Health,
    Johns Hopkins University,
    Baltimore, MD

Shelley L. Hearne
CityHealth, Bethesda, MD

Sabrina Hermosilla
Columbia University, New York, NY

Ilgaz Hisirci
School of Medicine, New York
    University, New York, NY

Christina Honeysett
Vital Strategies, New York, NY

Charity Hung
Vital Strategies, New York, NY

Barbara A. Israel
School of Public Health, University
    of Michigan, Ann Arbor, MI

Lei Jin
The Chinese University of Hong Kong,
    Shatin, Hong Kong

Chris Jones
Regional Plan Association,
New York, NY

Janisha Kamalanathan
Centre for Urban Health Solutions,
St. Michael's Hospital,
Toronto, Canada

Adam Karpati
Vital Strategies, New York, NY

Daniel Kass
Vital Strategies, New York, NY

Katie Keith
CityHealth, Bethesda, MD

Haneen Khreis
Center for Advancing Research in
Transport Emissions, Energy, and
Health, Texas A&M University,
College Station, TX

Patrick L. Kinney
School of Public Health, Boston
University, Boston, MA

Karen Lee
School of Public Health, University
of Alberta, Edmonton, Canada

Teng Ieng Leong
University of Macau, Taipa, Macau

Richard L. Lichtenstein
School of Public Health, University
of Michigan, Ann Arbor, MI

Russ Lopez
Northeastern University, Boston, MA

Thomas Matte
Vital Strategies, New York, NY

Blessing Mberu
African Population and Health Research
Center, Nairobi, Kenya

Layla McCay
Centre for Urban Design and Mental
Health, London, UK

Roshanak Mehdipanah
School of Public Health, University
of Michigan, Ann Arbor, MI

Steven F. Messner
University at Albany, State University
of New York, Albany, NY

Jennifer Karas Montez
Maxwell School of Citizenship and
Public Affairs, Syracuse University,
Syracuse, NY

Sandra Mullin
Vital Strategies, New York, NY

Mark Nieuwenhuijsen
ISGlobal, Centre for Research in
Environmental Epidemiology,
Barcelona, Spain

Patricia O'Campo
Centre for Urban Health Solutions,
St. Michael's Hospital, and
Dalla Lana School of Public
Health, University of Toronto,
Toronto, Canada

Danielle C. Ompad
College of Global Public Health,
New York University, New York, NY

Marisa Otis
School of Public Health, Boston
University, Boston, MA

Edith A. Parker
College of Public Health, University of
Iowa, Iowa City, IA

Catherine Patterson
de Beaumont Foundation, Bethesda, MD

Helen Pineo
Bartlett School of Environment, Energy
and Resources, University College
London, London, UK

Tahilia J. Rebello
Global Mental Health Program,
Columbia University, New York, NY

Angela G. Reyes
Detroit Hispanic Development
Corporation, Detroit, MI

Richard Rodger
School of History, Classics and
Archaeology, University of Edinburgh,
Edinburgh, UK

Ariella Rojhani
Vital Strategies, New York, NY

Zachary Rowe
Friends of Parkside, Detroit, MI

Abby E. Rudolph
College of Public Health, Temple
University, Philadelphia, PA

Jonathan M. Samet
Colorado School of Public Health,
University of Colorado, Colorado State
University, and University of Northern
Colorado, Aurora, CO

Amy J. Schulz
School of Public Health, University
of Michigan, Ann Arbor, MI

Amy Ellen Schwartz
Maxwell School of Citizenship and
Public Affairs, Syracuse University,
Syracuse, NY

Mandu Sen
Regional Plan Association,
New York, NY

Karen C. Seto
School of Forestry and Environmental
Studies, Yale University,
New Haven, CT

James M. Shultz
Center for Disaster and Extreme Event
Preparedness (DEEP Center), Miller
School of Medicine, University of
Miami, Miami, FL

Rohan Simkin
School of Forestry and Environmental
Studies, Yale University,
New Haven, CT

David Siscovick
The New York Academy of Medicine,
New York, NY

John D. Spengler
T. H. Chan School of Public Health,
Harvard University, Cambridge, MA

Shakira F. Suglia
Rollins School of Public Health, Emory
University, Atlanta, GA

Yesim Tozan
College of Global Public Health,
New York University, New York, NY

Alexander C. Tsai
Massachusetts General Hospital,
Boston, MA

Agis D. Tsouros
Imperial College London, Institute
 of Global Health Innovation,
 London, UK

Atheendar S. Venkataramani
Perelman School of Medicine, University
 of Pennsylvania, Philadelphia, PA

David Vlahov
School of Nursing, Yale University,
 New Haven, CT

Matt Vogel
University of Missouri–St. Louis,
 St. Louis, MO

Elizabeth Voyles
CityHealth, Bethesda, MD

Monica L. Wang
School of Public Health, Boston
 University, Boston, MA

Chenyu Ye
The Chinese University of Hong Kong,
 Shatin, Hong Kong

Jie Yin
T. H. Chan School of Public Health,
 Harvard University, Cambridge, MA

Nici Zimmermann
Bartlett School of Environment, Energy
 and Resources, Faculty of the Built
 Environment, University College
 London, London, UK

SECTION I

WHY CITIES, WHY HEALTH?

1

The Present and Future of Cities

SANDRO GALEA, CATHERINE K. ETTMAN, AND DAVID VLAHOV

1 What Is a City?

Cities occupy a special place in our popular imagination. Think of any number of movies—all set, evocatively, in some of the world's most prominent cities; remember the action movies set in New York City, Mumbai, and London, or the romantic comedies set in Casablanca, Paris, and Barcelona. Cities are exciting, dynamic places, populated with a broad range of humanity, where a babel of languages are spoken and food from all over the world is readily available. Cities are also magnets for new arrivals, for migrants from the nearby countryside, and from far flung parts of the world alike. Some of the world's most prominent cities are today populated by more people from other places than people who were born in the country where the city is itself. About 52% of Miami's residents, for example, were born outside the United States, and 46% of residents of Toronto, Canada's largest city, were born outside of Canada.[1,2] This makes cities rapidly evolving places, seats of financial and cultural power, places that set the pace for the rest of the world, places that occupy a particular place in our imagination. And yet, depending on one's perspective, cities are also unsettling, places with higher crime rates than less populated areas, where change happens quickly, upsetting the hard-fought status quo, and where newcomers have to fight to earn their place. Cities are characterized by deep inequalities, where extreme wealth often exists side by side with destitution that would not have been out of place centuries ago. Cultural works, going back to the time of, for example, Charles Dickens, have long captured this duality of cities—places of extraordinary opportunity and yet, at times, unspeakable hardship. More modern literary works—beautifully conveyed recently, for example, in award-winning books by Katherine Boo and Aravind Adiga—combine anthropologic observation with fiction to show much the same picture in rapidly growing Asian cities, where abject poverty exists side by side with gleaming new towers and conspicuous displays of consumption.

And these pictures, varied as they are, all represent the facets—sometimes contradictory, but all equally true—of cities. In many respects these pictures are ahead of the popular imagination. And although our view of cities in movies continues to center on Paris, London, New York City, and perhaps Tokyo, it is the cities of Asia and Africa that have for decades taken center stage as the world's largest, cauldrons of evolution for their populations, shaping the present and the future alike.

Embarking then on a book about cities and health, we start by orienting the reader to what a city actually is. At face value, this seems straightforward. We all have an idea of what a city is—it is a densely populated place, with a densely built environment, sometimes perhaps well planned, at other times characterized by informal urban settlements in lower income countries. These images are also, in their own way, accurate, and when one reflects on them for a moment, it is not hard to realize that any definition of cities must be richly varied and contend with the many ways in which urban settlements have evolved over the past century.

There is, in fact, no single definition of cities, and countries across the world define cities variously. For example, areas with 2,000 or more people are defined as cities in Argentina, with 1,000 or more people in New Zealand. Areas with 50,000 or more people are defined as cities in Japan, and in China, broadly speaking, cities are designated by State Councils as areas with a density of 1,500 or more per square kilometer. Cities are considerably smaller in more sparsely populated countries. In Norway, areas with more than 200 people are considered cities, and populated centers with 100 or more dwellings are considered cities in Peru.[3]

Aiming to better understand first what is a city, we turn to some definitions offered by the United Nations Human Settlements Program. As cities have gown worldwide, today's largest cities are those that have formed together as agglomerations of other cities, becoming mega-cities, or cities with a population of 10 million or more inhabitants.[4] These cities are listed in Table 1.1.

Table 1.1 **Ten most populous urban areas**

Rank	*Urban area*	*Country*	*Population*
1	Tokyo–Yokohama	Japan	38,050,000
2	Jakarta	Indonesia	32,275,000
3	Delhi	India	27,280,000
4	Manila	Philippines	24,650,000
5	Seoul-Incheon	South Korea	24,210,000
6	Shanghai	China	24,115,000
7	Mumbai	India	23,265,000
8	New York City	United States	21,575,000
9	Beijing	China	21,250,000
10	São Paulo	Brazil	21,100,000

Source: Cox W. *Demographia world urban areas*. 14th ed. Self-published. Available at http://demographia.com/db-worldua.pdf. Accessed August 1, 2018.

Table 1.1 lists the largest urban areas in the world. Urban areas include agglomerations of cities and densely populated adjoining regions. All of the five largest urban areas in the world are in Asia, including Tokyo (38.1 million), Jakarta (32.3 million), Delhi (27.3 million), Manila (24.7 million), and Seoul (24.1 million). Tokyo became the largest city in 1955, surpassing New York City, which was the largest city in the world at the time. Since then, Tokyo has topped the list. Japan's population is expected to decline in the coming century, with low immigration, an aging population, and a low birth rate, and, as such, Tokyo's population is expected to do the same. It is estimated that, by 2030, Delhi will surpass Tokyo, with an estimated 39 million living in Delhi compared to 37 million living in Tokyo.[5]

"Cities proper" are defined as municipal regions delineated by political and administrative boundaries.[6] The 10 largest cities are listed in Table 1.2. Half of the top 10 cities proper are in China (Chongqing at 30.2 million, Shanghai at 24.2 million, Beijing at 21.7 million, Guangzhou at 13 million, and Shenzhen at 12.5 million); the other half are in Asia and Africa (Lagos at 16 million, Istanbul at 15 million, Karachi at 15 million, Mumbai at 12.4 million, and Moscow at 12.2 million).

These cities remain, perhaps, the more classically defined conception of cities, with coherent urban agglomerations, well recognized globally as wholes. However, urban areas are also growing through mergers of contiguous urban settlements, and a variety of new configurations include *mega-regions, urban corridors,* and *city-regions.*[4] Examples include China's Hong Kong-Shenzhen-Guangzhou mega-region, with a population of 120 million people, and Japan's Tokyo-Nagoya-Osaka-Kyoto-Kobe mega-region, with a population of 60 million.[7]

Table 1.2 **Ten most populous "cities proper"**

Rank	City	Country	Population
1	Chongqing	China	30,165,500
2	Shanghai	China	24,183,300
3	Beijing	China	21,707,000
4	Lagos	Nigeria	16,060,303
5	Istanbul	Turkey	15,029,231
6	Karachi	Pakistan	14,910,352
7	Guangzhou	China	13,081,000
8	Shenzhen	China	12,528,300
9	Mumbai	India	12,442,373
10	Moscow	Russia	12,229,000

Source: https://en.wikipedia.org/wiki/List_of_cities_proper_by_population#cite_note-renamed_from_2015_on_20160214005959-6.

Table 1.3 shows the top five largest urban agglomerations in the world from 1950 through 2025. In 1950, three of the five largest cities were located in the Western Hemisphere (New York-Newark, London, and Paris). By 2025, none of the five largest urban agglomerations in the world will be in the Western Hemisphere.

With high populations relative to size, the largest urban areas in the world are extraordinarily dense. *Density* refers to the number of people occupying a given physical space, usually captured by the ratio of the total population to land mass. The physical shape of urban areas varies depending on topography, with some being located close to coasts and ports (Tokyo, Jakarta, Manila) and others being land-locked (Delhi, Beijing). A near ubiquitous factor across all populous urban areas, although to varying degrees, is density. The urban area Tokyo-Yokohama has a land area of 3,300 square miles—roughly two-thirds the size of New York City—with a population density of 11,500 people per square mile (New York-New Jersey-Connecticut has a density of 4,500 per square mile).[8] The second most populous urban area is Jakarta, which hosts 32.3 million people. It spans 1,275 square miles and has a population density of 25,300 per square mile.[8] Delhi is growing rapidly, currently the third most populous region, with 27.3 million. Delhi has a land area of 850 square miles, with a density of 32,100 people per square mile. Of the top 10 most populous urban areas, Mumbai, India, boasts the highest density, with 68,400 people per square mile.[8] And, at the extremes, the urban area with the largest density in the world is Dhaka, Bangladesh, with an average of 122,700 people per square mile (of 142 miles total).[8]

Having tightly packed, highly developed space provides both challenges and opportunities for population health. For example, high-density living can promote the rapid spread of vector-borne or infectious disease; similarly, their high density makes cities vulnerable to greater loss from terrorist attacks or mass violence. High-density living also provides opportunities for health: public transportation facilitates greater physical exercise and may reduce automobile use that contributes to air and noise pollution, high-density living can reduce social isolation, and cities can provide access to resources for their populations. Thus, density grows hand in hand with urbanization and will provide opportunities for health as cities continue to grow and expand.

Cities are remarkable in size and density, and their concentrated human capital provides a unique opportunity for business activity, generating wealth and global economic growth. It is estimated that 80% of global gross domestic product (GDP) is generated in cities.[9] Cities are disproportionate economic contributors to the wealth of countries. For example, New York City generates $1.5 trillion in economic activity, which is roughly the same size as the GDP of Canada or Spain and is around 9% of US GDP. Tokyo has an estimated GDP of $1.6 trillion, which is slightly smaller than the GDP of South Korea and, if a country, would be the fifteenth largest economy in the world.[10] Cities across the world generate GDP that is outsized compared to their land mass or populations.

Seeing these areas as economic generators, some countries have even provided special status to these areas to facilitate economic growth. For example, China has deemed the Pearl River Delta (including Guangdong, Shenzhen, Hong Kong, Macau, and other regions around the Pearl River) an economic zone, privy to more open trade and policy regulations than the rest of China. This economic zone creation was successful: while it covers less than 1% of China's land mass, the region generates more than a tenth of its

Table 1.3 **The five largest urban agglomerations ranked by population size at each point in time (1950–2025)**

Rank	1950		1975		2000		2025	
	City	Population (millions)	City	Population (millions)	City	Population (millions)	City	Population (millions)
1	New York-Newark	12.34	Tokyo	26.61	Tokyo	34.45	Tokyo	37.04
2	Tokyo	11.27	Osaka	16.30	Osaka	18.66	Delhi	34.67
3	London	8.361	New York-Newark	15.88	Mexico City	18.46	Shanghai	30.48
4	Osaka	7.01	Mexico City	10.73	New York-Newark	17.81	Dhaka	24.65
5	Paris	6.28	São Paulo	9.61	São Paulo	17.01	Cairo	23.07

Source: Department of Economic and Social Affairs. *World urbanization prospects: the 2018 revision.* New York: United Nations; 2018.

GDP and a quarter of China's exports.[11] With an annual GDP of $1.2 trillion, the Pearl River Delta has been called the "jewel in the crown" of China. The region has grown 12% annually for the past decade and is expected to continue increasing in population. Thus, urban areas attract populations for their economic and employment opportunities, fueling further growth in many regions.

Complementing this trend of urbanization, urban sprawl or suburbanization has also affected the evolution of cities. This includes the spread of populations to lower density regions surrounding high-density cities. Sprawling metropolitan areas may consume greater resources, such as metal, concrete, and asphalt, than compact cities because utilities, homes, and offices are farther apart.[12] As populations spread from urban areas, land is developed in a low-density configuration sometimes described as a "leapfrog" pattern.[13] Residential areas, work areas, and public areas such as parks, shops, and grocery stores are often separate from one another, often due to custom or local zoning. Regional planning may be weak in these areas, setting these spaces far apart and requiring more roads to connect them and higher car use to get from place to place. Lower density development is associated with increased automobile travel; increased car usage is linked with increased pollution, increased motor vehicle deaths, and heat island effects. Health effects associated with urban sprawl include decreased levels of physical activity (due to greater automobile use), increased exposure to road rage (reducing mental health), and potential social isolation.[13] Urban sprawl brings with it both protective and harmful health associations; as urban areas increase in population, the surrounding areas will continue to see increasing population growth and will be faced with its associated challenges.

Therefore, our conception of cities as single entities, readily defined and demarcated, has shifted over time. This then lends itself to some lack of clarity about what a city is across the world. What all these definitions do have in common, however, is that cities are characterized by denser population concentration than other surrounding areas and with commensurate physical development to accommodate their residents. In many respects, these features are the very characteristics that shall be discussed in depth in many chapters in this book and that create the potential for the study of urban health as the study of the forces that shape health in cities.[14]

2 Trends in Urban Living

Even as we start with a static picture of the state of cities today, central to any consideration of cities is their rapid growth and the rise in urban living worldwide. Importantly, the proportion of people living in cities has increased dramatically during the past century. At the turn of the twentieth century, approximately 10% of people lived in cities.[6] Urbanization in the second half of the twentieth century expanded at a rapid pace. In 1950, about 29% of the world's population lived in cities.[15] As seen in Figure 1.1, by 2007, more than half of the world's population lived in cities. In 2015, urban populations accounted for 54% of the world's population. It is projected that, by 2030, 60% of the world's population will reside in urban areas, and, by 2050, 68% of the world's population will live in cities.[6] In absolute terms, between 2000 and 2014, 1 billion additional people were added to cities, and the

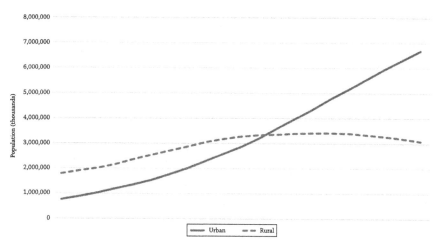

Figure 1.1 **Urban and rural population of the world, 1950–2050.** Source: Department of Economic and Social Affairs. *World urbanization prospects: the 2018 revision.* New York: United Nations; 2018.

world's urban population is expected to grow from 2.86 billion in 2000 to 4.94 billion in 2030.[15] Globally, the urban population is expected to grow approximately 1.5% per year between 2025 and 2030.[16] In absolute and relative terms, populations of urban dwellers have increased in the past century and will continue to increase in the coming 50 years. A variety of processes account for much of this urban growth, including, of course, native growth within cities themselves but also supplemented by growth from migration to cities.

Urbanization is increasing in all parts of the world. In 1950, Northern America, Oceania, and Europe had majority populations living in urban areas. By 2025, all continents except Africa will have majority populations living in cities, with Africa expected to have a majority urban population by 2035.[5]

While urbanization is occurring in all continents across the world, the largest number of people living in urban areas is in Asia. It is estimated that more than 2.1 billion people in Asia live in urban areas (Table 1.4). In Europe almost 550,000,000 people live in urban areas. Thus, Asia has 1.5 billion more people living in its urban areas than the next most populous urban continent; Asia's urban population is greater than the urban populations of all other continents combined. Asia accounts for 53% of the world's total urban population. From a population health perspective, understanding and addressing the health of urban dwellers, particularly in highly populated regions today and in the future, will be key.

In Figure 1.2, we see that urbanization is increasing at a more rapid rate in Africa and Asia relative to other continents. By 2025, 58.9% of Africa's population will live in cities, 66.2% in Asia, 72% in Oceania, 83.7% in Europe, and close to 90% in North America and Latin America.

Of central interest to anyone interested in understanding cities and their role in shaping human health in the coming decades is that much urban growth—estimated at approximately 90%—in the coming half century will take place in low- and

Table 1.4 **Urban populations by continent, 2015**

Continent	Population	Percent of total global urban population
Asia	2,119,873,000	53%
Europe	547,147,000	14%
Latin America and the Caribbean	505,392,000	13%
Africa	491,531,000	12%
Northern America	290,616,000	7%
Oceania	26,938,000	1%
Total	3,981,498,000	100%

Source: Department of Economic and Social Affairs. *World urbanization prospects: the 2018 revision.* New York: United Nations; 2018.

middle-income regions of the world (see Figure 1.3).[17] Over the past 70 years, the pace of urbanization in Asia has outpaced that in Europe. For example, it took London 130 years for the urban population to increase from 1 million to 8 million residents. Meanwhile, it took Bangkok, Dhaka, and Seoul 45, 37, and 25 years, respectively, to grow from 1 million to 8 million inhabitants.[18,19] Indeed, the absolute number of urban inhabitants in Asia in 2000 (1.36 billion) was already greater than the urban populations

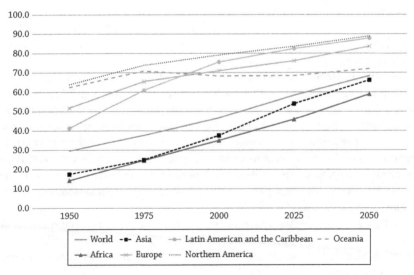

Figure 1.2 **Percentage of population at mid-year residing in urban areas, 1950–2050.**
Source: Department of Economic and Social Affairs. *World urbanization prospects: the 2018 revision.* New York: United Nations; 2018.

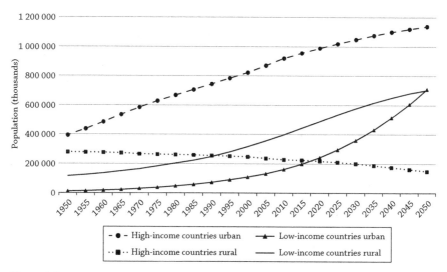

Figure 1.3 **Urbanization in high income versus low income countries, 1950–2050.**
Source: Department of Economic and Social Affairs. *World urbanization prospects: the 2018 revision.*
New York: United Nations; 2018.

in Europe (529 million) and North America (249 million) combined.[18] Between 2010 and 2015, Africa's annual urbanization rate was 1.11%, second only to Asia's (1.4%).[5] By 2050, 55% of the population in Africa will live in cities.[20]

The rate of population growth in low-income countries then is more rapid than that of high-income countries. While absolute urban populations remain higher in high-income countries, the rate of growth in low-income countries is higher. It is estimated that, by 2050, 1.1 billion people will live in urban areas in high-income countries, 4.8 billion people will live in urban areas in middle-income countries, and 700 million people will live in urban areas in low-income countries. Illegal and legal immigration will account for two-thirds of urban growth in high-income countries in the coming decades.[19]

Even as we note the overall trends in urban growth and development—recognizing that urban living is now the modal way of living worldwide—we recognize that there are substantial variations across regions, including urban and nonurban places, as well as within and across cities. While cities lead the world in economic development and in the provision of infrastructure that supports the well-being of their residents, it is estimated that today more than 880 million people live in slum conditions or informal settlements.[21] Projections suggest that, by 2050, closer to 2 billion people will live in slum-like conditions in urban areas if current circumstances remain uncahnged.[22]

3 Urban Health

Cities occupy and are going to increasingly occupy more of our human context. The rapid pace of urbanization is matched only by population aging as the most important human demographic shift over this century and likely going into the next. Simply put, we now live predominantly in cities, and cities shape how we live, where we live, and how we act on a daily basis. This sets the frame for our thinking about urban health and how cities may influence the health of urban populations. A consideration of cities and health does not mean thinking of cities as adverse to human health, nor as cities as generators of human health. Rather, an urban health approach considers cities as the modal form of human living and recognizes that such a commonly felt exposure must, by definition, influence much of what we do and how we do it. As we discuss more fully in Chapter 2, there are a number of conceptual frameworks that can help inform how we understand the influence of cities on our health. At core, however, and by way of framing, we note that we consider cities as one would any other ubiquitous exposure: the city inevitably has an influence on health through shaping all aspects of our context, influencing elements of our environment from the air we breathe to the water we drink, and including how we interact with these environments as we choose those behaviors ultimately influencing our health. Therefore, a concern with urban health is a concern with understanding the elements of the urban environment that may influence human health, drawing from all the various fields that offer insights into the questions at hand—from economics to urban planning, from sociology to epidemiology—and that enable us to understand how it is that cities ultimately *become health*. Importantly, understanding that cities are ubiquitous exposures means that a small change in cities stands to have a substantial change on the health of populations.[23] Thus, this presents an important opportunity to understand how cities shape human health, with the objective of shaping cities so that they can produce health. We consider the ends of urban health to be just that, and this book aims to be a step in that direction.

4 The Book's Approach

This book builds on previous work in the field, aiming to pull together insights from across disciplines to catalyze transdisciplinary interest in urban health.[18,24,25] Therefore, we approach the topic with due respect for the breadth of insight that resides in a number of disciplines that have, each in its own way, contributed to our understanding of how cities shape health. Toward this end, this book is divided into five sections. The first section simply sets the stage. We aimed in this chapter to ground the reader in an appreciation of the ubiquity of cities, setting the stage for a more formal understanding of how cities become health, as discussed in the next chapter. The second section tackles different urban exposures, aiming to elucidate how each of them contributes to health in cities. Therefore, Section II includes chapters about economics, education, housing, transportation, and population demographics. This section also discusses the processes that shape cities and shape health within them, including, for example, migration and the generation of health inequities. We hope that by the end of this section the reader will have a mental map of cities that no longer sees them as an undifferentiated whole when thinking about health, but rather sees the many elements of cities that influence health—positively or negatively—and that are centrally important determinants of urban health. Section III explicitly focuses on cross-disciplinary insights into urban health. Here, we bring together contributions from sociology, biology, urban design, history, and systems science among others to illustrate how each of these perspectives illuminates our understanding about how cities may influence health. Section IV turns its attention to case studies and examples. We aimed here to bring together contributions that talk about specific cities or movements that aspire to create healthier cities. The goal of this section is to illustrate what is possible in efforts to create healthier cities in the hope of motivating, through these examples, other cities' efforts toward building a healthier world. The last section looks forward to core issues in urban health and how we may think of preparing the next generation of scholars and leaders in the field by creating healthy governance and urban health curricula. Throughout, our aspiration was to create a comprehensive book that brings together the state of the science for a field that has been clarifying and emerging over the past two decades. We hope that this book will serve as a springboard for others who will innovate and push the field forward in coming decades. We hope our readers enjoy and learn from the book as much as we have enjoyed and learned from bringing it together.

References

1. Quick facts. Miami-Dade County, Florida. US Census Bureau website. Available at https://www.census.gov/quickfacts/fact/table/miamidadecountyflorida/PST045217. Accessed August 1, 2018.
2. 2016 Census highlights. Factsheet 8. Ontario Ministry of Finance website. Available at https://www.fin.gov.on.ca/en/economy/demographics/census/cenhi16-8.html. Accessed August 1, 2018.
3. What is a city? What is urbanization? Population Reference Bureau website. Available at https://www.prb.org/urbanization/ Accessed August 1, 2018.
4. United Nations. *State of the world's cities 2010/2011–cities for all: bridging the urban divide.* New York: UN-Habitat; 2010.
5. Department of Economic and Social Affairs. *World urbanization prospects: the 2018 revision.* New York: United Nations; 2018.
6. United Nations. *The world's cities in 2016.* New York: United Nations; 2016.
7. United Nations. *State of the world's cities 2004/2005: globalization and urban culture.* New York: UN-Habitat; 2004. Original source: McGee T. Metrofitting the emerging mega-urban regions of ASEAN: an overview. In: McGee T, Robinson I, eds. *The mega-urban regions of Southeast Asia.* Vancouver, Canada: University of British Colombia Press; 1995.
8. Cox W. *Demographia world urban areas.* 14th ed. Self-published. Available at http://demographia.com/db-worldua.pdf. Accessed August 1, 2018.
9. World Bank. Urban development. World Bank Group website. Updated June 22, 2018. Available at http://www.worldbank.org/en/topic/urbandevelopment/overview. Accessed August 18, 2018.
10. Florida R. The economic power of cities compared to nations. City Lab website. March 16, 2017. Available at https://www.citylab.com/life/2017/03/the-economic-power-of-global-cities-compared-to-nations/519294/. Accessed August 17, 2018.
11. Jewel in the crown: what China can learn from the Pearl River delta. *The Economist.* April 8, 2017.
12. McElfish JM. *Ten things wrong with sprawl.* Washington, DC: Environmental Law Institute; 2007.

13. Frumkin H. Urban sprawl and public health. *Public Health Rep.* 2002;117:201–217.

14. Vlahov D, Galea S. Urban health: a new discipline. *Lancet.* 2003;362(9390):1091–1092.

15. Department of Economic and Social Affairs. *World urbanization prospects: the 2003 revision, data tables and highlights.* New York: United Nations; 2004.

16. Department of Economic and Social Affairs. *World urbanization prospects: the 2009 revision.* New York: United Nations; 2010.

17. Department of Economic and Social Affairs. *World urbanization prospects: the 2014 revision highlights.* New York: United Nations; 2014.

18. Galea S, Vlahov D, eds. *Handbook of urban health: populations, methods, and practice.* New York: Springer; 2005.

19. United Nations. *Hidden cities: unmasking and overcoming health inequalities in urban settings.* Kobe, Japan: UN-Habitat; 2010.

20. Sow M. Africa in focus. Foresight Africa 2016: urbanization in the African context. Brookings website. December 30, 2015. Available at https://www.brookings.edu/blog/africa-in-focus/2015/12/30/foresight-africa-2016-urbanization-in-the-african-context/. Accessed August 1, 2018.

21. United Nations. *Millennium development goals report 2015.* New York: United Nations; 2015.

22. United Nations. *State of the world's cities 2012/2013: prosperity of cities.* New York: UN-Habitat; 2013.

23. Keyes K, Galea S. *Population health science.* New York: Oxford University Press; 2016.

24. Freudenberg N, Galea S, Vlahov D, eds. *Cities and the health of the public.* Nashville, TN: Vanderbilt University Press; 2006.

25. Vlahov D, Ivey Bufford JI, Pearson CE, Norris L, eds. *Urban health: global perspectives.* San Francisco, CA: John Wiley & Sons; 2010.

2

Why Cities and Health?

Cities as Determinants of Health

CATHERINE K. ETTMAN, DAVID VLAHOV, AND SANDRO GALEA

1 Cities and Health

In the first chapter, we summarized the increasing role that cities play in our lives, how cities are rapidly becoming the modal form of living worldwide, and how they will become even more so in coming decades. With this ubiquitous role of cities in mind, here we turn our attention to two questions that lie at the heart of urban health scholarship: How do cities influence the health of populations? And, as an equally important question, what is unique or uniquely interesting about urban health? That is, how does the study of urban health distinguish itself from other studies of population health? This chapter addresses these questions by way of providing a conceptual framework that can organize and guide thinking throughout the book, and it sets the stage for subsequent chapters.

1.1 Urban Health as a Population Health Science

We consider urban health to be a field of inquiry that draws on population health science, with an explicit focus on the urban setting. Population health science is concerned with the distributions of health in populations and with the determinants of these distributions.[1] Canonical to population health science is the recognition that it is the forces that influence whole populations that matter most to our collective health and that a focus on ubiquitous characteristics—the forces that shape how we live, what we eat, the air we breathe, and how we behave—stands to explain more about the health of groups than a focus on the individuals who constitute such groups. It is with this lens that we can see urban health as part of a broader intellectual agenda, one that is concerned with understanding the world around us in order to understand the production of health in populations so that we may do something to improve it.

Given this framing, it is then clear why cities matter for health. Given that the majority of the world's population is living in areas we call cities (as discussed in Chapter 1) and given that urban environments shape what we do, how we do it, what we consume, when and what we play, and generally how we behave, it is clear that cities will shape our health and that their very ubiquity makes them important forces to reckon with as we think about the health of populations. This then leads to the second question: How can we understand the influence of cities on health, and how do cities distinguish themselves—how does the study of urban environments stand apart from the study of other forces that shape the health of populations?

1.2 A Multilevel or Eco-Social Approach to Health

Addressing this latter question is well served by drawing on multilevel (also called *eco-social* and *social ecological*) frameworks of health. Over the past two decades, these frameworks have become established as important structures for shaping our views on the health of populations.[2] While there has been much written about these frameworks, multilevel thinking may be summarized simply as shown in Figure 2.1.

As shown in Figure 2.1, we can consider a number of "levels" of the forces that influence health.[3] These forces start with the "highest," "most distal," or "upstream" levels, such as global economic forces, and move on to "lower," "more proximal," or "downstream" levels, such as individual behavior. Features of urban environments reside somewhere midway through these levels. Importantly, the multilevel model, in positioning cities and their features as determinants of health and situating them within the full set of other levels, makes it clear that cities involve a complex set of forces that act on them and also a set of forces within them that act on individual and collective health.

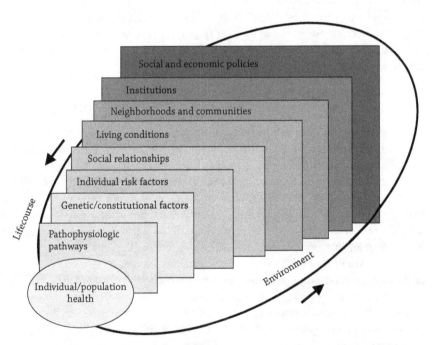

Figure 2.1 **Levels of influence on the health of populations.** Source: Modified from Kaplan, G. What's wrong with social epidemiology, and how can we make it better? *Epid Rev.* 2004; 26:124–135.

This book will present a range of topics that address the full range of levels that influence health. For example, at the highest levels, federal immigration policies shape access to cities at the broadest levels, affecting the health of immigrants and residents alike (Chapter 10). At an institutional level, practices such as predatory lending disproportionately affect minorities, perpetuating inequality and contributing to a host of negative health outcomes for those groups (Chapter 9). In the community, personal relationships matter; for example, studies show that a person's chance of being obese increases by 57% if she has a friend who becomes obese.[4] At the neighborhood level, safety and access to services influence health; Chapter 8 discusses the "popsicle test," which assesses whether children can safely walk to a grocery store and back home before the popsicle melts. The popsicle test includes in it the safety of neighborhoods and is able to capture neighborhood effects such as violence, walkable streets, and access to healthy foods. Closer to home, the houses in which we live affect our health, from the presence of lead in pipes reducing cognitive functioning in children to the presence of rodents contributing to higher rates of asthma (Chapter 5).[5,6] Individual risk factors are similarly affected by external forces: men who have sex with men who were exposed to financial hardship were more likely to engage in risky behavior (condomless sex) than their peers with financial stability (Chapter 24).[7] And finally, at the individual level, behavior is shaped by the options presented, by the context in which people live. For example, persons who live in cities with walkable sidewalks are more likely to walk and persons living in cities with smoking bans are less likely to smoke.[8,9] In all of these ways, health outcomes are shaped by the overlapping levels of influence of the forces that shape health; many of these forces are concentrated or amplified in cities, with urban living itself being a determinant of health at any given level.[10]

1.3 Cities Are Influenced by and Influence Other Drivers of Health

A full appreciation of cities and their contribution to population health requires us to examine cities in their context, to figure how cities are shaped by global and national forces, how cities in turn shape these forces, and how cities play a key role in modifying how these forces are experienced by residents of urban environments. Perhaps this is best understood by way of illustration. Forces such as immigration, changing roles of government, and cultural shifts toward suburbanization are all larger than any one city but they inexorably influence urban characteristics and eventually the health of urban residents.

Let us take immigration by way of example. In 2015, it is estimated that 984 million people—one in seven on the planet—migrated within their country of birth (740 million) or across international borders (244 million).[11,12] There were 19.5 million refugees—migrants who are forced to leave their country due to war or persecution—worldwide at the end of 2014.[13] Therefore, migration is a ubiquitous force worldwide, shaped by the economic, political, and social forces that drive it and in turn shaping these forces.

How then does migration intersect with urban living as a driver of health? Before considering this question, it is worth recognizing that the relation among migration, urban living, and health varies across cites worldwide and also varies for cross-border versus intranational migration. Therefore, in cities in low-income countries, migrants often (at least initially) reside in informal urban settlements (also called "slums," as discussed in Chapter 1) as they drift to urban environments in search of jobs in the formal economy, which are too often few and far between. These slums are characterized by poor infrastructure (i.e., housing, water, sanitation) and few resources and services, all contributing to a high prevalence of disease among residents. Intranational migrants are often marginalized populations who bear a disproportionate burden of the social and economic costs of rapid urbanization. For example, in China, although internal migration has fueled a substantial proportion of urban growth, until recently, the *hukou* registration system has limited the rights and options available to rural-urban migrants, limiting many to social marginalization and limited economic prospects.

The role of migrants to and within high-income countries can be quite different. In high-income countries, global immigrants can be an educated social and economic elite, drawn to rapidly growing urban areas by the prospect of economic gain, contributing to a city's growth, and benefitting from the economic opportunities (and attendant positive health) such cities afford. By contrast, however, cross-border immigrants to higher income countries can also constitute a substantial proportion of the low-skill low-wage workforce, taking on jobs that the native population is unwilling to do. Doha, Qatar, provides an example of international migration, where more than nine-tenths of the population is migrant, making migrants an ineluctable part of the local economy, even if they do not have the rights and endowments that are available to the minority native-born population. In western Europe and North America, migrants are disproportionately engaged in low-wage, physically demanding jobs, thus creating an economic and social underclass within cities that influences the health of these populations and the overall health of the population on aggregate.

Therefore, a quick summary amply illustrates that migrants occupy an important role in sustaining the urban economy, making them part of the urban ecosystem that, in part, sustains and promotes health in cities. At the same time, the urban conditions within which they live, work, and play shape the health of the migrants themselves. Therefore, urban health is inextricable from the forces of migration that are driven, in large part, by forces that are outside of cities themselves—and, just as importantly, these same forces influence other drivers of health in cities. In high-income countries, immigration has become over the past few years one of the defining political issues of our time, influencing elections, choice of elected leaders, and governance decisions. Several countries have elected populist leaders on anti-immigrant platforms, and, similarly, municipal leaders are elected in no small part based on their approach to immigration. The choice of leaders and governance decisions goes on to substantially influence the extent to which cities will influence the health of their resident populations, as we discuss later.

Therefore, cities shape health and are in turn shaped by—and shape—the forces across levels of influence that also produce human health. Importantly, while in this book we are focusing on urban health, we are aware that a full study of urban health requires examining the role of forces beyond cities. Several chapters in this book discuss these forces, aiming to provide the reader with the intellectual tools to consider cities as a part of the complex set of causes that create population health.

2 How Cities Influence Health

Using a multilevel framework, we have introduced political, cultural, and economic factors at more upstream levels that shape the characteristics of cities; here, we turn our attention to the second question posed at this chapter's outset: How is it that cities shape the health of urban populations? Several authors have proposed frameworks that are informative and potentially helpful to this end.[14-16] Some of these frameworks encompass a broad range of more "downstream" forces that intricately link cities to the health of the populations within them. By way of framing the book, we provide a simple formulation—building on published work—to guide the reader through subsequent chapters and illuminate how cities shape health.[16] This formulation emphasizes the consideration of how physical environments, social environments, and resource environments shape health in cities.

2.1 The Built and Physical Environment

We begin with the built environment simply because, in many respects, it accounts for how many of us interact with cities. Cities are a constructed place, and the built environment that surrounds us in cities inevitably shapes what we do in city living, how we live, and, in turn, our health. Think, for example, about obesity—one of the primary epidemics shaping noncommunicable disease health in the first part of the twenty-first century. At core an issue of energy imbalance, obesity represents the confluence of calorie-rich food intake coupled with limited energy expenditure in the form of exercise. Both of these forces—food available to us and opportunity to engage in physical activity—derive from where we live. Ample evidence exists that food environments within cities shape what residents eat and that built environments influence engagement in physical activity.[17,18] In one study, children in Seattle and San Diego who lived in neighborhoods with more access to healthy foods and a better "physical activity environment" were less likely than children living in worse neighborhoods to be obese after adjusting for individual, family, and neighborhood-level demographics.[19]

The urban physical environment includes air, water, and noise; the urban setting influences each of these factors, and they can influence individual and collective health. By way of example, motor vehicle density is much higher in cities than in less populated nonurban areas, contributing to air pollution that may influence health.[20] Globally, the World Health Organization recently linked 7 million premature deaths globally to air pollution.[21] Global air pollution deaths are a product of both outdoor pollution that comes from car exhaust and, especially in developing countries, indoor air pollution from poorly ventilated houses that rely on organic matter to provide heat and cooking fuel. The range of features of the physical environment that influence health are extensive and are covered in Chapters 12, 13, 14, 17, and 28.

2.2 The Social Environment

Cities shape how we interact with one another, what norms are socially acceptable, who we interact with on a regular basis, and who we do not associate with. That then creates features of the social environment that are integral to our behavior and, in turn, to our health. For example, one report documented an inverse association between high levels of neighborhood social cohesion and hypertension.[22] Several social theories have been proposed to account for how and why urban social environments shape health; these include *social disorganization theory*, which is focused on the forces that drive intraurban violence; *social contagion*, which treats patterning of behaviors by residents of densely populated urban areas; and *social stress theory*, which is focused on the insults of daily life in urban areas that have an effect on our health.[23] Chapters 24, 25, and 26 cover aspects of what we call the social environment, illustrating how these forces ultimately "get under the skin" and shape our health.

2.3 The Resource Environment

Ultimately, cities influence our health through the governmental, philanthropic, health service, and other resources that are available to residents. The health of urban populations is heterogenous and determined in no small part by the disparities in resource opportunities available or accessible to those of different socioeconomic status. In urban areas, formal local resources can complement or substitute for individual or family resources, particularly for highly transient urban populations. Therefore, urban stressors can be buffered by salutary resources (e.g., healthcare, social services) that are frequently more prevalent in urban compared to nonurban areas. We illustrate this in our Boston example presented later. This differential exposure to stressors and differential access to resources has been called the *differential vulnerability hypothesis*, and it posits that persons with lower socioeconomic status are both exposed to more stressors and also have fewer resources to help cope with them.[24] It then stands to reason that this may be particularly relevant to cities that are characterized by socioeconomic heterogeneity, an increasingly common feature of cities in the first half of the twenty-first century. Chapters 33, 35, and 38 provide concrete examples of how resource environments shape health in cities, particularly those chapters that focus on urban case studies.

3 A Case Example: The Health of Boston

Perhaps the abstraction of "urban health" becomes clearer by grounding it in an illustration from one city (where two of the editors live), Boston. While Chapter 34 provides more details about Boston as a case study seen through a historical lens, here we summarize briefly health in Boston as a way to introduce the chapters that follow.

Boston is characterized by substantial heterogeneity in health across the city. Life expectancy in this relatively small city varies by as much as 33 years between neighborhoods that are only a couple of miles away from each other, with a high of 91.9 in Back Bay and a low of 58.9 in Roxbury.[25] Premature mortality rates similarly vary across neighborhoods in Boston: Roxbury and South Boston have by far the highest rates of premature mortality, and Back Bay/Beacon Hill have the lowest.[26]

How do urban characteristics in Boston shape the health of the populations who live there? A spatial study by Duncan and colleagues compared open recreational space to neighborhood characteristics and found that neighborhoods with a high proportion of non-Hispanic black residents had significantly less green space, thus increasing the risk of obesity due to lack of physical activity.[27] Another study that focused on physical activity used the 2008 Boston Youth Survey to show a relationship between high social fragmentation in a neighborhood and lower physical activity among adolescents. Consistent with research in other cities, study after study showed that many of the indictors associated with poor health cluster together.[28] The lowest income neighborhoods in Boston coincide with those that have less open green space and worse health outcomes. In many studies, area-level poverty serves as a ready marker for the accumulation of factors that adversely affect health in urban areas. In the study by Chen and colleagues, the authors found that the incidence of premature mortality rates was 1.4 times higher in the most economically deprived census tracts compared to those in the least impoverished tracts. They also found an attributable fraction of 25–30% excess deaths due to living in high-poverty census tracts. These census tracts with the highest poverty have also consistently been found to have the highest proportion of black residents and the lowest levels of education.[29]

Therefore, a quick overview of Boston and its health provides a concise example of how we may approach urban health. Descriptively health in Boston varies tremendously. This variability can in turn be associated with specific aspects of the physical and resource environment that are responsible for these differences. A full study of the determinants of health in Boston requires a grasp of a range of approaches taken from economics, sociology, health services, and epidemiology to name a few—all discussed in other chapters in this book.

4 In Summary: Cities as Determinants of Health

There is ample theoretical reason to suggest that cities influence the health of populations. A multilevel framework helps frame how cities influence the health of populations and also how cities are shaped by other "higher level" forces that shape cities themselves and, in turn, the health of urban residents. Cities then in turn influence the physical, social, and resource environments, and these environments influence the health of urban residents. This framing can help inform inquiry into urban health and practice that aim to improve health in cities. We hope that it also helps organize the reader's thinking throughout the rest of the book as different chapters touch on the elements of this framing.

References

1. Keyes KM, Galea S. *Population health science*. New York: Oxford University Press; 2016.
2. Galea S, Vaughan R. Multilevel thinking and life course perspectives inform public health practice. A public health of consequence. 2018. *Am J Publc Health*. In press.
3. Kaplan, G. What's wrong with social epidemiology, and how can we make it better? *Epid Rev.* 2004; 26:124–135.
4. Christakis NA, Fowler JH. The spread of obesity in large social networks over 32 years. *N Engl J Med.* 2007; 357:370–379.

5. Canfield RL, Jusko TA, Kordas K. Environmental lead exposure and children's cognitive function. *Riv Ital Pediatr.* 2005 Dec; 31(6):293–300.

6. Matsui EC. Environmental exposures and asthma morbidity in children living in urban neighborhoods. *Allergy.* 2014; 69:553–558.

7. Duncan DT, Park SH, Schneider JA, et al. Financial hardship, condomless anal intercourse and HIV risk among men who have sex with men. *AIDS Behav.* 2017; 21(12):3478–3485.

8. Handy SL, Boarnet MG, Ewing R, Killingsworth RE. How the built environment affects physical activity: views from urban planning. *Am J Prev Med.* 2002; 23(2S):64–73.

9. Kilgore EA, Mandel-Ricci J, Johns M. Making it harder to smoke and easier to quit: the effect of 10 years of tobacco control in New York City. *Am J Public Health.* 2014; 104(6): e5–e8. doi: 10.2105/AJPH.2014.301940

10. Vlahov D, Freudenberg N, Proietti F, et al. Urban as a determinant of health. *J Urban Health.* 2007; 84(S):16–26.

11. International Organization for Migration. *World migration report 2018.* Geneva: International Organization for Migration; 2017.

12. United Nations. *International migrant stock: the 2017 revision.* United Nations website. 2017. Available at http://www.un.org/en/development/desa/population/migration/data/estimates2/estimates17.shtml. Accessed May 1, 2018.

13. United Nations High Commissioner for Refugees (UNHCR). Website. Available at http://www.unhcr.org/uk/. Accessed August 1, 2018.

14. Andrulis DP. Community, service, and policy strategies to improve health care access in the changing urban environment. *Am J Public Health.* 2000; 90:858–862.

15. Galea S, Freudenberg N, Vlahov D. Cities and population health. *Soc Sci Med.* 2005; 60(5):1017–1033.

16. Galea S, Vlahov D. Urban health: evidence, challenges, and directions. *Annu Rev Public Health.* 2005; 26:341–365.

17. Belon AP, Nieuwendyk LM, Vallianatos H, Nykiforuk CIJ. Perceived community environmental influences on eating behaviors: a Photovoice analysis. *Soc Sci Med.* 2016; 171:18–29.

18. Giles-Corti B, Giles-Corti R. The relative influence of individual, social and physical environment determinants of physical activity. *Soc Sci Med.* 2002; 54:1793–1812.

19. Saelens BE, Sallis JF, Frank LD, et al. Obesogenic neighborhood environments, child and parent obesity: the Neighborhood Impact on Kids study. *Am J Prev Med.* 2012; 42(5):e57–e64. doi: 10.1016/j.amepre.2012.02.008

20. Fleisch AF, Gold DR, Rifas-Shiman SL, et al. Air pollution exposure and abnormal glucose tolerance during pregnancy: the project Viva cohort. *Environ Health Perspect.* 2014; 122(4):378–383.

21. World Health Organization. 7 million premature deaths annually linked to air pollution. World Health Organization website. 2014. Available at http://www.who.int/mediacentre/news/releases/2014/air-pollution/en/#.UzD4e3UCm-o.twitter. Accessed August 1, 2018.

22. Mujahid MS, Diez Roux AV, Morenoff JD, et al. Neighborhood characteristics and hypertension. *Epidemiol.* 2008; 19(4):590.

23. Galea S, Bresnahan M, Susser S. Mental health in the city. In Freudenberg N, Galea S, Vlahov D, eds. *Cities and the health of the public.* Nashville, TN: Vanderbilt University Press; 2006: 247–276.

24. Pearlin L. Stress and mental health: a conceptual overview. In: Horwitz A, Scheid T., eds. *A handbook for the study of mental health.* Cambridge, UK: Cambridge University Press; 1999: 161–175.

25. Center on Human Needs. *Social capital and health outcomes in Boston. Technical report.* Richmond, VA: Virginia Commonwealth University; 2009.

26. Chen JT, Rehkopf DH, Waterman PD, et al. Mapping and measuring social disparities in premature mortality: the impact of census tract poverty within and across Boston neighborhoods, 1999–2001. *J Urban Health.* 2006; 83(6):1063–1084.

27. Duncan DT, Kawachi I, White K, Williams DR. The geography of recreational open space: influence of neighborhood racial composition and neighborhood poverty. *J Urban Health.* 2013; 90(4):618–631.

28. Pabayo R, Molnar BE, Cradock A, Kawachi I. The relationship between neighborhood socioeconomic characteristics and physical inactivity among adolescents living in Boston, Massachusetts. *Am J Public Health.* 2014; 104(11):e142–e149. doi: 10.2105/ AJPH.2014.302109

29. Boston Public Health Commission. *Health of Boston report 2016–2017.* Available at http:// www.bphc.org/healthdata/health-of-boston-report/Pages/Health-of-Boston-Report.aspx Accessed August 1, 2018.

HEALTH CHALLENGES AND OPPORTUNITIES IN CITIES

Economic Conditions

ATHEENDAR S. VENKATARAMANI AND ALEXANDER C. TSAI

1 Introduction

For centuries, cities have been critical engines for economic development.[1] Urbanization has enabled societies to achieve rapid growth by capturing economies of scale and by allowing efficient coordination of the production and delivery of goods and services.[2] Cities have attracted large, dense populations comprised of individuals with diverse sociocultural backgrounds, thus allowing for the free exchange of ideas necessary for expanding knowledge and human capital, both of which further stimulate growth.[3,4]

The central role of cities in organizing and catalyzing economic activity, along with their rapid growth, have long shaped the economic conditions within them. These conditions have been intimately tied to public health.[5–7] At the broadest level, economic growth is associated with better living conditions.[8] However, economic fortunes have varied both across and within cities.[9] Technological advances and globalization have led to economic inequality, which can create inequality in health outcomes.[10–13] Moreover, the very forces in cities that spur human capital accumulation and economic growth may also generate conflict and instability—which can in turn further influence health.[9]

In this chapter, we discuss connections between economic conditions and health in cities. We start with a historical overview because many parallels can be drawn between the relationships of economic conditions and health in the past and the present. We then discuss the modern context, starting with a statistical portrait of economic and health trends across and within cities. We conclude with a discussion about the critical forces currently shaping economic conditions in today's cities and the implications for health moving forward. Throughout, we will use the example of the United States as it provides a useful case study with which to illustrate the key mechanisms by which economic conditions influence health. Where appropriate, we will also draw on international examples to broaden the scope of discussion.

2 Historical Perspective

Rapid urbanization began during the Industrial Revolution in the nineteenth century. The production of goods were both labor- and capital-intensive, growth in a competitive economy required the generation of new ideas to spur innovation, and transportation costs were high—all of which necessitated agglomerations with high population densities. Individuals flocked to cities, motivated by the promise of upward mobility.

Rapid population growth—along with poor living standards and inadequate infrastructure—created the conditions for poor health to emerge within cities, namely the rapid spread of infectious diseases such as typhoid, cholera, yellow fever, and tuberculosis.[14] The use of fossil fuels such as coal to power both manufacturing and housing in the early Industrial Revolution raised the burden of disease from respiratory illness.[7,15] The elevated burden of disease was disproportionately borne by the poor as richer individuals were able to migrate to safer enclaves, even as the cost of living rose.

Left unattended, worsening public health could have limited the pace of urbanization. However, the early to mid-twentieth century saw dramatic improvements in public health, and the so-called urban (health) penalty disappeared. Some historians suggest that rising living standards—associated with greater access to nutrition, improving education, and improvements in housing—played the dominant role in improving population health.[5,6]

However, the economic conditions of cities also contributed to public health improvements, in two indirect, yet substantial, ways. First, explicit investments in public health infrastructure, such as municipal water disinfection and sewage, appear to have had dramatic impacts on reducing mortality.[7,16] These investments were motivated in part by a growing recognition that the private sector had limited capacity and incentive to provide these services at scale and realized due to innovations in municipal financing.[17] Second, rising inequality and concentrated poverty led to highly visible and dramatic accounts of urban squalor and disease outbreaks. These events precipitated social movements and political responses that were critical in expanding public health investments and regulation.[7,18]

3 Economic Conditions and Health in Modern Cities: The Data

The economic conditions of cities remain strongly linked to health even in the present day. Here, we examine some broad trends from the United States as a means to illustrate this point. Since the mid to late twentieth century, economic inequality in the United States has grown both *between* cities and *within* them.[9] Focusing between cities, Figure 3.1 depicts trends in inflation-adjusted gross domestic product (GDP) per capita over time and across US cities during the twenty-first century. Trends are stratified by GDP per capita in 2001 (highest quartile vs. lowest quartile of GDP per capita). The figure reveals two relevant patterns. First, the economic inequality across cities is vast; average GDP per capita is nearly twice as high in the richest versus poorest sets of cities. Second, these gaps widened over time; the cities richest at baseline grew faster than the poorest cities. This divergence accelerated after the Great Recession (end of 2007 to mid-2009) due to stagnant economic performance in the poorest cities.

The variation in economic conditions across cities and increasing divergence over time is mirrored by similar differences in health outcomes. Figure 3.2 depicts 2001–2014

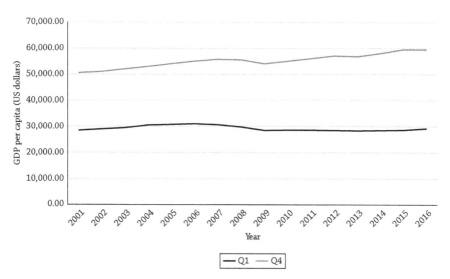

Figure 3.1 **Economic divergence across US cities.** Trends in gross domestic product (GDP) per capita for US metropolitan areas separately for cities in the bottom and top quartiles of per capita GDP in 2001. Source: Bureau of Economic Analysis website. Available at https://www.bea.gov/regional/. Accessed August 25, 2018.

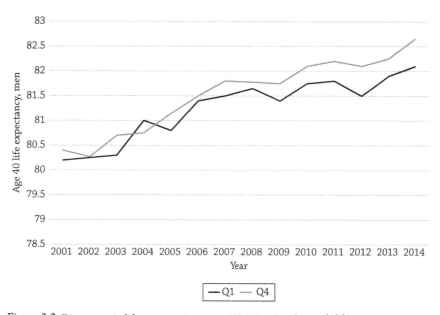

Figure 3.2 **Divergence in life expectancies across US cities.** Trends in male life expectancy at age 40 for US metropolitan areas, separately by commuter zones in the bottom and top quartiles of per capita GDP in 2001. Source: Chetty R, Stepner M, Cutler D, et al. The health inequality project. 2016. Available at https://healthinequality.org/data/. Accessed August 25, 2018.

trends in one measure of population health—overall life expectancy at age 40 (among men)—focusing again on cities in the top and bottom quartiles of GDP per capita in 2001. While the trend lines for the two groups tracked closely with each other through 2006, gaps opened up after the Great Recession, coincident with the increasing rate of divergence in economic fortunes seen in Figure 3.1. Put together, these data suggest that the relationship between economic conditions in cities and health may have grown stronger over time, a point that has been noted in more formal analyses.[13]

The congruent patterns in cities' economic fortunes and life expectancy are consistent with well-known relationships between living standards and health.[5,6,8] However, such comparisons mask substantial heterogeneity *within* city populations. In economic terms, some cities are characterized by much more economic inequality than others. For example, the ratio of the average income of the top 5% of city residents to the ratio of the average in the bottom 20% ranges from 4.5 (Daytona, Florida) to more than 17 (Washington, DC). Recent work suggests that within-city inequality has grown over time, paralleling the diverging fortunes of cities considered as a whole.[19]

Within-city inequalities in health are also substantial. For example, life expectancy gaps between the rich and poor range from under 1 year in Miami, Florida, to more than 16 years in Memphis, Tennessee.[20] These gaps have also grown over time, increasing most sharply in cities that are increasingly lagging in economic performance (Figure 3.3). The growth in life expectancy gaps across cities is largely driven by more sluggish increases in life expectancy among the poor. In addition to differences across the

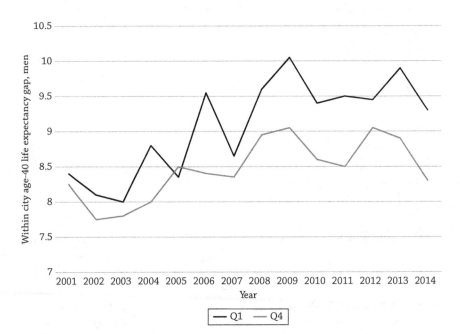

Figure 3.3 **Life expectancy gaps within US cities.** Trends in rich–poor gaps in male life expectancy at age 40 for US metropolitan areas, separately by commuter zones in the bottom and top quartiles of per capita GDP in 2001. Source: Chetty R, Stepner M, Cutler D, et al. The health inequality project. 2016. Available at https://healthinequality.org/data/. Accessed August 25, 2018.

income distribution, another way to quantify within-city variation in health outcomes is by looking across neighborhoods. The variation here, too, is substantial. For example, average life expectancy at birth is nearly 14 years greater in the Loop neighborhood of Chicago, Illinois, versus the Washington Park neighborhood.[21]

These data suggest that economic conditions in cities play an important role in shaping health. We can test this hypothesis more formally. Using data from 2014, we find that just a few coarse economic measures—average household income per capita, percentage of college graduates (a marker of human capital), income inequality, social mobility (as measured by the probability that a child born into a household in the bottom income quintile would ascend to a higher income quintile during adulthood), labor force participation, and population density—explain more than half of the cross-city variation in differences in life expectancy among individuals in the poorest income quartile in the United States.[1,9,22] Greater social mobility, higher college graduation rates, and lower rates of segregation by income are most strongly associated with higher life expectancy among the poor. By contrast, economic measures collectively explain less than 5% of variation in life expectancy in the highest income quartile.

These data yield a set of stylized facts that are helpful in understanding the importance of economic conditions as a driver of health. They also provide insights on key underlying mechanisms, particularly those that are most likely to influence health in the coming decades. We discuss these in detail in the following section.

4 Drivers of Economic Conditions in Cities and Their Implications for Health

Economic inequality both across and within cities is a cardinal feature of the urban environment. This inequality is driven by a number of forces, each of which has important implications for population health.

Research in economics has shown that areas with higher concentrations of educated, highly skilled workers are more productive and will continue to attract more skilled workers, creating a divergence in economic opportunities and outcomes across metropolitan areas over time.[9,23] This self-reinforcing process occurs because skill-driven technological change accelerates economic growth and further raises the monetary returns to additional skills.[3,4] Similarly, cities with higher rates of poverty and unemployment—who therefore cannot benefit from this virtuous cycle—have languished (as we see in Figure 3.1).

Differences in economic fortunes across cities also reflect differences in how skills are rewarded. These monetary returns to high skill have grown over time. Modern economic growth is driven by technological change, which requires knowledge and human capital.[10,24] Cities with a higher concentration of educated workers are best poised to take advantage of these trends. Similarly, technological change has brought increasing automation and routinization to the economy. This, too, has raised the premium for workers in fields that require greater cognitive skills or those working in service-oriented industries.[25] Globalization has exacerbated these trends. Cities with more skilled workers have the opportunity to achieve higher returns to these skills through trade, while cities with a smaller proportion of skilled workers are subject to greater competition from low-wage workers elsewhere in the world.[26]

The patterns described in the previous section—diverging incomes and health outcomes and the strengthening relationship between income, education, and health in cities—speak to the broader importance of these economic forces in driving population health. More directly, a growing body of research demonstrates linkages between economic inequality, social mobility, and a wide range of health behaviors and outcomes.[27–29] Other work has directly linked employment loss from globalization-related exposure to trade to rising mortality.[30] With economic projections suggesting that large numbers of current employment opportunities may eventually succumb to continued automation, either through job loss or declines in real wages, it is likely that health outcomes will continue to diverge across and within cities.[11,27,31–34] Loss of wages or work can jeopardize self-esteem; diminish hope and future expectations; reduce access to pensions, health insurance, and financial resources to invest in health; reduce access to health care; and restrict the ability to preferentially locate to areas free of pollution and disease. Even outside the loss of work, rising income inequality may directly influence health by diminishing the motivation to engage in health behaviors.[35,36]

Rising inequality within cities can substantively affect public health through more indirect channels. Increasing financialization of the economy, regressive tax policies, and the reemergence of monopolies have increased the concentration of wealth among small subsets of the population.[8,12,37] This may lead to the concentration of political power and the subsequent implementation of policies that serve to further wealth concentration at the expense of investments (such as in public health, housing, transportation, or safety-net institutions) that may be consequential for health and well-being among poorer individuals.[38]

These dynamics also are relevant at more local levels. Increasing residential segregation by income within cities follows from income inequality. This may in part be driven by the preferences of more resourced individuals to move within and across cities even with higher costs of living. In addition, residential segregation by income may stem from the maturation of new sectors of the economy (e.g., software development) and the need to leverage economies of scale from close concentrations of skilled workers.[39] The creation of these inevitably richer neighborhoods, which may increasingly become located in more choice areas of the city where environmental and other determinants of health are more favorable, can lead to the concentration of tax resources that allow for higher quality schooling opportunities.[38,40] Further, the high concentration of skilled, resourced workers in these neighborhoods could lead to peer effects that encourage and reinforce human capital accumulation.[41] On the other side, poorer neighborhoods lack these attributes; they would be disadvantaged by poverty and an inability to raise funds to support human capital accumulation and thus experience erosion of social capital.[9] This increasing divergence would serve to exacerbate existing economic inequalities. The strong relationship between neighborhood of residence during childhood and long-run health and economic outcomes observed in recent economic studies suggests that these local inequalities can extend across generations.[42]

Wide within-city variation in socioeconomic status may also generate social unrest. Economic theory suggests that crime and rioting may be viewed as intrinsic consequences of the same forces that make cities critical for economic growth. The close proximity of poor and rich individuals may increase the anticipated return to criminal activity among some individuals.[9] Also, in the same way that innovations in technology and production spread rapidly through cities, so, too, can innovations in criminality or social movements precipitate social unrest or rioting. In an economic framework, criminal organizations or gangs can arise and develop in the same way that cadres of highly skilled professionals can arise. Crime, unrest, and the resulting loss of social cohesion from these processes can also negatively influence health through increasing stress as well as disrupting investments in key health and social services.[43,44]

Importantly, these economic dynamics may most strongly undermine health in traditionally vulnerable populations, such as racial and ethnic minorities. These groups have long had lower access to social and economic opportunities and may thus be more vulnerable to the negative effects of these broader economic forces.[45]

Rapid population growth in cities may exacerbate these general trends, as well as influence health through other pathways. The starkest examples come from low- and middle-income countries. Migrants in these countries arrive in cities for their promise of upward mobility but often do so with low levels of education and employment prospects typically found in low-skilled, low-pay (and sometimes transitory or dangerous) work. Not surprisingly, urban population growth in these areas has come with increasing numbers of workers in the "informal sector," a set of industries that are not regulated or taxed by government authorities, and the rapid proliferation of slums, within which an estimated 30% of urban dwellers in low-income countries now reside.[46,47] Consequently, many new migrants in these cities are exposed to heightened risks of infectious disease and pollution due to living and working conditions while lacking fringe benefits (such as social security, paid sick leave, or insurance).[48] These risks are exacerbated by older infrastructure (such as dilapidated piped water and sanitization facilities) that increasingly are stretched thin by population growth.[49]

However, it is important to note that the continued evolution of the economic forces described in this chapter may have positive consequences for health as well. This is revealed by taking a political perspective. In the United States and Britain, for example, appalling inequality in cities in the early twentieth century spurred dramatic changes to economic and public health policy that resulted in improved population health, particularly among the poor.[7,18] Thus, the tendency for cities to house and exacerbate the extremes of the human condition may also precipitate corrective action. Having populations in close proximity makes it likely that the plight of the impoverished is noticed. Currently, decades of stagnant or diminishing economic fortunes have led to increased agitation from poor and working-class individuals.[12] Subsequently, there has been greater discussion around the plight of these individuals, as well as the need for innovative social policies (e.g., the implementation of a basic income grant) to address growing economic insecurity.[50] In India and China, there have been important developments around environmental regulation brought forth by the exceptionally high burden of disease from air pollution, which is disproportionately borne by the poor.[51] The United Nations includes as one of its Sustainable Development Goals the imperative to make "cities and human settlements inclusive, safe, resilient, and sustainable," motivated specifically by slum conditions in low-income countries.

The experience of the mid-twentieth-century United States offers still other, more positive, clues. Rapid technological progress during this period improved economic circumstances for a broad segment of the population. Indeed, income inequality was falling relative to the early twentieth century. This broadly shared prosperity was driven by large-scale investments in education, the economic and political organization of labor through unions, and the implementation social and financial policies (e.g., expansions of the safety net and progressive taxation) that promoted the growth of a vast middle class.[37,52,53] It is argued that the erosion of these forces may have contributed to the notable rise in income inequality since the 1980s. Moving forward, innovative social policies that allow broader segments of the population to participate in the modern economy and that reduce financial risk from the loss of employment opportunities due to technological change may help decouple the increasingly robust relationship between income distribution and health. Such policies may be particularly salient when taking an intergenerational perspective; for example, boosting early childhood investments can yield high returns in long-run economic well-being and health.[54]

5 Conclusion

An additional 2.5 billion individuals are projected to join the world's cities by 2050.[55] This remarkable projection underscores the central role of cities as engines of economic growth. While economic growth generally leads to improved health, technological change and globalization will create inequality in both economic and health outcomes across and within cities. These changes may particularly threaten health outcomes among vulnerable urban populations—with potential spillover effects on more advantaged populations as well. Population growth driven by the prospects for upward mobility granted by cities will additionally challenge health through stretching existing infrastructure beyond capacity. To address these challenges, policymakers and public health practitioners will have to consider a broad set of interventions, including social and labor market policies, political action, and financial innovations to raise capital for critical infrastructure investments.

References

1. Glaeser EL. *Triumph of the city: how our greatest investment makes us richer, smarter, greener, healthier, and happier.* New York: Penguin; 2011.
2. Krugman P. *Geography and trade.* Cambridge, MA: MIT Press; 1991.
3. Lucas R. On the mechanics of economic development. *J Monet Econ.* 1988; 22:3–42.
4. Romer P. Increasing returns and long run growth. *J Political Econ.* 1986; 90:1257–1278.
5. Costa D. Health and the economy in the United States, from 1750 to the present. *J Econ Lit.* 2015; 53(3):503–570.
6. McKeown T. *The modern rise of population.* New York: Academic Press; 1976.
7. McMichael AJ. The urban environment and health in a world of increasing globalization: issues for developing countries. *Bull World Health Organ.* 2000; 78(9):1117–1126.
8. Deaton A. *The great escape: health, wealth, and the origins of inequality.* Princeton, NJ: Princeton University Press; 2013.
9. Glaeser EL, Resseger M, Tobio K. Inequality in cities. *J Reg Sci.* 2009; 49(4):617–646.
10. Autor D. Skills, education, and the rise of earnings inequality among the "other 99%." *Science.* 2014; 344(6186):843–851.

11. Acemoglu D, Restrepo P. *Robots and jobs: evidence from US labor markets.* Cambridge, MA: National Bureau of Economic Research; 2017. doi:10.3386/w23285

12. Stiglitz J. *The great divide: unequal societies and what we can do about them.* New York: WW Norton & Company; 2016.

13. Bor J, Cohen GH, Galea S. Population health in an era of rising income inequality; USA, 1980-2015. *Lancet.* 2017; 389:1475–1490.

14. Floud R, Fogel RW, Harris B, Hong SC, eds. *Health, mortality, and the standard of living in Europe and North America since 1700, vols. 1 and 2.* Northampton, MA: Edward Elger; 2015.

15. Hanlon WW, Tian Y. Killer cities: past and present. *Am Econ Rev.* 2015; 105(5):570–575.

16. Cutler D, Miller G. The role of public health improvements in health advances. *Demography.* 2005; 42(1):1–22.

17. Cutler D, Miller G. Water, water, everywhere: municipal finance and water supply in American cities. In Glaeser EL, Goldin C, eds. *Corruption and reform: lessons from America's economic history.* Chicago, IL: University of Chicago Press; 2006.

18. Szreter S. Economic growth, disruption, deprivation, disease, and death: on the importance of the politics of public health for development. *Pop Dev Rev.* 1997; 23(4):693–728.

19. Baum-Snow N, Pavan R. Inequality and city size. *Rev Econ Stat.* 2013; 95(5):1535–1548.

20. Chetty R, Stepner M, Lin S, et al. The association between income and life expectancy in the United States, 2001-2014. *JAMA.* 2016; 315(16):1750–1766.

21. Does where you live affect how long you live? Robert Wood Johnson Foundation website. Available at https://www.rwjf.org/en/library/interactives/whereyouliveaffectshowlongyoulive.html. Accessed April 15, 2018.

22. Chetty R, Hendren N, Kline P, Saez E. Where is the land of opportunity? The geography of intergenerational mobility in the United States. *Q J Econ.* 2014; 129(4):1553–1623.

23. Berry CR, Glaeser EL. The divergence of human capital levels across cities. *Pap Reg Sci.* 2005; 84(3):407–444.

24. Autor D, Levy F, Murnane R. The skill content of recent technological change: an empirical exploration. *Q J Econ.* 2003; 118:1279–1333.

25. Autor D, Dorn D. The growth of low-skill service jobs and the polarization of the US labor market. *Am Econ Rev.* 2013; 103(5):1553–1597.

26. Autor D, Dorn D, Hanson GH. The China syndrome: local labor market effects of import competition in the United States. *Am Econ Rev.* 2013; 103(6):2121–2168.

27. Berkman L, Kawachi I, Glymour M, eds. *Social epidemiology.* 2nd ed. New York: Oxford University Press; 2014.

28. Venkataramani A, Chatterjee P, Kawachi I, Tsai A. Economic opportunity, health behaviors, and mortality in the United States. *Am J Public Health.* 2016; 106(3):478–484.

29. Case A, Deaton A. Rising morbidity and mortality in midlife among white non-Hispanic Americans in the 21st century. *Proc Natl Acad Sci U S A.* 2015; 112(49):15078–15083.

30. Pierce J, Schott P. *Trade liberalization and mortality: evidence from U.S. counties.* Cambridge, MA: National Bureau of Economic Research; 2017. doi:10.3386/w22849

31. Cutler D, Huang W, Lleras-Muney A. *Economic conditions and mortality: evidence from 200 years of data.* Cambridge, MA: National Bureau of Economic Research; 2016. doi:10.3386/w22690

32. Ross C, Mirowsky J. Does employment affect health? *J Health Soc Behavior.* 1995; 36(3):230–243.

33. Turner JB. Economic context and the health effects of unemployment. *J Health Soc Behavior.* 1995; 36(3):213–229.

34. Marmot M. *The health gap: the challenge of an unequal world.* London: Bloomsbury Publishing; 2015.

35. Kearney MS, Levine PB. Income inequality, social mobility, and the decision to drop out of high school. *Brookings Pap Econ.* 2016: 333–396.

36. Pickett K, Wilkinson R. Income inequality and health: a causal review. *Soc Sci Med.* 2015; 128:316–326.

37. Hacker J, Pierson P. *Winner-take-all politics: how Washington made the rich richer and turned its back on the middle class.* New York: Simon and Schuster; 2010.

38. Boustan L, Ferreira F, Winkler H, Zolt EM. The effect of rising income inequality on taxation and public expenditures: evidence from US municipalities and school districts, 1970-2000. *Rev Econ Stat.* 2013; 95(4):1291–1302.

39. Berkes E, Gaetani R. Income segregation and the rise of the knowledge economy. Mimeo, Northwestern University. 2018. Available at https://events.barcelonagse.eu/live/files/2127-berkespdf. Accessed August 25, 2018.

40. Hearey O. The effect of rising income inequality across neighborhoods on local school funding and enrollment. Mimeo, University of California, Los Angeles. 2015. Available at https://www.anderson.ucla.edu/Documents/areas/ctr/ziman/2016-15WP.pdf.   Accessed August 25, 2018.

41. Durlauf S. A theory of persistent income inequality. *J Econ Growth.* 1996; 1:75–93.

42. Chetty R, Hendren N. The impacts of neighborhoods on intergenerational mobility II: county-level estimates. *Q J Econ.* 2018; 133(3):1168–1228.

43. Wilkinson R, Pickett K. *The spirit level: why greater equality makes societies stronger.* New York: Bloomsbury; 2010.

44. Wilson M, Daly M. Life expectancy, economic inequality, homicide, and reproductive timing in Chicago neighborhoods. *BMJ.* 1997; 314(7089):1271–1274.

45. Chetty R, Hendren N, Jones MR, Porter SR. Race and economic opportunity in the United States: an intergenerational perspective. Mimeo, Stanford University. 2018. Available at https://scholar.harvard.edu/files/hendren/files/race_paper.pdf. Accessed August 24, 2018.

46. *Women and men in the informal economy: a statistical picture.* 3rd ed. Geneva, Switzerland: International Labor Organization; 2018.

47. Department of Economic and Social Affairs. *Back to our common future: sustainable development in the 21st Century (SD21) Project.* New York: United Nations; 2012.

48. Vlahov D, Freudenberg N, Proietti F, et al. Urban as a determinant of health. *J Urban Health.* 2007; 84(S1):16–26.

49. Bhalotra S, Diaz-Cayeros A, Miller G, Miranda A, Venkataramani AS. *Urban water disinfection and mortality decline in developing countries.* Cambridge, MA: National Bureau of Economic Research; 2017. doi:10.3386/w23239

50. Devarajan S. Three reasons for universal basic income. *Brookings.* February 15, 2017; Available at https://www.brookings.edu/blog/future-development/2017/02/15/three-reasons-for-universal-basic-income/. Accessed April 3, 2018.

51. Catching up with China. *The Economist.* October 10, 2015. Available at https://www.economist.com/news/asia/21672359-prime-minister-wants-india-grow-fast-over-next-20-years-china-has-over-past-20. Accessed September 2, 2018.

52. Goldin C, Katz LF. *The race between education and technology.* Cambridge, MA: Harvard University Press; 2008.

53. Piketty T. *Capital in the twenty-first century.* Cambridge, MA: Harvard University Press; 2014.

54. Heckman JJ. Skill formation and the economics of investing in disadvantaged children. *Science.* 2006; 312(5782):1900–1902.

55. Department of Economic and Social Affairs. *World urbanization prospects: the 2014 revision, highlights.* New York: United Nations; 2014.

4

Reducing Poverty, Improving Health

SANJAY BASU

1 Introduction

Poverty reduction approaches may improve health by addressing the most persistent and central correlate to morbidity and mortality: low income.[1] There is substantial evidence that higher income is correlated to better health outcomes and lower income to worse health outcomes, often because material resources essential for health—nutritious food, safe housing, and the education to make healthy decisions—require adequate income.[2] Hence, numerous actors—governments, international organizations, and community groups—have sought to reduce poverty as a strategy to improve health. In this chapter, I review key historical lessons from efforts to reduce poverty and improve health worldwide.

2 Modesty in the Face of History

In his seminal book on the history of public health, George Rosen catalogues the many ways public health academics and practitioners have attempted to reduce poverty as a strategy to improve health.[3] Rosen catalogues European public health thinkers as far back at the 1840s, who vigorously proposed radical changes to society to address the deep linkage between poverty and disease. The physician Rudolph Virchow in Germany, for example, argued that social inequality ultimately caused the typhus epidemic in Poland and suggested that more democratic government could help avert unequal allocation of resources to poor neighborhoods and associated epidemics of the disease. Similarly, in France, the economist-physician Louis-René Villermé statistically correlated poverty with illness in Paris neighborhoods and proposed radical economic redistribution to allay ailments he considered a consequence of urban overcrowding fueled by poverty. To the dismay of Virchow and Villermé, actual policies implemented were far less ambitious. In Germany, reforms were generally limited to sanitation improvements. In France, local public health councils were formed that had no enforcement powers. The next 100 years did little to improve the reputation that governments often failed to address poverty as a root cause of disease.

In more recent history, public health intellectuals and practitioners have written less radical proposals to address the twin burdens of poverty and disease. Debates following World War II centered around whether it was possible to provide limited and temporary assistance to the poor instead of perpetual assistance.[4] Following the Marshall Plan in Europe and the decline of colonialism in India and Africa, a key question around the concept of economic "development" (a term previously reserved for discussions of a child's growth into puberty) was whether poor countries could lift themselves out of conflict and into prosperity. The Bretton Woods conference that followed World War II established the World Trade Organization (WTO), International Monetary Fund (IMF) and World Bank. The WTO opened up borders to increased import-export business as a strategy for economic growth, while the latter two institutions provided temporary loans premised on the goal of reducing poverty by encouraging business and building infrastructure for roads, power systems, and industry. The debates around war and inequality in the 1960s gave rise to the criticism that poverty was, in fact, persisting despite (or perhaps sometimes because of) such efforts, fueling conflict and indebtedness, with poverty relief programs often serving as a bandage or even political disguise for nefarious profiteering. Popular protests argued that loans were often given to dictators or corporations that exploited or displaced the poor.[4]

The "Decade of Development" declared by the United States in response to such criticism focused international attention on child nutrition and the provision of larger, longer term equipment, drugs, vehicles, and training stipends to organizations such as the United Nations Children's Program (UNICEF) to address concerns about a population explosion and the importance of family planning and childhood vaccination (resulting in the awarding of the Nobel Peace Prize in 1965 to UNICEF).[5] Domestically, the "War on Poverty" in the United States and parallel movements in Europe expanded social welfare legislation, with education and job training programs, food aid, and housing, often in direct response to dire ethnographic descriptions of rural poverty and nutritional deficiencies. Yet the failure of sustained government support and the fickleness of shifting political priorities rendered such interventions temporary, and their health effects were often not formally evaluated.[6]

Some fiscal conservatives grew concerned about their obligations to perpetually spend on lower income groups. Out of their concern grew the formalization of "neoliberalism," spearheaded into policy by Ronald Reagan in the United States, Helmut Kohl in Germany, and Margaret Thatcher in the United Kingdom. The neoliberal mantra stated that private markets would provide a fair alternative to politically fraught state governments; capitalism and free trade would provide a meritocratic basis upon which to grow economies, provide jobs, and lift hard workers out of poverty. The IMF and World Bank occupied a central role in instituting neoliberal policies worldwide, particularly in low-income countries where they conditioned loans on cuts to government spending for social safety-net programs, expecting that such cuts would reduce the risk of inflation and enable private companies to more efficiently fulfill the obligations of public-sector programs. Domestically, in the United States and much of western Europe, similar cuts to social safety nets were accompanied by the encouragement of private equity and large multinational corporate consolidation.[4]

Public health academics and practitioners documented the rise of both poverty and disease, in concert, during the neoliberal era. Far from reducing poverty, the period of neoliberalism was instead characterized by deepening and entrenched poverty, and with it, HIV and tuberculosis. For example, in southern Africa, failures to build public housing and education programs were accompanied by the expansion of private mineral mining initiatives, producing massive seasonal migration of low-wage, unskilled laborers from both cities and rural areas to gold, diamond, and other mineral mines. In this context, prostitution among women increased as a means for subsistence around the mines, spreading HIV. Tuberculosis spread in the crowded hostels occupied by miners, and again spread when the miners returned home.[7-10] In many countries affected by neoliberalism, increased mental illness and substance dependence, including tobacco smoking, alcoholism, and injection drug use, were observed among populations experiencing rising levels of unemployment and low-wage work. The privatization initiative in the former Union of Soviet Socialist Republics (USSR) dramatically cut education and job opportunities for Russian men, corresponding to an incredible rise in alcoholism and in street crimes, incarceration, and tuberculosis among vast Siberian prisons.[11-13] Rapid privatization in East Asia and Latin America was associated with the development of manufacturing sectors that left few options to leave poverty and led to the spread of infectious diseases along migration routes and morbidities (e.g., lung disease, cancers) associated with abundant pollution by the industrial sector.[4,14] Additionally, as global food markets transformed toward processed foods that were easier for large companies to ship across borders, local farming systems collapsed from inadequate support, and agricultural conglomerates made use of surplus corn by converting it to high-fructose corn syrup and transformed palm oil to trans-fat. Cheap processed foods saturated markets worldwide.[15,16] In turn, chronic diseases such as heart disease and type 2 diabetes mellitus began to overlap with infectious disease epidemics in both higher income and, increasingly, lower-income urban populations.

In light of this depressing history, we can ask the question: Can we modestly, but still hopefully, reduce poverty and in turn reduce poverty-related disease?

3 Redistribution-Based Poverty Reduction

Returning to the work of Virchow and Villermé may help us to recalibrate our perspective on poverty and health. In particular, we can revisit their claim that fundamental social and economic forces can be addressed to reduce both poverty and disease.

While the history of neoliberalism is discouraging, recent literature on redistribution programs and health provide hope that fundamental government forces can be aligned to address poverty and related disease. In particular, many communities in Latin America began experimenting during the 1990s and early 2000s with programs to directly redistribute money from wealthier to poorer populations, moving beyond the narrow focus of prior poverty relief programs on material aid or private sector growth. Among the most cited of these efforts is Mexico's PROGRESA program (later called Oportunidades), which redistributed cash to low-income households. As with many of the programs that followed, PROGRESA was a "conditional" cash transfer (CCT) program, meaning that cash was provided as long as families continued to meet certain requirements. For example, children had to be brought to regular health checkups, and mothers had to attend pre- and postpartum health checks and counseling programs.

PROGRESA was associated both with reduction in poverty as well as improvements in a range of metrics for child's growth and nutrition.[17,18] Similar programs in other countries have been associated with improvements in broad metrics of preventive health service utilization and vaccination coverage.[19-22]

One dilemma posed by CCT programs is the question of whether the conditions imposed on participants in such programs are essential or even necessarily beneficial. In some instances, the conditions imposed by transfer programs have led to worse health outcomes. For example, a program in Honduras was associated with increased fertility rates because women needed to be pregnant to receive cash.[23] Similarly, a program in Brazil was associated with problematic weight loss among children because beneficiaries incorrectly thought that at least one malnourished child had to be in each household to continue receiving money from the program.[23] These perverse outcomes highlight the importance of carefully working with community members to ensure that CCT programs have their intended effects. Additionally, CCT programs that require people to attend health clinics or other services require sufficient access to such services. It is perverse to require a mother to attend prenatal care to receive a poverty-relieving cash transfer if adequate prenatal care is not made available. Evaluators of CCT programs have had difficulty understanding which conditions produce good outcomes and which may limit effectiveness because multiple requirements are often entangled together. In many cases, the complex web of requirements may make it difficult to generalize the results of one transfer program to other settings.[21]

To improve redistributive programs, newer studies have examined the impact of unconditional cash transfers. Unconditional transfers remain a rare and early-stage phenomenon at the time of this writing yet emerging data from careful evaluations have already found improvements in the proportion of children receiving necessary medications, attending school, experiencing common illnesses, and incurring high healthcare spending.[24] One of the most important factors that can be addressed with an unconditional transfer is the need for low-income families to have flexibility around how they deal with unanticipated problems. A limitation of traditional material support programs, such as food aid, is that families in poverty often have very volatile incomes and savings, often transferring between informal jobs and having unpredictable debts. For example, poor families may have a surplus of food in one month but not enough money to pay rent. Another month, unexpected illness may lead to medical debts or avoidance of necessary healthcare services to ensure that enough money remains to pay for food and other routine costs.[25] Unconditional cash transfers allow for greater flexibility to address the inherent volatility that often comes with poverty. Nevertheless, it remains unclear how to decide what an appropriate amount of money is to transfer to a family; ongoing work is trying to identify a so-called *threshold effect*, to determine the critical minimum amount of cash that is needed to help buffer poverty-related adversity.[21]

4 Participatory Budgeting

As direct redistribution programs proliferate, an important question is whether it is possible to address not only individual poverty but also systemic neighborhood-level poverty. A key feature of poverty and disease since the time of Virchow and Villermé is the failure of governments to enact policies that fundamentally address the lack of material resources in low-income neighborhoods. Many of the problems that must be addressed to decouple poverty and disease are related to the lack of community resources. Among these are collective resources that would be too expensive for any one individual to purchase for the community based on cash transfer programs alone, such as sanitation infrastructure, clean water resources, environmental cleanups at sites with hazardous waste, improved electrification, building standards that reduce the risk of injury or lung disease, and communal resources, such as markets with healthier food.

One approach to address the challenge of building collective resources for community-level poverty is *participatory budgeting*. Participatory budgeting refers to the process by which community members decide how public funds are spent. In particular, citizens deliberate in groups among themselves and often with government officials during the funding allocation process. Effectively, government meetings where elected representatives previously decided budgets through the closed-door process are instead opened to members of the public and to committees formed by citizens actively and routinely engaging in the budget deliberation process.[26] In Brazil, where participatory budgeting was first codified as a concept, municipalities engaging in participatory budgeting experienced major reallocations of public expenditures toward sanitation and health services and associated declines in infant mortality.[27] Following the Brazilian example, participatory budgeting has expanded to other countries in recent years. Subsequent studies have observed reductions in poverty rates, improvements in education and housing, and associated reductions in morbidity and mortality.[26]

One limiting assumption of participatory budgeting, however, is that there is a sufficient tax base to redistribute wealth. Recent analyses suggest that tax policies are among the most important public policies affecting health funding and associated healthcare coverage; public health funding through a strongly redistributive tax base has in turn been linked to declines in preventable deaths.[26,28] It is important to have a tax base to subject to the participatory budgeting process. Public health academics have yet to comprehensively investigate what strategies may ensure sustained public health funding.

5 Future Efforts to Reduce Poverty and Improve Health

Although the history of public health highlights numerous failures to address the deep linkage between poverty and disease, recent history provides an opportunity for hope. Public health academics and practitioners nevertheless have many challenging questions to address to ensure that early signs of hope can be translated into sustained movement toward reducing poverty and its associated ailments.

One leading question that must be addressed through careful study is the question of what should be measured across the numerous programs and policies enacted simultaneously around the world. Recent reviews of cash transfer programs, for example, have highlighted that different investigations have used very different metrics to measure key outcomes such as child growth and nutrition.[21] Consistently measuring the same

quantity across many different programs and locations will help us to rigorously understand which programs are truly the most effective and in what contexts. Inconsistent
or unreliable measures may prevent potentially successful programs from being widely
adopted.

Related to the problem of measurement is the challenge of communicating how
programs are actually implemented. Anecdotally, we know that the ways in which a program is instituted on the ground is often critical to its actual measured performance. For
example, maintaining a friendly staff and short waiting lines to sign up for a program
may critically affect whether that program has high enrollment and positive outcomes,
even if it transfers less material resources than an alternative program with long waiting
lines and daunting staff. We must create a systematic way to describe how a project or
policy was executed, both to ensure that we understand the health effects of the poverty reduction program and to replicate it widely. Given the extensive online communications infrastructure now available, it should be possible to systematically catalog
the experiences of program participants and administrators online, in repositories that
help to make program details more transparent and thereby facilitate wider knowledge
dissemination—analogous to the strategies used by computer programmers to share
their code, not simply their results.

Finally, as public health remains a relatively elite profession, we must address the
issue of power. Virchow and Villermé are exceptional role models, but they did not ultimately come from the poverty that they described. Enhancing the ability of people
who actually experience poverty and disease to describe their experiences and to engage
in the work of designing and evaluating programs that are intended to address those
experiences may ultimately serve to prevent future catastrophic policy proposals such
as those experienced in the neoliberal era.

Although poverty and disease remain intricately entwined, we now have unique
opportunities to learn across communities worldwide. This potential, and the renewed
desire to address the twin epidemics of poverty and disease, may help us overcome
long-standing challenges to actively addressing our most persistent societal ailments.

References

1. *Poverty and health.* Geneva, Switzerland: World Health Organization; 2003.
2. Sachs J. *Macroeconomics and health: investing in health for economic development: report of the commission on macroeconomics and health.* Geneva, Switzerland: World Health Organization; 2001.
3. Rosen G. *A history of public health.* Baltimore, MD: Johns Hopkins University Press; 1958.
4. Kim JY, Millen J, Irwin A, Gershman J, eds. *Dying for growth: global inequality and the health of
the poor.* Monroe, ME: Common Courage Press; 2000.
5. Bellamy C. *The state of the world's children 1996.* Oxford: Oxford University Press; 1996.
6. Harrington M. *The other America: poverty in the United States.* New York: MacMillan; 1962.
7. Basu S, Stuckler D, Gonsalves G, Lurie M. The production of consumption: addressing the
impact of mineral mining on tuberculosis in southern Africa. *Global Health.* 2009; 5(1):11.
8. Stuckler D, Basu S, McKee M, Lurie M. Mining and risk of tuberculosis in sub-Saharan Africa.
Am J Public Health. 2011; 101(3):524–530.
9. Stuckler D, Steele S, Lurie M, Basu S. "Dying for gold": the effects of mineral mining on HIV,
tuberculosis, silicosis, and occupational diseases in Southern Africa. *Int J Health Serv.* 2013;
43(4):639–649.

10. Basu S. AIDS, empire, and public health behaviorism. *Int J Health Serv*. 2004; 34(1):155–167.

11. Stuckler D, Basu S, McKee M, King L. Mass incarceration can explain population increases in TB and multidrug-resistant TB in European and central Asian countries. *Proc Natl Acad Sci USA*. 2008; 105(36):13280–13285.

12. Stuckler D, King L, Basu S. International monetary fund programs and tuberculosis outcomes in post-communist countries. *PLoS Med*. 2008; 5(7):1079–1090.

13. Stuckler D, King L, McKee M. Mass privatisation and the post-communist mortality crisis: a cross-national analysis. *Lancet*. 2009; 373(9661):399–407.

14. Bello W, Cunningham S, Li KP. *A Siamese tragedy: development and disintegration in modern Thailand*. Oakland, CA: Food First Books; 1998.

15. Patel R. *Stuffed and starved: the hidden battle for the world food system*. New York: Melville House Publishing; 2012.

16. Popkin B. *The world is fat: the fads, trends, policies, and products that are fattening the human race*. New York: Penguin Group; 2009.

17. Gertler P. Do conditional cash transfers improve child health? Evidence from Progresa's control randomized experiment. *Am Econ Rev*. 2004; 94(2):336–341.

18. Rivera JA, Sotres-Alvarez D, Habicht J-P, Shamah T, Villalpando S. Impact of the Mexican program for education, health, and nutrition (Progresa) on rates of growth and anemia in infants and young children. *JAMA*. 2004; 291(21):2563.

19. Karlan D, Appel J. *More than good intentions: how a new economics is helping to solve global poverty*. New York: Penguin Group; 2011.

20. Banerjee AV, Duflo E. *Poor economics: a radical rethinking of the way to fight global Poverty*. New York: Public Affairs; 2011.

21. Lagarde M, Haines A, Palmer N. Conditional cash transfers for improving uptake of health interventions in low- and middle-income countries. *JAMA*. 2007; 298(16):1900.

22. Cohen J, Easterly W, eds. *What works in development? Thinking big and thinking small*. Washington, DC: Brookings Institution Press; 2009.

23. Morris S, Olinto P, Flores R, Nilson E, Figueiró A. Conditional cash transfers are associated with a small reduction in the rate of weight gain of preschool children in northeast Brazil. *J Nutr*. 2004; 134(9):2336–2341.

24. Pega F, Liu SY, Walter S, Pabayo R, Saith R, Lhachimi SK. Unconditional cash transfers for reducing poverty and vulnerabilities: effect on use of health services and health outcomes in low- and middle-income countries. *Cochrane Database Syst Rev*. 2017; 11. doi:10.1002/14651858.CD011135.pub2

25. Basu S. Income volatility: a preventable public health threat. *Am J Public Health*. 2017; 107(12):1898–1899.

26. Gilman HR. *Democracy reinvented : participatory budgeting and civic innovation in America*. Washington, DC: Brookings Institution Press; 2016.

27. Gonçalves S. The effects of participatory budgeting on municipal expenditures and infant mortality in Brazil. *World Dev*. 2014; 53:94–110.

28. Reeves A, Gourtsoyannis Y, Basu S, McCoy D, McKee M, Stuckler D. Financing universal health coverage—effects of alternative tax structures on public health systems: cross-national modelling in 89 low-income and middle-income countries. *Lancet*. 2015;386(9990):274–280.

5

Housing

ROSHANAK MEHDIPANAH, ALEXA K. EISENBERG, AND AMY J. SCHULZ

1 Housing and Health Overview

Housing is a multidimensional determinant of health. Affordability, access, and the conditions of housing all contribute to health independently and jointly. Understanding the relationship between housing and health requires consideration of the policy-, community-, and individual-level factors that operate independently and collectively to pattern population health outcomes. Socioecological models of housing, as shown in Figure 5.1, illustrate multiple layers of influence shaping dimensions of housing and their effects on health.

Much of the literature to date has focused on understanding housing and health at the two innermost layers of this conceptual model: community or neighborhood and individual levels. For example, place-based research has focused on health effects of housing location in terms of the physical (e.g., access to healthy foods and parks, exposure to pollutants), social (e.g., race-based segregation, crime, social capital), and economic (e.g., poverty, employment opportunities, educational investment) contexts or neighborhoods in which people live.[1,2] Research at the individual level has examined the health implications of housing access and conditions. Historically, most studies have focused on overcrowding and physical conditions (e.g., dampness, mold, toxins, energy efficiency) and found associations with health such as asthma, heart disease, and mortality.[3-6] More recent research has increasingly focused on access, which includes affordability and instability (e.g., foreclosures and evictions), and its consequences for the health of those affected.[7,8] Only rarely have these studies encompassed examination of the social, historical, and geographic contexts in which these processes take place.

Extending studies to consider the political and economic systems (macro-level) as well as housing policies and real estate markets (meso-level) shown in Figure 5.1 can expand our understanding of housing as a public health issue. Specifically, situating housing within the context of macro- and meso-levels of a social ecological model shifts the lens more explicitly to a health equity framework that links housing systems to health inequities through multiple, intersecting pathways. At the macro level, political and economic systems vary across cities, with implications for democratic decision-making and market-based economies.[9] At the local level, housing systems shape neighborhood inequalities including, for example, racial residential segregation and the resulting misdistribution of

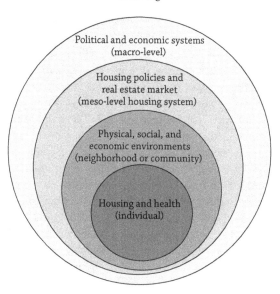

Figure 5.1 **Socio-ecological model of housing.**

access to resources.[1] As described herein, historical and contemporary patterns of housing discrimination have led to disproportionate representation of people of color and other ethnic minorities in neighborhoods with older and poorly maintained homes, resulting in disparities across neighborhoods and, ultimately, health inequities.[10,11]

Expanding research on housing and health examines the relationship between housing and various mental and physical health outcomes. Much of the literature considering affordability and access has examined the acute impact on mental health, including symptoms of depression and anxiety, and the long-term effects on stress manifested through outcomes like blood pressure.[7,8,12,13] In addition to mental health outcomes, the implications of poor housing conditions and asthma, allergies, poisoning (e.g., lead and asbestos), and pest–related diseases have been discussed.[14-16] In some studies, the increase of infectious diseases like tuberculosis has been studied in relation to overcrowded conditions.[17] Throughout this chapter, we discuss how the multiple dimensions of housing systematically affect these and other outcomes and ultimately influence health equity at the population level.

While the issue of housing and health is an international one, this chapter draws primarily on examples from the United States, returning later to the global context for the discussion of next steps. First, guided by the social-ecological framework described earlier, we briefly review the literature linking housing with health and health inequities, organized in three overarching dimensions: housing affordability, access, and condition.

2 Housing Affordability

Housing affordability is a critical urban health issue, particularly as increasing proportions of the world's population migrate to urban areas.[18] In the United States, the

Department of Housing and Urban Development (HUD) defines affordable housing as that for which households spend no more than 30% of their income on housing costs, including rent or mortgage, property taxes, utilities, and other costs associated with their homes.[19] While definitions vary across countries, the underlying concept—high housing expenditure leaves less money for other basic needs—is generally accepted globally. When households face difficulties keeping up with these costs, they are considered *housing insecure* and at greater risk for losing their homes. Furthermore, households that pay more than this are considered *cost burdened* and at greater risk for inability to afford other necessities like food, medical care, clothing, and transportation.

According to HUD, a family living on one full-time minimum wage income is no longer able to afford local fair-market rent for a two-bedroom apartment in any urban area across the United States.[19] As urban populations continue to grow, inequities may widen as the shortage of affordable housing increases. Across the world, cities like Bogota, Beijing, and Moscow are facing similar trends.[20] The global housing crisis is characterized not just by a chronic shortage of affordable housing for the least advantaged but also, increasingly, for the working and middle classes as well. Unaffordable housing can result in food and medication insecurity and the fear or experience of being evicted or foreclosed, as well as frequent moving, "doubling-up," and homelessness—all of which are associated with negative health outcomes. In a 2017 study by the Center for Disease Control and Prevention, researchers showed that individuals reporting housing insecurity (defined here as feeling worried or stressed about having enough money to pay the rent/mortgage) were about twice as likely to report poor or fair self-rated health or postpone medical treatment due to costs compared to housing secure participants.[12] In another study by Desmond and Kimbro in 2015, urban mothers who had experienced eviction were more likely to report depression, poorer health for themselves and their children, and more parenting stress 1 year later compared to those who had not been evicted.[7]

Much of the literature considering housing affordability and urban health has compared owners to renters. Several such studies have reported better health outcomes among homeowners, a finding that some have attributed to the stability and wealth accumulation homeownership can provide.[21–23] However, the health benefits of homeownership may vary across subgroups of the population, as highlighted by the 2008 housing crisis in the United States, when predatory lending targeting low-income communities of color resulted in disproportionate rates of default and dispossession.[8,24] These circumstances, combined with other strong evidence that historic and contemporary exclusion within the US housing market results in differential opportunities for homeownership and the characteristics of neighborhoods in which homes are purchased, raise important questions about the extent to which the health benefits of homeownership vary across population subgroups: for example, racialized groups in the United States continue to experience discrimination in housing markets and may be less likely to realize the social, economic, and health-related gains associated with homeownership in nonracialized populations.

There is also evidence to suggest that the health implications of housing affordability extend beyond individuals to influence the health of affected urban communities. For instance, foreclosures have been shown to disrupt neighborhood social networks, degrade the physical environment as a form of blight, and encourage violent crime, all being documented health risk factors.[4,25] In the aftermath of the Great Recession in the United States, studies linked measures of foreclosure at the neighborhood level with increased hospital visits, poorer self-reported health, and higher blood pressure.[5,13,25] Among groups and places that are disproportionately affected by housing affordability problems, the physical, social, and economic costs of housing instability may intersect with existing neighborhood inequalities to exacerbate health inequities. These intersections warrant further examination into the ways that the social and spatial patterning of housing instability may operate directly and indirectly to create, perpetuate, and amplify health inequities in urban areas.

3 Access to Housing

Beyond affordability and the financial barriers just described, housing policies and the real estate market disproportionately benefit certain groups over others. For example, in the United States, the Federal Housing Administration (FHA) of 1934 was intended to make homeownership more accessible to middle-class Americans by providing low-interest, long-term mortgages.[26] However, the FHA also instituted the practice of "redlining," in which neighborhoods consisting largely of people of color were categorized as a financial risk and excluded from attaining mortgages. By restricting access to affordable homeownership in these communities, such policies constrained housing choice among people of color and contributed to the long-term disinvestment in urban communities.[26] Although policies like the Fair Housing Act of 1968 have since made it illegal to discriminate based on characteristics like race, color, sex, disability, and national origin at the time of purchase, rent, lease, sale or finance of a residence, present-day housing discrimination perpetuates segregated housing patterns across the United States.[27]

Housing discrimination has been linked to barriers in education, employment, and economic growth, as well as to an increased likelihood of residing in neighborhoods characterized by higher segregation and limited access to healthy foods, high-quality schools, and healthcare centers.[1,27,28] A recent study in Philadelphia found a significant negative association between perceived housing discrimination and self-reported health among individuals living in neighborhoods with higher housing values.[29] Another study in southeastern Wisconsin found that black women experienced reduced colorectal cancer survival rates in neighborhoods that had higher racial bias in the mortgage lending process.[30] Such studies, combined with substantial empirical evidence linking education and employment opportunities to health, suggest the profound public health implications of ongoing housing discrimination, operating through multiple pathways to affect multiple health outcomes.[28]

With a projected increase in urban populations globally over the next decade, along with continued shortages of affordable housing, there is a critical need to better understand these linkages to inform initiatives that reduce and prevent housing discrimination and its adverse health effects. Understanding neighborhood dynamics, including how changing patterns of housing discrimination correspond with shifts in racial, economic, or educational patterns as well as changes in housing values, local businesses, and financial investment, is essential to develop intervention and prevention efforts, with a focus on neighborhoods at higher risk of housing discrimination incidents.

4 Housing Conditions

In 2010, the World Health Organization released international guidelines on healthy housing with the goal of promoting better housing to prevent injuries and various diseases.[31] Poor housing conditions include inadequate ventilation, lack of protection from extreme temperatures, pest infestation, exposure to toxics, and poor infrastructure.[29] These conditions are firmly linked to multiple adverse health outcomes. For example, black mold buildup due to poor air ventilation has been linked to respiratory diseases including asthma and allergies.[29] Extreme weather conditions (e.g., cold, heat) and older or poorly maintained heating or cooling systems have been linked to increased mortality, particularly among the elderly, homebound, and other vulnerable populations.[32] Overcrowding has been linked to increased exposure to various communicable diseases including tuberculosis, while pest infestations have been linked to numerous diseases and disorders including asthma and allergies.[17,31] Exposure to lead-based paint is linked to lead poisoning and developmental problems among children, while structural deficiencies can exacerbate some of these conditions by posing hazardous threats (e.g., roof or wall collapse, flooding) that result in home-based injuries.[32,33]

Repairs to address these conditions can be expensive and may be unexpected. Low-income households are more likely to have poorer housing conditions and fewer resources available to address them, forcing them to decide between living under potentially harmful conditions and paying for necessities such as rent, mortgage, food, or medications.[34] Housing affordability and conditions can therefore interact to widen health inequities. For example, fuel poverty, defined as the inability to keep a home at a comfortable temperature and/or meet energy consumption needs at a reasonable cost, may be more common among homes that are older and less well maintained, and thus less expensive to buy or rent.[32] Fuel poverty has been linked to poor physical health including increased exposure to cold or warm temperatures; deteriorating housing conditions leading to increased dampness, mold, and allergens; and poor mental health due to physical and psychosocial stress induced by extreme temperatures and overcrowding to reduce energy costs.[32,35] While policies exist to address fuel poverty (e.g., programs to improve energy efficiency), the burden often falls on individual households to make those changes.[35] This is further complicated in the case of renters, who may be excluded from retrofitting programs or who may rely on landlords' willingness to pay for upgrades. Even when landlords agree, costs associated with home upgrades or retrofits may be passed along to the renters and can result in financial burdens that disproportionately affect low-income households.[9]

5 Next Steps

In this chapter, we have applied a socioecological approach to describe three interrelated housing dimensions—affordability, access, and conditions—and their implications for health equity. While our examples have largely been drawn from the US context, housing affordability and access to safe and secure housing, particularly for those with fewer economic resources, continues to be an issue of critical concern as urban populations increase and the economic and social inequalities among population subgroups continue to grow. We have attempted to illustrate how systemic differences in the ability to attain and maintain safe and stable housing shape the distribution of population health risk, with disparate impacts for socially marginalized groups. These inequalities reflect social and economic processes that position housing as a commodity symbolizing social and economic success rather than as a basic human right to shelter.[24] The global context in which housing is considered a commodity and access is driven by markets creates systematic differentials in housing opportunities shaped by differential access to economic resources and by racial, ethnic, or other forms of discrimination. Together, these processes create systematic differences in health across population subgroups or health inequities.

As urban populations continue to grow globally and gaps in income continue to expand, housing is likely to present new and pressing challenges for cities worldwide. Those with lower incomes are likely to find it increasingly challenging to afford and maintain housing, more likely to experience housing insecurity, and more likely to live in substandard housing conditions. Without intentional and informed interventions, these processes are likely to exacerbate current health inequities.

Thoughtful and innovative interventions to address these challenges exist but must be met with political will and economic investment. First, strategies to develop and retain affordable housing stock for low- and moderate-income households must be prioritized and widely adopted. Municipal Housing Trust Funds (which provide a dedicated source of funding for developing and rehabilitating affordable housing units), inclusionary zoning ordinances (which require new development to designate a proportion of its units as affordable), and rent control laws are effective strategies already in use in some areas. Shared equity homeownership models—including community land trusts (CLTs) and limited equity housing cooperatives—can help low- and moderate-income residents gain access to affordable homeownership, stabilize property values, promote community-based development, and preserve affordable units in the long-term. Education and public outreach are needed for both consumers and providers to ensure that laws like the Fair Housing Act are followed to prevent housing discrimination and the further marginalization of specific populations. Policies and programs to improve housing conditions should consider the broader social and economic inequalities in which these housing inequities are embedded, address issues of affordability and fuel poverty simultaneously, and create funding and remedial measures that account for complex landlord–tenant relationships. A clear understanding of housing as a public health issue, including the specific pathways through which housing systems affect access to safe and affordable housing while simultaneously influencing access to other social, economic, and political resources necessary to maintain health, must be embraced across disciplines and incorporated into public and private decision-making. A socioecological approach to housing and health can enable analyses that look beyond individual and neighborhood solutions to develop programs and policies that can address the root causes of these inequities.

References

1. Schulz AJ, Williams DR, Israel BA, Lempert LB. Racial and spatial relations as fundamental determinants of health in Detroit. *Milbank Q.* 2002; 80(4):677–707.

2. Ross CE, Mirowsky J. Neighborhood disadvantage, disorder, and health. *J Health Soc Behav.* 2001; 42(3):258.

3. Sharpe RA, Thornton CR, Nikolaou V, Osborne NJ. Higher energy efficient homes are associated with increased risk of doctor diagnosed asthma in a UK subpopulation. *Environ Int.* 2015; 75:234–244.

4. Downing J. The health effects of the foreclosure crisis and unaffordable housing: a systematic review and explanation of evidence. *Soc Sci Med.* 2016; 162:88–96.

5. Currie J, Tekin E. *Is there a link between foreclosure and health?* Cambridge, MA: National Bureau of Economic Research; 2011. doi:10.3386/w17310

6. Aylin P. Temperature, housing, deprivation and their relationship to excess winter mortality in Great Britain, 1986-1996. *Int J Epidemiol.* 2001; 30(5):1100–1108.

7. Desmond M, Kimbro RT. Eviction's fallout: housing, hardship, and health. *Soc Forces.* 2015; 94(1):295–324.

8. Burgard SA, Seefeldt KS, Zelner S. Housing instability and health: findings from the Michigan recession and recovery study. *Soc Sci Med.* 2012; 75(12):2215–2224.

9. Marí-Dell'Olmo M, Novoa AM, Camprubí L, et al. Housing policies and health inequalities. *Int J Health Serv.* 2016; 47(2):207–232.

10. Saegert S, Fields D, Libman K. Mortgage foreclosure and health disparities: serial displacement as asset extraction in African American populations. *J Urban Health Bull N Y Acad Med.* 2011; 88(3):390–402.

11. Mehdipanah R, Schulz AJ, Israel BA, et al. Neighborhood context, homeownership and home value: an ecological analysis of implications for health. *Int J Environ Res Public Health.* 2017; 14(10):1098.

12. Stahre M, VanEenwyk J, Siegel P, Njai R. Housing insecurity and the association with health outcomes and unhealthy behaviors, Washington State, 2011. *Prev Chronic Dis.* 2015; 12:140511.

13. Arcaya M, Glymour MM, Chakrabarti P, Christakis NA, Kawachi I, Subramanian SV. Effects of proximate foreclosed properties on individuals' systolic blood pressure in Massachusetts, 1987 to 2008. *Circulation.* 2014; 129(22):2262–2268.

14. Krieger J, Higgins DL. Housing and health: time again for public health action. *Am J Public Health.* 2002; 92(5):758–768.

15. Wang C, El-Nour MMA, Bennett GW. Survey of pest infestation, asthma, and allergy in low-income housing. *J Community Health.* 2008; 33(1):31–39.

16. Rabito FA, Shorter C, White LE. Lead levels among children who live in public housing. *Epidemiology.* 2003; 14(3):263–268.

17. Antunes JLF, Waldman EA. The impact of AIDS, immigration and housing overcrowding on tuberculosis deaths in São Paulo, Brazil, 1994–1998. *Soc Sci Med.* 2001; 52(7):1071–1080.

18. Knowledge Network on Urban Setting. *Our cities, our health, our future: acting on social determinants for health equity in urban settings.* Kobe, Japan: World Health Organization; 2008.

19. *Affordable housing: who needs affordable housing?* US Department of Housing and Urban Development (HUD) website. Available at https://www.hud.gov/program_offices/comm_ planning/affordablehousing/. Accessed May 1, 2018.

20. Brodie C. These cities have the least affordable housing. World Economic Forum website. Available at https://www.weforum.org/agenda/2017/11/affordable-housing-is-a-big-problem-in-these-cities/. Published September 7, 2017. Accessed April 14, 2018.

21. Ellaway A, Macintyre S. Does housing tenure predict health in the UK because it exposes people to different levels of housing related hazards in the home or its surroundings? *Health Place.* 1998; 4(2):141–150.

22. Pollack CE, Griffin BA, Lynch J. Housing affordability and health among homeowners and renters. *Am J Prev Med*. 2010; 39(6):515–521.

23. Rohe WM, Zandt SV, McCarthy G. Home ownership and access to opportunity. *Hous Stud*. 2002; 17(1):51–61.

24. Marcuse P, Madden D. *In defense of housing: the politics of crisis*. New York: Verso; 2016.

25. Schootman M, Deshpande AD, Pruitt SL, Jeffe DB. Neighborhood foreclosures and self-rated health among breast cancer survivors. *Qual Life Res Int J Qual Life Asp Treat Care Rehabil*. 2012; 21(1):133–141.

26. Gotham KF. Racialization and the state: the Housing Act of 1934 and the creation of the Federal Housing Administration. *Sociol Perspect*. 2000; 43(2):291–317.

27. Relman JP. Foreclosures, integration, and the future of the Fair Housing Act Symposium—The Fair Housing Act after 40 Years: continuing the mission to eliminate housing discrimination and segregation. *Indiana Law Rev*. 2008; 41:629–652.

28. de Leeuw MB, Whyte MK, Ho D, Meza C, Karteron A. *Residential segregation and housing discrimination in the United States: violations of the international convention on the elimination of all forms of racial discrimination. A report to the U.N. Commission on the Elimination of All Forms of Racial Discrimination*. The Poverty & Race Research Action Council & The National Fair Housing Alliance; 2007. Available at http://www.prrac.org/pdf/FinalCERDHousingDiscriminationReport.pdf. Accessed January 23, 2017.

29. Yang T-C, Chen D, Park K. Perceived housing discrimination and self-reported health: how do neighborhood features matter? *Ann Behav Med*. 2016; 50(6):789–801.

30. Zhou Y, Bemanian A, Beyer KMM. Housing discrimination, residential racial segregation, and colorectal cancer survival in southeastern Wisconsin. *Cancer Epidemiol Biomarkers Prev*. 2017; 26(4):561–568.

31. *Health impact assessment: housing and health*. World Health Organization website. Available at http://www.who.int/hia/housing/en/. Published 2010. Accessed May 1, 2018.

32. Howden-Chapman P, Viggers H, Chapman R, O'Sullivan K, Telfar Barnard L, Lloyd B. Tackling cold housing and fuel poverty in New Zealand: a review of policies, research, and health impacts. *Energy Policy*. 2012; 49:134–142.

33. Runyan CW, Perkis D, Marshall SW, et al. Unintentional injuries in the home in the United States: part II: morbidity. *Am J Prev Med*. 2005; 28(1):80–87.

34. Novoa AM, Ward J, Malmusi D, et al. How substandard dwellings and housing affordability problems are associated with poor health in a vulnerable population during the economic recession of the late 2000s. *Int J Equity Health*. 2015; 14(1):120.

35. Camprubí L, Malmusi D, Mehdipanah R, et al. Façade insulation retrofitting policy implementation process and its effects on health equity determinants: a realist review. *Energy Policy*. 2016; 91:304–314.

6

Transport and Health

MARK NIEUWENHUIJSEN AND HANEEN KHREIS

1 Introduction

Transport is instrumental in today's urban areas and the economic activity surrounding them and is often envisioned as a driver of urban development and a key contributor to economic returns. Through supporting labor markets, allowing businesses to harvest the benefits of larger catchment areas, and providing "the right connections in the right places," urban transport networks facilitate the economic competitiveness and social progress of cities.[1,2] Urban transport networks provide some people with options for getting around, allowing them to access needs, opportunities, and social contacts and to participate in their societies. Transport also has direct (negative and potentially positive) impacts on the health of populations, especially in urban areas.[3] These impacts are particularly connected to the use and prevalence of motorized transport. In high-income countries, there is a cultural and economic dependence on motor vehicles as the primary mode of transport that dominates urban transport planning and policy.[4] Although mass motorization started later in low-income countries, it is growing rapidly with heavy marketing from the car industry, causing similar problems in many emerging economies.[5,6]

When considered at a global level, the adverse health impacts of motor vehicle traffic are striking. Each year, more than 1.5 million deaths and 79.6 million injuries are due to motor vehicle crashes (MVC).[7] Traffic-related exposures including air pollution, greenhouse gases, noise, dwindling green space, and urban heat islands have resulted in stressors on the environment and, in turn, on the population's health.[8,9] By conservative estimates, 184,000 deaths globally were attributed to traffic-related air pollution (TRAP), including 91,000 deaths from ischemic heart disease, 59,000 deaths from stroke, and 34,000 deaths from lower respiratory infections, chronic obstructive pulmonary disease, and lung cancer.[7] Mass motorization and the associated lack of active travel reduce opportunities for physical activity and increase sedentary behavior.[10–12] Current urban forms are furthermore reinforcing the use of motorized transport for short-distance trips, further increasing traffic-related environmental exposures and reducing opportunities for physical activity.[13,14] These trends are associated with a significant burden of disease and increased premature mortality. For example, air pollution and lack of physical activity, both to a great extent caused by motorized transport, are associated with an annual 7 million and 2.1 million global deaths, respectively.[15]

At the level of urban areas and cities, the impacts are also substantial. In a recent health impact assessment study in Barcelona, Spain, urban and transport planning–related exposures such as air pollution, noise, heat islands, and the lack of green space and physical activity were responsible for nearly 3,000 premature deaths, 5,000 disease cases, and 50,000 disability-adjusted life-years (DALYs).[16,17] The adverse health impacts associated with urban transport and the potential solutions that a change in transport design and planning could offer reinforce the need to develop and implement effective policies that delineate, consider, and address health consequences.[3] To this end, a clear scoping of traffic-related health impacts and the provision of usable tools to identify and quantify these effects are needed.

2 A Framework for Understanding the Impact of Transport on Health

Urban and transport planning, environment exposures, physical activity, and health are linked (Figure 6.1). These linkages have been discussed in detail elsewhere.[8] In general, large investment in infrastructure for cars has led many cities and urban areas to become car dominated. These investments have often happened at the expense of investments in public and active transport. The catering to motor vehicle traffic led to more infrastructure such as roads and parking spaces, which in turn led to greater use of motor vehicles and changing land use patterns that go hand in hand with increasing traffic mobility. These changes resulted in higher levels of TRAP, noise, and heat island effects. Additionally, they led to less active travel and physical activity, as well as increased premature mortality and morbidity across a wide variety of health indicators. Furthermore, infrastructure for cars takes up a large amount of public space in cities that can be used for other purposes like green space or public space for people to meet and relax. A move away from car infrastructure to infra-structure for public and active transport could lead to an increase in the use of public and/or active transport, reducing air pollution, noise, heat island effects, and stress. Additionally, increased use of public and/or active transport would increase physical activity, thus re-ducing morbidity and premature mortality.[18] Investment in cycling infrastructure could lead to an increase in the number of cyclists and thereby reduce premature mortality.[19] Such changes can turn a city that is detrimental to health into one that is promoting health.

3 Health Effects of Transport in Urban Areas

Transport planning and policy can affect health through nine main pathways, each of which provides a helpful framing to understand the link between transport and health.[20] These are:

1. MVCs
2. TRAP
3. Noise
5. Increased local heat exposures

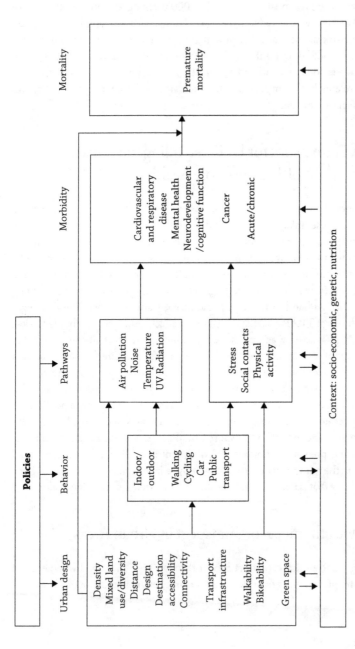

Figure 6.1 **Interlinkages between urban and transport planning, environment, physical activity, and health.** Source: Nieuwenhuijsen MJ. Interlinkages between urban and transport planning, environment, physical activity and health. *Environ Health.* 2016; 15(S1):38.

6. Reduced green space exposures and biodiversity loss
7. Lack of physical activity
8. Climate change
9. Social exclusion and community severance

MVCs have been associated with premature mortality, injuries, traumas, posttraumatic stress, and other indirect impacts, including less active travel and outdoor play/physical activity due to perceived safety threats. Air pollution has been associated with premature mortality, cardiovascular and respiratory disease, lung cancer, diabetes, obesity, reduced lung and cognitive function in children, low birth weight, and premature birth. Noise has been associated with cardiovascular mortality and morbidity, annoyance and sleep disturbance, type 2 diabetes, high blood pressure in children, and reduced cognitive function in children. Heat islands have been associated with premature mortality, cardiorespiratory morbidity, hospital admissions, children's mortality, and hospitalization. The lack of green space has been associated with premature mortality, cardiovascular disease, poor mental health, poorer cognitive function, and behavioral problems in children. The lack of physical activity has been associated with premature mortality, cardiovascular disease, dementia, breast cancer, diabetes, and colon cancer. Climate change has been associated with extreme weather events; adverse effects on the ecosystem and species; sea level rise; salination of coastal land and sea water; thermal stress; premature deaths (150,000–250,000 annually); illness and injury from floods; food poisoning; unsafe drinking water; changes in vector–pathogen host relations and in infectious disease geography/seasonality; impaired crop, livestock, and fisheries yield and impaired nutrition; changes in air pollution; loss of livelihoods; and displacement leading to poverty and adverse mental and physical health. Social exclusion and community severance have been associated with poorer mental health and well-being, premature mortality, lack of physical activity, and stress.[20]

These pathways and the health impacts associated with them are broader than previously documented and continue to expand.[3,21] Specifically, the health effects of community severance, noise, local heat exposures, and green space exposures (beyond mental health and stress) are all matters of emerging research and have not been common inquiries in contemporary transport and health research. However, the evidence base has strengthened, and further research and syntheses are under way, supporting the inclusion and consideration of these pathways and their health outcomes in practice. For example, emerging evidence suggests that the impact of noise on premature mortality is comparable to and independent of the impacts of air pollution on premature mortality.[16,22,23] Furthermore, when morbidity is considered, the health burden attributable to noise is even higher than that attributable to air pollution or physical inactivity.[17] In comparison, very little quantitative evidence is currently available for the health impacts of traffic-related heat, green space, social exclusion, and community severance. More research is needed on these pathways.

4 Future Directions

Mass motorization has been detrimental to health. Recently, new technological solutions such as electric cars and autonomous vehicles have been suggested to reduce the adverse health impacts associated with transport. However, these technological fixes can only reduce some of the adverse exposures generated by the air pollution, noise, and MVC issues, but they do not address many of the other pathways linking transport and health. Autonomous vehicles will be rapidly introduced into the market, but it is unclear how the technology will be used and adopted and how people's behavior may change as a result. Therefore, the impacts of these technologies on public health are difficult to foresee and estimate. Will autonomous vehicles be individual or shared? Will people continue to live in the same locations, or will they move farther from their workplaces (for cheaper living) because they can now commute in autonomous vehicles? With so many uncertainties, and with these technologies being largely driven by markets that have not been considerate of public health, we probably should not rely on these technological solutions but instead get people out of their cars and into public and active transport, a change that has already shown substantial health benefits.[24]

Urban and transport planning and policies, such as more compact planning, providing mixed land use, greater street connectivity, street furniture, safe urban environments, and pedestrian-friendly and cyclist-friendly amenities, could promote positive active commuting behavior and physical activity, eventually building these into daily routines.[20,25-27] It is important to overcome contemporary physical inactivity, which is a major health problem and a particularly important issue at times when people are generally too busy to be physically active during their leisure time. The role of transport planning in providing opportunities for physical activity is similarly important. Furthermore, getting people to use public transport, walk, and/or cycle to their destinations would not only make them physically more active and thus healthier, but would also have positive environmental effects such as reducing their carbon footprint, local air pollution, and noise levels.[20,28] Public and active transport also take up less space than cars and could free up public space to be used by people rather than by cars.

5 Conclusion

Current transport practices produce unwanted side effects and adverse environmental exposures such as air pollution, noise, heat island effects, MVCs, decreasing green space and physical activity, climate change, social exclusion, and community severance, all of which increase morbidity and premature mortality. An urgent shift is needed from motorized private vehicles to public and active transport to create cities that promote health. A more holistic approach to our cities bringing together urban and transport planners, architects, and environmental and public health professionals can make our cities more sustainable, more livable, and healthier.

References

1. Eddington R. *The Eddington transport study. Main report: transport's role in sustaining the UK's productivity and competitiveness.* London: Department for Transport; 2006.
2. Hall RP, Gudmundsson H, Marsden G, Zietsman J. *Sustainable transport.* Thousand Oaks, CA: Sage; 2014.

3. Khreis H, Warsow KM, Verlinghieri E, et al. The health impacts of traffic-related exposures in urban areas: understanding real effects, underlying driving forces and co-producing future directions. *J Transp Health.* 2016; 3(3):249–267.

4. Jeekel MH. *The car-dependent society: a European perspective.* London: Routledge; 2013.

5. Dargay J, Gately D, Sommer M. Vehicle ownership and income growth, worldwide: 1960–2030. *Energy J.* 2007; 143–170.

6. Douglas MJ, Watkins SJ, Gorman DR, Higgins M. Are cars the new tobacco? *J Public Health.* 2011; 33(2):160–169.

7. Bhalla K, Shotten M, Cohen A, et al. *Transport for health: the global burden of disease from motorized road transport. Global Road Safety Facility.* Washington, DC: World Bank Group; 2014.

8. Nieuwenhuijsen MJ. Urban and transport planning, environmental exposures and health-new concepts, methods and tools to improve health in cities. *Environ health.* 2016; 15(1):S38.

9. *Traffic-related air pollution: a critical review of the literature on emissions, exposure, and health effects, Special Report 17.* Boston, MA: Health Effects Institute; 2010.

10. Audrey S, Procter S, Cooper AR. The contribution of walking to work to adult physical activity levels: a cross sectional study. *Int J Behav Nutr Phys Act.* 2014 (11): 37. doi:10.1186/1479-5868-11-37

11. Mackett RL, Brown B. *Transport, physical activity and health: present knowledge and the way ahead.* London: Centre for Transport Studies; 2011.

12. Wanner M, Götschi T, Martin-Diener E, Kahlmeier S, Martin BW. Active transport, physical activity, and body weight in adults: a systematic review. *Am J Prev Med.* 2012; 42(5):493–502.

13. Cervero R, Duncan M. Walking, bicycling, and urban landscapes: evidence from the San Francisco Bay Area. *Am J Public Health.* 2003; 93(9), 1478–1483.

14. Giles-Corti B, Donovan RJ. Socioeconomic status differences in recreational physical activity levels and real and perceived access to a supportive physical environment. *Prev Med.* 2002; 35(6):601–611.

15. Forouzanfar MH, Alexander L, Anderson HR, et al. Global, regional, and national comparative risk assessment of 79 behavioural, environmental and occupational, and metabolic risks or clusters of risks in 188 countries, 1990–2013: a systematic analysis for the Global Burden of Disease Study 2013. *Lancet.* 2015; 386(10010):2287–2323.

16. Mueller N, Rojas-Rueda D, Basagaña X, et al. Urban and transport planning related exposures and mortality: a health impact assessment for cities. *Environ Health Perspect.* 2017; 125(1):89.

17. Mueller N, Rojas-Rueda D, Basagaña X, et al. Health impacts related to urban and transport planning: a burden of disease assessment. *Environ Int.* 2017; 107:243–257.

18. Nieuwenhuijsen MJ, Khreis H. Car free cities: pathway to healthy urban living. *Environ Int.* 2016; 5(94):251–262.

19. Mueller N, Rojas-Rueda D, Salmon M, et al. Health impact assessment of cycling network expansions in European cities. *Prev Med.* 2018; S0091-7435(17):30497–30498.

20. Khreis H, May AD, Nieuwenhuijsen MJ. Health impacts of urban transport policy measures: a guidance note for practice. *J Transp Health.* 2017; 6:209–227.

21. Cohen JM, Boniface S, Watkins S. Health implications of transport planning, development and operations. *J Transp Health.* 2014; 1:63–72.

22. Stansfeld SA, Berglund B, Clark C, et al. Aircraft and road traffic noise and children's cognition and health: a cross-national study. *Lancet.* 2005; 365(9475):1942–1949.

23. Tétreault LF, Perron S, Smargiassi A. Cardiovascular health, traffic-related air pollution and noise: are associations mutually confounded? A systematic review. *Int J Public Health.* 2013; 58:649–666.

24. Mueller N, Rojas-Rueda D, Cole-Hunter T, et al. Health impact assessment of active transport: a systematic review. *Prev Med.* 2015; 76:103–114.

25. Scheepers CE, Wendel-Vos GCW, den Broeder JM, van Kempen EEMM, van Wesemael, Schuit AJ. Shifting from car to active transport: a systematic review of the effectiveness of interventions. *Transport Res Part A.* 2014; 70:264–280.

26. Heinen E, Panter J, Mackett R, Ogilvie D. Changes in mode of travel to work: a natural experimental study of new transport infrastructure. *Int J Behav Nutr Phys Act.* 2015; 12:81.

27. Giles-Corti B, Vernez-Moudon A, Reis R, et al. City planning and population health: a global challenge. *Lancet.* 2016; 388:2912–2924.

28. Sallis JF, Cerin E, Conway TL, Adams MA, Frank LD, Pratt M. Physical activity in relation to urban environments in 14 cities worldwide: a cross-sectional study. *Lancet.* 2016; 387:2207–2217.

7

Aging Populations

KATHLEEN A. CAGNEY

1 Introduction

Rapid urbanization combined with an increasingly older age structure means that cities around the world and in the United States will need to consider age and aging as a key factor in urban planning and resource allocation, particularly related to health.[1] The physical and social spaces of cities may need to be rethought and reconfigured as the population ages and as more people age in place.[2] How do aging populations affect cities, and how should cities view age and aging?

This chapter reviews how urban population composition is changing with respect to age. It lays out key attributes of both the physical and social infrastructure of cities as they relate to older adults and their well-being. It then examines potential implications of an older age structure, acknowledging its challenges but also drawing out possible opportunities. The chapter suggests new measurement approaches that have the potential to provide insight into how older adults navigate urban space and closes with a brief set of comments on future directions to consider. To provide focus, this chapter draws primarily on examples from the United States circumstance, with the aim of generalizing these observations to aging and urban context globally.

2 Cities and Age

Population aging is evident in cities of the United States and across the globe. The United States Census Bureau reports that the population of those 65 and older is projected to be 83.7 million in 2050, which is nearly double the 2012 count of 43.1 million.[3] Globally, there are approximately 962 million people 60 years and older, with Europe having the greatest percentage of older adults at 25%. By 2050, all regions of the world are expected to have nearly one-quarter of their populations at age 60 or older.[4] Falling fertility and rising life expectancy have been described as the key drivers.[1]

Concomitant with this changing age structure is the continued migration to urban areas. Currently, more than half the global population lives in a city, reaching 66% by 2050.[4] In the United States, rural and suburban areas are composed of more older adults, but the age structure in urban areas in changing markedly as well. For instance,

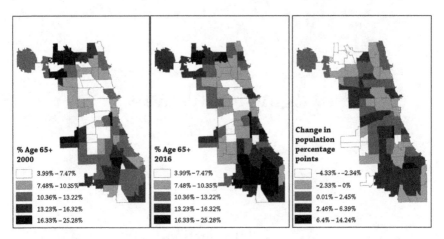

Figure 7.1 **Chicago and its 77 community areas. Population composition for those 65 and older.**

the median age in Scottsdale, Arizona, is 46.3 years while in Santa Fe, New Mexico, it is 42.9. The median age in Chicago, Illinois, by contrast, is 33.9 years.[5]

Chicago provides an interesting case study, since its median age may mask important variation at the community level. Attention to micro-level population processes is less common but potentially important for understanding aging in the context of urban space.[6] The nature of the micro-environment may more readily determine where residence is feasible. That is, some communities may have a greater or lesser number of older adults, and this may influence whether older persons stay in the community, choose to move to another one, or whether the social and physical infrastructure is amenable to those with physical vulnerabilities.

Figure 7.1 indicates that Chicago as a whole is aging but that there are important differences by neighborhood. Communities tend to be older around the edges of the city and in areas with lower levels of in-migration. Older adults may age where they initially settled, or they may choose neighborhoods based on age-specific needs. The structure of housing, such as the presence of an elevator or a single-floor layout, may also make older adults gravitate toward certain neighborhoods (if, for instance, housing types cluster by neighborhood). The extent to which certain neighborhoods hold the physical and social resources appealing to older adults may also shape the patterns observed here. Older adults are remaining community-resident until later ages, so part of what we are observing is that the neighborhood is aging collectively.[7]

To take a closer look, Figure 7.2 shows the age structure of three neighborhoods in Chicago—Bridgeport, Brighton Park, and North Lawndale—using the 2010 Census and the 2016 American Community Survey. We see distinct differences in the shapes of these population pyramids over the course of 16 years. Bridgeport, on Chicago's south side and an initial destination for Irish immigrants, is aging but also has an influx of younger population groups. Brighton Park, located on the southwest side of the city, was originally a destination for European immigrants, particularly those from Poland, Lithuania, and Italy. It is aging, too, but has experienced a significant population loss in those 20–40 years. North Lawndale, on Chicago's west side and an initial destination for

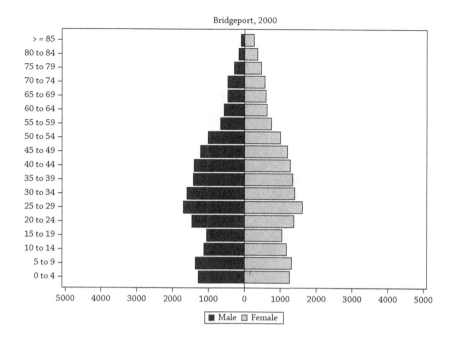

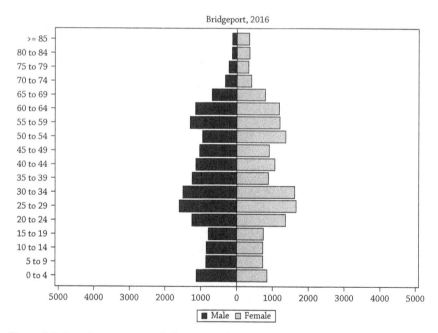

Figure 7.2 **Population pyramids for three Chicago neighborhoods: 2000 and 2016.**

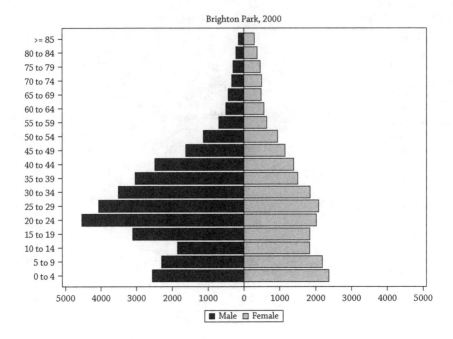

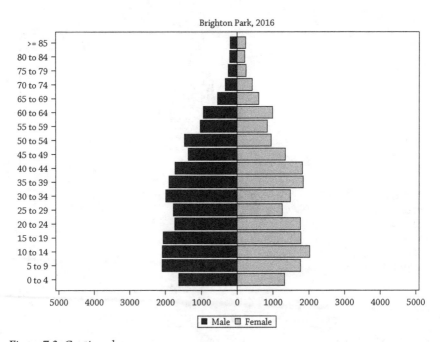

Figure 7.2 Continued

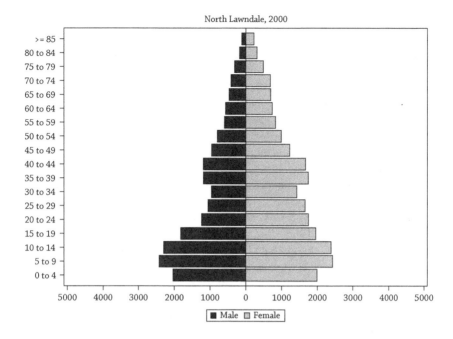

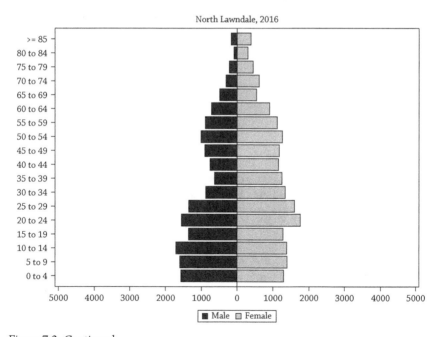

Figure 7.2 Continued

Bohemian immigrants, also is aging but, perhaps more important, is experiencing significant population loss. These descriptive data do not incorporate salient information related to in- and out-migration, but they do suggest, at these two different time points, that the neighborhoods' age compositions have changed.

These descriptive data also suggest that our communities exhibit some segregation with respect to age. Age segregation may be due to a number of factors but may indeed be increasing.[6,8,] It may result because a subset of older adults have greater resources, allowing them access to buildings and neighborhoods with more amenities. Or, a community may not have employment opportunities for those in younger age strata, leading to population loss in those age ranges. Implications for increasing age segregation include a lack of information exchange across generations and limited opportunities to engage in informal assistance, such as childcare or older adult healthcare and social support. The lack of opportunity for interaction may be detrimental for both the young and the old, which is addressed in more detail later in the chapter.

Naturally occurring retirement communities (NORCs) are a related phenomenon and one that may confer benefits to older adults given their typically smaller scale and, in some instances, more intentional nature.[9] Aging in a particular place, with little residential shift or population in-migration from younger age groups, may result in a NORC. Relatedly, NORCs also include spaces where older adults move when they retire. NORCs have been identified in cities across the country, and, in some instances, they are formalized and equipped with supportive services. Indeed, some are designated as NORC Supportive Service Programs; these may incorporate social workers, nurses, and caregivers and also may facilitate interaction between the residents and their respective communities.[10] Policy initiatives for NORCs more broadly may include property tax concessions, pedestrian interventions (e.g., increasing duration of time for yellow and green traffic lights), and senior-led voluntary activities.[9]

3 The Structure of the City

The physical and social attributes of urban areas arguably affect older adults more readily given that physical vulnerabilities may make navigating urban areas more challenging. Yen et al.'s comprehensive review suggested that neighborhood context matters for the health and functioning of older adults, yet it can be difficult to discern whether the physical, the social, or their interplay matter more or less for residential tenure and subsequent health and well-being.[11] Theory from sociology and related disciplines has been instructive in guiding analyses that attempt to examine the impact of a community's structural features—that may impact particular outcomes such as health—from the social processes that emerge in neighborhood or community context. What follows is a description of how each component may affect the lives of older urban residents.

3.1 Physical Infrastructure

Aspects of the built environment may make an urban center not only more or less appealing, but actually determine its feasibility and practicability as a living space.

Disordered physical spaces may be harder for older adults to traverse and engage in the routine activities necessary for independent living. Cracked sidewalks, poor lighting, and the absence of curb cuts may mean that older adults hesitate to walk outside. This limits both physical exercise and also the opportunity to informally engage with neighbors and foster social connections over time. Balfour and Kaplan, for instance, found that older adults who reported problems in the neighborhood environment had a greater risk of functional deterioration over the course of 1 year compared to those in neighborhoods with fewer problems.[12] Aspects of the community may also be protective. For example, older adults who lived in neighborhoods with active business districts were much less likely to die during the 1995 Chicago heat wave.[13] The availability of resources and services where routine needs could be met, the authors surmised, set the stage for social connections to take hold. Architects and urban planners have long viewed the physical environment as central to social interaction and its potential benefits, and it is to this topic that we now turn.

3.2 Social Infrastructure

A large body of evidence suggests that older adults fare better physically and socially when embedded in rich and interconnected social networks. Social engagement matters for both physical and mental health and has an impact on both chronic and acute illnesses.[14] Recent research indicates that those who reside in urban spaces have networks that are larger and denser, but pockets of isolation may exist that act as a significant risk factor for depressive symptomatology.[15,16]

Research focused on the social processes that emerge from social engagement suggests that meso-level factors such as trust and norms of reciprocity may buffer the deleterious effects of a disordered space. Collective efficacy, or the ability of the community to come together for the common good, has been shown to be associated with a range of health outcomes.[17] Social cohesion and informal social control, its attendant properties, may have independent effects on the well-being of older adults. For example, Latham and Clarke, in new work with the National Health and Aging Trends Study, found that low social cohesion was associated with a decreased odds of visiting friends and family and participating in organizations.[18] Moreover, they found that disorder was associated with a decreased odds of visiting friends and family, participating in organizations, and going out for enjoyment.

Social network interaction at the individual level and the social context of the surrounding community appear important for urban-dwelling older adults. Increasing connections at both of these levels may facilitate physical and emotional well-being and increase the likelihood of older adults remaining in their respective communities until later ages.

In Jacobs's seminal work, the notion of "eyes on the street" was largely invoked with the image of an older adult surveying the block, noting who did and did not belong based on everyday patterns and providing a generalized sense of security for neighbors.[19] This form of contribution is articulated in a broad range of urban scholarship, but the extent to which older adults may be central to this aspect of informal social control is typically not established. Older adults can make important contributions to the fabric of the community and may supply a unique form of capital.

4 Age as Capital

The implications of an aging population are generally referred to with caution, citing, for instance, fewer workers in the labor market and additional resource demands, particularly around healthcare and long-term care service provision. These are all significant concerns as the dependency ratio shifts dramatically. That said, we rarely consider what attributes are conferred with age and how these may be tapped in novel ways to address unmet needs.

Older adults may come to their later life stage with significant training and employment experience and may have the time and financial resources not realized at earlier stages of the life course. Older adults may choose to retire from the employment circumstance that dominated their middle years but still wish to pursue paid and unpaid activities that are of interest, draw on their skills, and provide opportunities for social engagement.

In the context of cities, drawing from such a resource might be particularly advantageous. Urban school systems, for example, may not be uniformly able to provide the forms of instruction and support necessary for primary and secondary school children. Enhancement activities led by older adults could augment conventional pedagogical programs and lead to important social interaction that benefits both groups. For example, Experience Corps, developed in Baltimore and now in place in several cities, places older volunteers in elementary schools for tutoring and other academic enhancement activities.[20] For students, evaluation results suggest selective improvements in reading and classroom behavior.[21] For volunteers, modest improvements in physical and social activity were documented 1 year after initial participation and, after 2 years, some protection against dementia.[22,23] The larger model draws on concepts of social capital and the transmission of wisdom as frameworks for the research.[24]

Experience Corps and other programs of its kind recognize that conventional retirement timing coupled with increased longevity could lead to unprecedented opportunity for a cohort of individuals who, in the general case, will have many active years of generativity. Initial engagement may be contingent on health, but that engagement could further stave off health decline.

5 Novel Data and Measurement App--roaches

New data resources, sometimes described as "big data" or "found data," allow for a richer understanding of the context of older adult lives. The ability to precisely track and document population movements, transit, air quality, and congestion, for instance, is now possible and the resulting data analyzable. Data of this form will allow for a detailed description of the micro-environment, which, as discussed earlier, is critical for older adults who wish to remain in their urban environments. And traditional social surveys, when coupled with these data, can allot the greater share of a questionnaire to questions about perceptions rather than direct recall.

New measurement approaches also have implications for how we understand older adult lives in urban physical and social spaces. Measurement techniques that allow for global positioning system (GPS) tracking capture what sociologists and geographers describe as "activity spaces." Activity spaces encompass the social environments that individuals encounter during their routine activities in everyday life.[25] Accordingly, activity spaces likely include but are not limited to residential neighborhoods.[26] Examining exposure spaces, arguably more important than data from one residential location, will provide novel insights into the range and type of spaces that older adults traverse and how and why those spaces might matter for their health. It also may help answer whether lives constrict as we age, a common adage but not one typically examined empirically.

6 Conclusion and New Directions

Attention to age in urban context is compelling in its own right, but the rapidly changing age structure indicates a more immediate need to examine its implications. This chapter described the changing age structure as it relates to urban context and the physical and social characteristics that affect older adults in urban space. A more general case was made that we need to recognize those aspects of urban living that may be health enhancing. Opportunities afforded from living in close social space—a serendipitous exchange with a neighbor, a sharing of a roof or walls in a cooperative living arrangement, informal assistance provided in time of crisis—may not be fully appreciated, nor the extent to which older adults enhance our ability to make use of these resources.

How do we address the health needs of an aging urban population? How do we recognize the human and social capital that may be untapped? This chapter does not address the likely increases in healthcare costs in an urban context but rather the precursors that might maintain health. Nor does this chapter incorporate the ever-increasing influences of virtual space. It will be important to understand how virtual interactions impact health because, even in a densely populated city, transit or health limitations may mean that face-to-face interaction is not feasible. These forms of communication may not only alter how we describe and enumerate social networks, they may indeed provide some form of clinical counsel and, potentially, healthcare. Fundamentally, they may buffer the deleterious effects of social isolation.

This chapter has relied primarily on findings from the sociological and epidemiological literatures. Research in other fields, such as architecture and urban planning, may provide promising insights for those engaged in research on health. Of note, the United States pavilion at the 2018 Biennale, Dimensions of Citizenship, featured the work of seven architecture practices to "explore how citizenship may be defined, constructed . . . or expressed in the built environment . . . about issues including belonging, sovereignty, and ecology."[27] One could imagine that work of this form could suggest novel approaches to creating a physical environment that enhances social engagement and a sense of belonging and that is attentive to the needs of more vulnerable urban-dwelling populations, young or old.

This chapter also has relied on the United States as an exemplar, with a focus on the micro-environment. Taking the United States example and looking outward, we can imagine that many of the principles discussed—communities that allow for intergenerational interaction, that are socially rewarding and physically accommodating—are important across regions and nations. An initiative through the World Health Organization (WHO), Age-Friendly World, lays out a series of programs that aim to foster an inclusive environment for older adults; it now includes 600 cities and communities across the globe.[28] This network of cities acts as a platform for exchange and advice provision and recognizes the roles of social integration and social cohesion as central to older adult well-being. The commonalities among nations and cultures are numerous with respect to accommodating and enhancing older adult lives; novel initiatives such as this allow for ready exchange of information that more quickly leads to innovation.

References

1. Harper S. Economic and social implications of aging societies. *Science.* 2014; 346(6209):587–591.
2. Pynoos J. The future of housing for the elderly: four strategies that can make a difference. *Public Policy Aging Rep.* 2018; 28.
3. Ortman J, Velkoff, VA, Hogan, H. *An aging nation: the older population in the United States.* Washington, DC: US Census Bureau; 2014.
4. Department of Economic and Social Affairs. *World population prospects: the 2017 revision.* New York: United Nations; 2017.
5. American fact finder: community facts 2018. US Census Bureau website. Available at https://factfinder.census.gov/faces/nav/jsf/pages/community_facts.xhtml. Accessed June 11, 2018.
6. Cagney KA. Neighborhood age structure and its implications for health. *J Urban Health.* 2006; 83(5):827–834.
7. Young Y, Kalamaras J, Kelly L, Hornick D, Yucel R. Is aging in place delaying nursing home admission? *J Am Med Dir Assoc.* 2015; 16(10):900.e901–900.e906.
8. Hagestad G, Uhlenberg, P. The social separation of old and young: a root of ageism. *J Soc Issues.* 2005; 61:343–360.
9. Masotti PJ, Fick R, Johnson-Masotti A, MacLeod S. Healthy naturally occurring retirement communities: a low-cost approach to facilitating healthy aging. *Am J Public Health.* 2006; 96(7):1164–1170.
10. Vladeck AA, A. The future of the NORC-Supportive Service Program Model. *Public Policy Aging Rep.* 2015; 25(1):20–22.
11. Yen IH, Fandel Flood J, Thompson H, Anderson LA, Wong G. How design of places promotes or inhibits mobility of older adults: realist synthesis of 20 years of research. *J Aging Health.* 2014; 26(8):1340–1372.
12. Balfour JL, Kaplan GA. Neighborhood environment and loss of physical function in older adults: evidence from the Alameda County Study. *Am J Epidemiol.* 2002; 155(6):507–515.
13. Browning CR, Wallace D, Feinberg SL, Cagney KA. Neighborhood social processes, physical conditions, and disaster-related mortality: the case of the 1995 Chicago heat wave. *Am Sociol Rev.* 2006; 71(4):661–678.
14. Cornwell EY, Waite LJ. Social disconnectedness, perceived isolation, and health among older adults. *J Health Soc Behav.* 2009; 50(1):31–48.
15. Baernholdt M, Yan G, Hinton I, Rose K, Mattos M. Quality of life in rural and urban adults 65 years and older: findings from the National Health and Nutrition Examination Survey. *J Rural Health.* 2012; 28(4):339–347.
16. Aneshensel CS, Wight RG, Miller-Martinez D, Botticello AL, Karlamangla AS, Seeman TE. Urban neighborhoods and depressive symptoms among older adults. *J Gerontol B Psychol Sci Soc Sci.* 2007; 62(1):S52–S59.
17. Sampson RJ, Raudenbush SW, Earls F. Neighborhoods and violent crime: a multilevel study of collective efficacy. *Science.* 1997; 277(5328):918–924.
18. Latham K, Clarke PJ. Neighborhood disorder, perceived social cohesion, and social participation among older Americans: findings from the National Health & Aging Trends Study. *J Aging Health.* 2018; 30(1):3–26.
19. Jacobs J. *The death and life of great American cities.* New York: Vintage; 1961.

20. Fried LP, Carlson MC, McGill S, et al. Experience Corps: a dual trial to promote the health of older adults and children's academic success. *Contemp Clin Trials*. 2013; 36(1):1–13.

21. Rebok GW, Carlson MC, Glass TA, et al. Short-term impact of experience Corps® participation on children and schools: results from a pilot randomized trial. *J Urban Health*. 2004; 81(1):79–93.

22. Parisi JM, Kuo J, Rebok GW, et al. Increases in lifestyle activities as a result of Experience Corps® participation. *J Urban Health*. 2015; 92(1):55–66.

23. Carlson MC, Kuo JH, Chuang Y-F, et al. Impact of the Baltimore Experience Corps Trial on cortical and hippocampal volumes. *Alzheimers Dement*. 2015; 11(11):1340–1348.

24. Parisi JM, Rebok GW, Carlson MC, et al. Can the wisdom of aging be activated and make a difference societally? *Educ Gerontol*. 2009; 35(10):867–879.

25. Cagney K, Browning, CR, Jackson, AL, Soller, B. Networks, neighborhoods, and institutions: an integrated "Activity Space" approach for research on aging. In Waite LJ, Plewes TJ, ed. *New directions in the sociology of aging*. Washington, DC: National Academies Press; 2013:151–174.

26. York Cornwell E, Cagney KA. Assessment of neighborhood context in a nationally representative study. *J Gerontol B Psychol Sci Soc Sci*. 2014; 69 S2:S51–S63.

27. Kubek D. US pavilion at Biennale Architettura 2018 announces details of architects' projects for dimensions of citizenship. School of the Art Institute of Chicago website. Available at http://www.saic.edu/press/us-pavilion-announces-details-architects-projects-dimensions-citizenship. Accessed June 10, 2018.

28. Age-friendly world. World Health Organization website. Available at https://extranet.who.int/agefriendlyworld/. Accessed June 12, 2018.

8

Children and Adolescents in Cities

SHAKIRA F. SUGLIA

1 Introduction

Healthy child development, including social, cognitive, emotional, and physical development, is critical for health and well-being across the life course because the early years of childhood can set the course for children's ability to mature into healthy adults. Childhood is a time of rapid neurodevelopment; play, social interactions, physical activity, and safe and nurturing environments are necessary for optimal child development. The various contexts within which children are developing, including family, childcare/school, and neighborhood, can promote or hinder child development. While the family environment is the first and most proximate environment influencing child development, as children grow their interactions with other contexts change and become perhaps equally influential. Neighborhood environments can promote healthy child development by facilitating play in recreational spaces, contact with nature in green spaces, and interactions with caretakers and peers.

With the rise of the global obesity epidemic, the influence of the neighborhood environment, particularly the built environment in cities, and its impact on child health has been, appropriately, the focus of much attention. However, cities can affect child health in several other areas of development, including social, cognitive, and emotional. Urban environments are experienced differently by children and adolescents compared to adults because they interact with features of the social and physical environment in distinct ways across various developmental stages. Almost half of the world's children live in urban areas, presenting opportunities to develop cities that are friendly to children and adolescents, as well as some particular challenges that could hinder child development.[1]

2 The Urban Environment and Child and Adolescent Health

Urban environments have both positive and negative dimensions that can affect child health and development. Several factors prevalent in cities are particularly detrimental to child health. Numerous studies have documented associations between features of the urban built environment—such as lower housing density, access to parks and recreational facilities, walkable paths, and access to green spaces—and greater physical activity among children and adolescents and, consequently to some extent, with lower risk of obesity. The built environment, however, can promote more than just physical activity and lower levels of body mass index (BMI). While not as extensively studied, research suggests that features of the built environment can influence child development.[2] Traffic congestion, in addition to increasing risk for pedestrian injuries, can also limit access to educational and recreational spaces. Air pollution has been shown to affect respiratory health, particularly asthma, as well as cognition among children.[3]

The neighborhood social environment, or the socioeconomic composition of the neighborhood and its residents, as well as the "relationships, groups, and social processes that exist between individuals who live in a neighborhood," has been shown to affect child and adolescent health.[4–6] For example, a relation between urbanicity and child mental health symptoms has been attributed to low social cohesion and high crime.[7,8] In disadvantaged neighborhoods, lack of structural opportunities (i.e., safe parks) for social interaction can result in limited social networks. Lack of neighborhood safety, defined as perceptions of unsafe neighborhoods as well as objectively measured high-crime neighborhoods, increases risk of injury to children and mental stress which can alter sleep patterns, increase distress and consequent mental health outcomes, and affect cardiometabolic health.[9,10] Preschool children in New York City were found to have a 22% higher prevalence of obesity if they resided in zip codes with high homicide rates, independent of neighborhood socioeconomic status and other characteristics.[11] In a recent review of neighborhood factors and child adiposity, of the four studies that examined constructs of social capital, collective efficacy, and social disorder, all noted that lower neighborhood social capital was associated with higher BMI and higher odds of being overweight or obese.[12] Social cohesion and social capital have been positively associated with physical activity among adolescents and with healthy child development and behavioral outcomes among young children.[13,14] Among children in the Fragile Families and Child Well-being study, neighborhood collective efficacy was associated with more hours of outdoor play and more trips to a park or playground.[15]

In addition to the social and built dimensions of the urban environment, access to medical, educational, and recreational facilities is crucial to the health and well-being of children and adolescents. In urban environments, access to these vital resources may be difficult for lower socioeconomic households. In urban areas with high poverty concentrations, early childhood programs are often unavailable. In low-income countries, it is estimated that 200 million children under the age of 5 do not reach their full cognitive potential. These inequalities persist into school age, with an estimated 67 million primary school-aged children not enrolled in school in 2008.

Features of the urban environment can promote healthy child development. Cities can facilitate children's interaction with diverse cultural experiences; cities' dense housing composition and variety of commercial and recreational establishments can foster social and emotional development; access to green spaces, transportation, and walkability can promote play, exploration, and physical activity as well as social interactions. Child-friendly cities often meet "the popsicle test," a simple measure of whether a child can go somewhere safely, buy a popsicle, and return home before the popsicle melts. This simple "test" conveys a number of factors of the environment (walkability, safety, connectedness) in addition to proximity to resources. Given the impact that urban environments can have on child health and development across the life course, it is critical to consider how the multiple dimensions of cities can be improved to be child-friendly.

3 The Urban Environment, Early- and Mid-Childhood, and Adolescence

A consideration of the urban environment and how it affects child health must consider that childhood encompasses multiple developmental periods. In infancy and early childhood, a period of rapid brain development, the environment is largely experienced through parental and caretaker's interactions. Direct experiences with the urban environment are more limited and focused on interactions at home or in childcare facilities. Thus, the urban environment indirectly impacts child health through its impact on parents and caretakers.[16] For example, in the US-based Early Childhood Longitudinal Study (ECLS), children whose parents perceived their neighborhoods to be unsafe watched more television and engaged in less physical activity. Parents who perceive an unsafe neighborhood may be more likely to keep their children indoors, leading children to engage in less outdoor play and more sedentary indoor activities such as TV watching.[17] As children reach school age, the school becomes an important component in how children interact with their environment. Getting to and from school, accessing green spaces and recreational spaces while at school, breathing clean air, and drinking clean water become part of how children interact with their environment. In adolescence, increasing autonomy opens the door for exposure to aspects of the environment that may not be guided by parents or caretakers but highly influenced by peers. The environment potentially widens beyond residences, parks, and schools to include residences of friends, movie theaters, sports venues, shopping centers, and other recreational venues. Adolescents' interactions in urban environments encompass a new dimension that younger children don't experience, given adolescents' ability to choose which activity spaces they interact with and how they choose to navigate those spaces. Unfortunately, adolescent interactions can often be viewed as unsafe and disruptive, particularly in areas of high poverty, and these are often discouraged by neighborhoods and government entities. Considerations of how adolescents interact with the urban environment is often overlooked by city planners and developers. Playgrounds and play spaces are targeted to younger children, with spaces for adolescents to gather and socialize not generally developed.

In addition, parents and caretakers may also limit the scope and breadth of the environment their children experience based on the child's developmental stage. Recent research suggests that, among several factors, the age of a child determines the activities and environment that are sought out by parents, with families of younger children limiting their activities and families of older children broadening their activities spaces, willing to travel farther so that older children and adolescents can access resources such as schools, sports, and other recreational activities.[16] Those designing spaces for children and adolescents need to consider how children at different developmental stages use their environment and how they experience their environment through their caretakers and peers.

4 Optimizing Urban Environments to Promote Healthy Childhood and Adolescence

Opportunities abound to promote health and well-being among children and adolescents in urban spaces. Much of the existing work on building healthier cities for children has focused on the promotion and development of the physical environment through the addition of parks, playgrounds, and recreational facilities that promote physical activity and potentially reduce the risk for obesity. However, these interventions will not reach their full potential if not integrated with other features of the social environment, such as safety, social trust, and cohesion.[18] A recent review of 33 intervention studies focusing on developing healthy urban environments for children found only weak evidence of the effectiveness of public health interventions that focused on features of the built environment.[19]

A focus on improving neighborhood social conditions as a way of promoting physical activity and likely other positive health outcomes suggests the need for engagement with municipal agencies, business associations, and civic groups that might not typically self-identify with health promotion. Strategies to improve neighborhood social environments require systems-level and multisectoral approaches encapsulated in the "Health in All Policies" approach to municipal government, which incorporates health considerations into decision-making across sectors, policy areas, and governmental agencies that typically have not focused on health as a major part of their mission.[20]

Child Friendly Cities Initiative (CFCI), launched in 1996 by the United Nations International Children's Emergency Fund (UNICEF) and UN-Habitat, is an initiative that "supports municipal governments in realizing the rights of children at the local level using the UN Convention on the Rights of the Child as its foundation." Under this initiative, a child-friendly city is defined as any city that is committed to improving the lives of children within its jurisdiction. This encompasses many aspects of the environment, including but not limited to access to quality services; a safe and clean environment; safety from violence, abuse, and exploitation; access to quality educational opportunities; and access to green spaces. Several local government organizations in various countries have partnered with UNICEF to develop child-friendly cities. In Costa Rica, for example, 32 municipalities were recognized in 2017 for demonstrating improvements in five areas: (1) child and adolescent participation, (2) child rights awareness-raising, (3) a child-friendly legal framework and policies, (4) regular reporting, and (5) coordinating mechanisms to promote cross-sectoral planning.

Other cities have focused on structural changes that can be made to make cities more child-friendly. In 2006, after being labeled the worst Dutch city in which to raise a child, Rotterdam invested US$24 million, largely in one neighborhood, to create play spaces, widen sidewalks, convert parking lots to playgrounds, and develop housing more suitable for families. The second phase of this initiative expanded to other neighborhoods and, along with improvements in public spaces and housing, targeted improvements in education. The investment has to an extent met its goals, with more families moving into Rotterdam. Two major considerations when municipalities and government agencies invest in these revitalization projects are (1) the potential for other neighborhoods to be left behind or (2) that the influx of families to more friendly cities does not come at the cost of pushing out lower income families. These unintended consequences should be carefully evaluated so as not to further harm the very population of children that could benefit most from improvements in urban environment design.

5 Conclusion

It is well recognized that both positive and negative experiences in early childhood and adolescence have an impact on health across the life course. Early life experiences, which can be shaped by the social and physical attributes of urban environments, can influence health behaviors as well as mental and physical health in childhood and, in turn, affect adult health. Thus, urban environments as experienced early in life have the potential to shape adult health.

Optimizing the multiple dimensions of the urban environment to promote child and adolescent health and well-being requires a conceptual framework that recognizes that children interact with urban spaces differently based on developmental stage; that how parents interact with urban environments indirectly affects child health; and that, given the vulnerability of children, all aspects of the urban environment have the potential to impact child and adolescent health. Given that health and well-being in childhood sets the stage for health across the life course, an approach that focuses on optimizing interactions with urban environments in early life is warranted.

References

1. *The state of the world's children 2012 executive summary*. New York: United Nations Children's Fund; 2012.
2. Villanueva K, Badland H, Kvalsvig A, et al. Can the neighborhood built environment make a difference in children's development? Building the research agenda to create evidence for place-based children's policy. *Acad Pediatr.* 2016; 16(1):10–19.
3. Suglia SF, Gryparis A, Schwartz J, Wright RJ. Black carbon associated with cognition among children in a prospective birth cohort study. *Epidemiology.* 2007; 18(5):S163–S163.
4. Carroll-Scott A, Gilstad-Hayden K, Rosenthal L, et al. Disentangling neighborhood contextual associations with child body mass index, diet, and physical activity: the role of built, socioeconomic, and social environments. *Soc Sci Med.* 2013; 95:106–114.
5. Sampson RJ, Morenoff JD, Earls F. Beyond social capital: spatial dynamics of collective efficacy for children. *Am Sociol Rev.* 1999; 64:633–660.
6. Yen IH, Syme SL. The social environment and health: a discussion of the epidemiologic literature. *Annu Rev Public Health.* 1999; 20:287–308.
7. Newbury J, Arseneault L, Caspi A, Moffitt TE, Odgers CL, Fisher HL. Why are children in urban neighborhoods at increased risk for psychotic symptoms? Findings from a UK longitudinal cohort study. *Schizophr Bull.* 2016; 42(6):1372–1383.
8. Newbury J, Arseneault L, Caspi A, Moffitt TE, Odgers CL, Fisher HL. Cumulative effects of neighborhood social adversity and personal crime victimization on adolescent psychotic experiences. *Schizophr Bull.* 2018; 44(2):348–358.
9. Suglia SF, Staudemayer J, Cohen S, Wright RJ. Relationships between community violence and posttraumatic stress on children's diurnal cortisol rhythms. *Am J Epidemiol.* 2007; 165(11):S103–S103.

10. Suglia SF, Ryan L, Bellinger DC, Bosquet Enlow M, Wright RJ. Children's exposure to violence and distress symptoms: influence of caretakers' psychological functioning. *Int J Behav Med.* 2010; 18(1):1–4.

11. Lovasi GS, Schwartz-Soicher O, Quinn JW, et al. Neighborhood safety and green space as predictors of obesity among preschool children from low-income families in New York City. *Prev Med.* 2013; 57(3):189–193.

12. Carter MA, Dubois L. Neighbourhoods and child adiposity: a critical appraisal of the literature. *Health Place.* 2010; 16(3):616–628.

13. Cradock AL, Kawachi I, Colditz GA, Gortmaker SL, Buka SL. Neighborhood social cohesion and youth participation in physical activity in Chicago. *Soc Sci Med.* 2009; 68(3):427–435.

14. Drukker M, Kaplan C, Feron F, van Os J. Children's health-related quality of life, neighbourhood socio-economic deprivation and social capital. A contextual analysis. *Soc Sci Med.* 2003; 57(5):825–841.

15. Kimbro RT, Brooks-Gunn J, McLanahan S. Young children in urban areas: links among neighborhood characteristics, weight status, outdoor play, and television watching. *Soc Sci Med.* 2011; 72(5):668–676.

16. Wolf JP, Freisthler B, Kepple NJ, Chavez R. The places parents go: understanding the breadth, scope, and experiences of activity spaces for parents. *GeoJournal.* 2017; 82(2):355–368.

17. Brown BB, Werner CM, Smith KR, Tribby CP, Miller HJ. Physical activity mediates the relationship between perceived crime safety and obesity. *Prev Med.* 2014; 66:140–144.

18. Suglia SF, Shelton RC, Hsiao A, Wang YC, Rundle A, Link BG. Why the neighborhood social environment is critical in obesity prevention. *J Urban Health.* 2016; 93(1):206–212.

19. Audrey S, Batista-Ferrer H. Healthy urban environments for children and young people: A systematic review of intervention studies. *Health Place.* 2015; 36:97–117.

20. Rudolph L, Caplan J. *Health in all policies: a guide for state and local governments.* Washington, DC: Public Health Institute; 2013.

9

Inequities in Cities and in Urban Health

BEN BRISBOIS, PATRICIA O'CAMPO, AND JANISHA KAMALANATHAN

1 Cities and Inequities

From the early stages of industrialization, the burdens of urbanization have been shouldered disproportionately by the urban poor. In his seminal work on the conditions of the working class in England, Friedrich Engels describes his walk through London, contrasting impressive urban development with the unfavorable living conditions of the poor.[1] Centuries later, increases in the gross domestic product (GDP) generated by cities often do not correspond to increased participation in the labor force or improvements in the well-being of the majority of city residents.[2] As documented in the United Nations World Cities Report, income inequality in most countries is at its highest level in 30 years.[3] In 2015, the 62 richest people in the world had the same amount of wealth as the 3.6 billion people at the bottom. Over the course of five years, these 62 individuals accumulated more than a half a trillion dollars while, at the same time, the wealth of the bottom half fell by a trillion dollars.[4]

Such global inequities have a notably urban character. The financial sectors driving global economic activity operate out of cities, and the industries and working (or underemployed) classes affected by inequity-generating economic processes are primarily urban.[5] Indeed, for centuries, urbanization has played a major role in helping to resolve societal economic crises, often to the detriment of the marginalized majority.[6] The subprime mortgage and subsequent global financial crises of 2008, for example, were triggered by high-risk predatory lending to promote largely urban and suburban housing development in the United States.[6] This strategy temporarily propped up the US economy, but in ways that were notoriously unsustainable, exploitative, and disastrous for health equity in cities (and rural areas) around the world.[7,8]

In this chapter, we explore the health consequences of such city-associated inequities as well as their causes and potential solutions. We first present a framework for understanding health inequities in relation to cities. We next apply that framework to two illustrative urban health equity issues—extreme heat and epidemic obesity—highlighting the importance of structural (i.e., power-related) explanations. We end by discussing the implications for responses such as policies, programs, and social movements.

2 Documenting and Explaining Urban Health Inequities

Inequalities are qualified as *inequities* when they are systemic, socially produced, and therefore avoidable and unjust.[9] These include inequities in health, or *health inequities,* which reflect differentials in class, gender, racialization, ability, age, and other axes of inequality.[5,10] In low- and middle-income countries, the largest urban disparities in health between rich and poor include mortality (i.e., maternal mortality, child under-5 mortality, and mortality due to noncommunicable diseases) and infectious diseases such as tuberculosis and HIV.[11] In middle- and high-income countries, we see income disparities in adverse health behaviors (e.g., smoking), diabetes, and infectious diseases such as HIV and other sexually transmitted infections.[5] Environmental justice scholarship similarly shows disproportionate exposures of racialized and other marginalized communities to toxic pollution in cities around the world.[12]

2.1 A Framework for Understanding the Production of Urban Health Inequities

Figure 9.1 presents a framework for understanding how such inequities are produced, adapted from common frameworks for understanding urban health, urban health inequities, and political economic drivers of health determinants.[13–16] In this framework, domains toward the left represent root causes of urban health inequities at wide spatial and temporal scales, such as colonialism/imperialism, militarism, and rules governing global finance. In order of more or less decreasing spatial scale and level of governance, the framework then presents factors such as national and municipal institutions. These institutions structure the experiences of urban living conditions that generate health outcomes and constrain individual agency to make healthy choices.[8,16] The crosscutting role of the biophysical environment is recognized as interacting with governance and health determinants at all scales, from global environmental change to housing conditions and even "internal ecologies" within human bodies. Importantly, exposures to inequities are influenced by aspects of identity such as race, gender, socioeconomic status, and other characteristics shaped by the uncontrollable circumstances in which people live, work, grow, and age. Such "axes of inequality" interact with institutions and other structures at all scales, from the symbiosis of racism and imperialism to the role of sexism in gendered household-level interactions such as intimate partner violence.[10]

Space limitations preclude a detailed explanation of all specific determinants of urban health represented in Figure 9.1, many of which are amply described in other chapters of this book. We next apply the framework to two illustrative urban health issues, showing the necessity of engaging with large-scale structural influences on health inequity in cities.

2.2 Gaps in Existing Research on Urban Health Inequities

Scholarship on urban health and inequities typically focuses primarily on the more "proximal" (right hand side) boxes depicted in Figure 9.1. For example, most studies of social determinants of health (SDOH) and inequalities almost exclusively focus on such proximal determinants as psychosocial factors (e.g., social support); health behaviors, such as diet or physical activity; income levels; employment status; and healthcare access.[17] A small but growing subset of SDOH scholarship looks upstream at structural and political forces that are increasingly recognized as the root causes of health inequalities. One framework we drew from in designing Figure 9.1 omits "national or international wider factors" in explaining the causes of urban health inequalities, while another acknowledges them but suggests that "the most promising strategies for improving urban health are those that seek to make specific and targeted changes in [local, urban] living conditions."[15(p. 389),13(p. 12)] But while such targeted health interventions might produce improvements in health equity, too often we see their effectiveness limited by dominant—but not inevitable or unmodifiable—political and economic dynamics at national and global levels. Thus, a framework to inform evidence needs and solutions for growing urban health inequities must meaningfully consider a broader set of drivers.

3   Politicizing Explanations of Urban Health Inequities: Extreme Heat and Epidemic Obesity

In this section, we show the implications of urban health inequities as understood through the framework presented in Figure 9.1, especially when dynamics in the structural boxes on the left-hand side are foregrounded. We do this using one urban health issue strongly linked to global and local environmental change and often considered a "natural" disaster (extreme heat) and another (epidemic obesity in cities) typically linked to moralistic emphases on personal responsibility. Politicized explanations of these issues uncover important causal factors and injustices that are often neglected in common urban health approaches. Through this explicitly political lens, parallels can also be drawn with many other health inequities found in cities.

3.1   Extreme Heat and Obesity Through an Explicitly Political Lens

3.1.1   Extreme Heat, Climate Change, and Environmental Injustice in Cities

Extreme heat is a major urban health issue linked to anthropogenic climate change. The 2003 European heat wave—described by the Intergovernmental Panel on Climate Change (IPCC) as "likely" attributable to climate change—caused an estimated 15,000 deaths in France alone, with elderly Parisians living in isolation and with preexisting illnesses especially vulnerable.[18] In the 1995 Chicago heat wave, elderly, isolated, low-income, and African American men were disproportionately represented in mortality statistics.[19] In a classic depoliticizing explanation, the mayor of Chicago initially called the 1995 heat wave a "natural" disaster and actually blamed the victims for not seeking help.[19] The IPCC's 2014 report does slightly better, pointing out that "Black Americans have been reported to be more vulnerable to heat-related deaths than other racial groups in the USA. This may be due to a higher prevalence of chronic conditions such as overweight and diabetes, financial circumstances (e.g., lower incomes may restrict access to

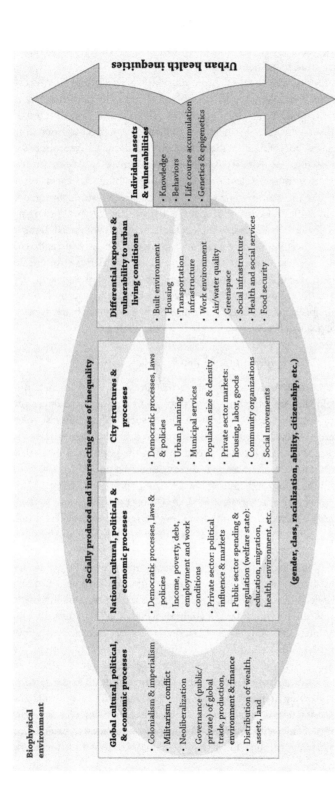

Figure 9.1 **A framework for understanding the political and intersectional production of urban health inequities.** Source: Adapted extensively from (1) Galea S, Freudenberg N, Vlahov D. A framework for the study of urban health. In: Freudenberg N, Galea S, Vlahov D, eds. *Cities and the health of the public.* Nashville, TN: Vanderbilt University Press; 2006:3–18; (2) Friel S, Hancock T, Kjellstrom T, McGranahan G, Monge P, Roy J. Urban health inequities and the added pressure of climate change: an action-oriented research agenda. *J Urban Health.* 2011; 88(5):886–889; (3) Borrell C, Pons-Vigués M, Morrison J, Díez È. Factors and processes influencing health inequalities in urban areas. *J Epidemiol Community Health.* 2013; 67(5):389–391; and (4) Birn A-E, Pillay Y, Holtz TH. *Textbook of global health.* 4th ed. New York, NY: Oxford University Press; 2017.

air conditioning during heat-waves), or community-level characteristics such as higher local crime rates or disrupted social networks."[18(p. 718)]

The IPCC, however, stops well short of identifying the power relations driving differential vulnerability. For example, what are the historical causes of black Americans' lower incomes and "disrupted social networks?" As Klinenberg's "social autopsy" demonstrates, mortality in the Chicago heat wave resulted from political decisions such as municipal service cuts, fragmentation, and privatization, all disproportionately experienced in low-income African American neighborhoods.[19] Such institutional changes interacted with and exacerbated cumulative "ethnoracial exclusion in the metropolis."[19(p. 254)] The most affected neighborhoods had been historically defined by "ethnoracially driven battles for control of space," such as urban renewal programs, segregated social housing, and race riots in which black Chicagoans who tried to move into white neighborhoods were physically attacked. Such dynamics, of course, extend centuries-long material and cultural (racist) processes affecting African Americans and originating in colonialism, from slavery through Jim Crow to the present day. The Chicago heat wave thus shows how the intersection of natural and built urban environments, questionable public policies, and long-standing racialized patterns of social exclusion can have deadly effects.

3.1.2 Epidemic Obesity and Behaviors

Obesity—abnormal or excessive fat accumulation that presents a risk to health—and its dramatic rise globally are among the top concerns of health practitioners and policymakers. A major contributor to the leading killers such as heart disease, obesity shows clear patterned urban inequities.[20] In the United States, obesity rates are the highest in North America, with more than one-third of the population older than 20 years of age obese. Rates are highest among African American populations, at close to 50% of the over-20 population, and, among low-income populations (those ≤130% of the federal poverty level), the obesity rate is 39%.[21,22] Common explanations for such patterns emphasize lifestyle factors, and the World Health Organization's (WHO) calls for action emphasize strategies to reduce high-calorie diets and promote greater physical activity.[20]

To identify interventions that will be most effective, we must instead consider the historical, social, political, and economic forces that shape urban development and constrain or promote lifestyle choices and behaviors.[23,24] Such explanations link obesity to the growth of households living with financial strain or poverty, falling wages for low- and middle-income families, and rising costs of housing, transportation, and nutritious meals. A *chronic social stress* pathway—due to increasingly precarious employment, unaffordable housing, and growing environmental threats—also alters the distribution of body fat and leads to unhealthy behaviors such as "craving of nutrient-dense comfort foods."[25(p. 16)] As a growing literature demonstrates, the influence of agri-food and advertising industries, retraction of social services, and urban planning play key roles in generating such "obesogenic" city settings.[23,25] Thus, a comprehensive explanation for obesity places major responsibility for action with industry, urban planners, and politicians at all levels.

3.2 Looking Upstream: Neoliberalism and Political Determinants of Urban Health Inequities

Politicized explanations of the structural determinants of inequities related to extreme heat and obesity are required to make full use of the framework in Figure 9.1, especially the left-hand boxes. While common explanations for urban health disparities implicate the populations most affected by those disparities, more perceptive research notes that the public's health has suffered drastically because politicians at multiple levels support "economic policy decisions [that] favor business at the expense of others in society."[26(p. 274)] Such decisions prominently include implementation of "neoliberal" austerity measures that restrict access to social determinants of health or delegate responsibility for addressing urban crises or running public services to the private sector.[8,27] "Neoliberalism" is a heuristic term for the globally dominant political and economic ideology and reforms of the time period beginning in approximately the mid-1970s—reforms that reproduce and sustain the injustices of colonialism and imperialism.[7,16] This ideology extols the power of unrestricted markets to increase societal well-being, views government "interference" in the economy as inherently inefficient, and promotes individual responsibility for solving health and other social problems.[27]

A focus on neoliberalism rounds out our explanations of obesity and racialized vulnerability to extreme heat. In the latter half of the twentieth century, North American cities lost secure middle- and working-class jobs as manufacturing declined and left the continent.[28] Mirroring the macroeconomic drivers of this urban decline (i.e., "globalization"), neoliberal reforms have reduced municipal budgets and personnel for housing, transportation, and social services, including public health activities; reduced support for labor and increased precarious work; and promoted costly private sector provision of basic city services.[8] In the case of the Chicago heat wave, therefore, the reduction, privatization, and fragmentation of city services that proved so specifically deadly to racialized communities were thoroughly consistent with broader neoliberal trends, driven by the quite purposeful national and international neoliberal "class project" to redistribute wealth *upward*.[6] These same policy changes at global, national, and municipal levels have simultaneously served to produce obesogenic environments and chronic stress pathways to obesity.[24] Thus, looking upstream from both extreme heat and obesity—and, we would add, urban health more generally—implicates neoliberal policy changes at multiple levels, making them important targets for action to reduce urban health inequities.

4 Strategies to Address Urban Health Inequities

In this section, we briefly outline the kinds of solutions our framework leads to when applied in an explicitly politicized manner to explain urban health inequities. Cities continue to be shaped by elite interests, creating and maintaining social, economic, political, and health inequalities and impoverishing a larger majority of urban dwellers.[6,23] Yet these interests can be and are being challenged as urban populations pressure governments at all levels to create inclusive cities through policies that explicitly disrupt unfair power relationships and prioritize the well-being of residents. Urgent action should be taken to raise the quality of life for the lowest income urban residents who often reside in economically and racially segregated neighborhoods lacking high-quality employment and services.

Cities with redistributive welfare policies are generally more equal and produce better population health outcomes than those that rely on markets for distribution.[16] Such democratic and inclusive policies and planning include electoral reform, participatory governance (e.g., neighborhood budgeting), or support for advocacy coalitions that strengthen civil society and give residents a voice in the making of public policies.[16] For example, density-based agreements (DBAs) in some Canadian cities force real estate developers to fund infrastructure and community services in neighborhoods where development takes place, simultaneously giving voice to grassroots groups by encouraging city staff to consult with neighborhood residents.[29] Wage rates and levels of governmental assistance that make it arithmetically impossible to afford both housing and healthy diets indicate that measures to promote decent work and a living wage are also essential.[4,8]

Complementing—and often spurring—such progressive policies, citizen-led social movements that are explicitly committed to structural transformation often pursue disruptive strategies to challenge inequities in their communities.[6] For example, the New Orleans Worker's Center for Racial Justice was formed after Hurricane Katrina to expose systemic inequities in New Orleans, organizing for labor and immigrant justice and undertaking several significant lawsuits against employer labor abuse.[30] The US-based Poor People's Campaign continues Martin Luther King Jr.'s movement to expose racialized injustices in economic, political, and social systems.[31] Today's campaign documents policies that contribute to inequities, and pursues electoral, health system, and prison reform through teach-ins, protests, rallies, and planned acts of civil disobedience.[31]

Moving beyond local campaigns, taking national and global structures as legitimate intervention points suggests a need to join up disparate urban social movements to challenge the power dynamics driving large-scale phenomena such as neoliberal capitalism and the ongoing impacts of colonialism and imperialism.[6] An analogue for such a globally organized collection of local movements is provided by the global movement for food sovereignty and its major organizational home, La Via Campesina. The food sovereignty movement brings together organizations such as small farmer cooperatives in the Global South with Global North movements for food justice and local food and seeks to influence global structures such as trade agreements and transnational corporations.[32] While the results of this coming-together are often messy and not always successful, the fundamental challenge posed by the multiscalar food sovereignty movement to inequitable global power structures provides a promising model for research-informed actions to challenge both local and global drivers of urban health inequities.

5   Moving Forward

While academic research, public policy, and social movements can fall prey to depoliticizing tendencies, such as individualizing emphases on personal responsibility and acceptance of inequitable power relations, alternatives are possible and urgently needed. Social movements that are grounded in an awareness of the contextual/structural causes of social problems, for example, have the power to inspire solidarity and make visible experiences of injustice that are shared by so many in cities. It is vital that upstream causes of health inequities be brought to the forefront of academic and popular discourse to create more aware, politically active, and mobilized communities that are better equipped to demand equality through participation in the shaping of cities. This collective struggle could be informed and inspired by a more robust field of evidence and research and pushed forward by researchers, policymakers, advocates, and activists across all sectors.

References

1. Wischnewetzky FK, Engels F, eds. The great towns. In Engels F. *The condition of the working-class in England in 1844.* Cambridge: Cambridge University Press; 2010: 23–74.
2. OECD. *Making cities work for all: data and actions for inclusive growth.* Paris: OECD Publishing; 2016. doi:10.1787/9789264263260-en
3. *Urbanization and development: emerging futures.* Nairobi: UN-Habitat; 2016.
4. Hardoon D, Ayele S, Fuentes Nieva R. *An economy for the 1%: how privilege and power in the economy drive extreme inequality and how this can be stopped.* Oxford: Oxfam International; 2016.
5. Hodgetts D, Stolte O. *Urban poverty and health inequalities: a relational approach.* New York: Routledge; 2017.
6. Harvey D. *Rebel cities: from the right to the city to the urban revolution.* London: Verso; 2013.
7. Ottersen OP, Dasgupta J, Blouin C, et al. The political origins of health inequity: prospects for change. *Lancet.* 2014; 383(9917):630–667.
8. Schrecker T, Bambra C. *How politics makes us sick: neoliberal epidemics.* New York: Palgrave MacMillan; 2015.
9. Braveman PA, Kumanyika S, Fielding J, et al. Health disparities and health equity: the issue is justice. *Am J Public Health.* 2011; 101(S1):S149–S155.
10. Gkiouleka A, Huijts T, Beckfield J, Bambra C. Understanding the micro and macro politics of health: inequalities, intersectionality and institutions—a research agenda. *Soc Sci Med.* 2018; 200:92–98.
11. World Health Organization. *10 facts on health inequities and their causes.* World Health Organization website. Available at http://www.who.int/features/factfiles/health_inequities/en/. Accessed May 25, 2018.
12. Brulle RJ, Pellow DN. Environmental justice: human health and environmental inequalities. *Annu Rev Public Health.* 2006; 27(1):103–124.
13. Galea S, Freudenberg N, Vlahov D. A framework for the study of urban health. In Freudenberg N, Galea S, Vlahov D, eds. *Cities and the health of the public.* Nashville, TN: Vanderbilt University Press; 2006:3–18.
14. Friel S, Hancock T, Kjellstrom T, McGranahan G, Monge P, Roy J. Urban health inequities and the added pressure of climate change: an action-oriented research agenda. *J Urban Health.* 2011; 88(5):886–895.
15. Borrell C, Pons-Vigués M, Morrison J, Díez È. Factors and processes influencing health inequalities in urban areas. *J Epidemiol Community Health.* 2013; 67(5):389–391.
16. Birn A-E, Pillay Y, Holtz TH. *Textbook of global health.* 4th ed. New York: Oxford University Press; 2017.
17. Berkman L, Kawachi I, Glymour M, eds. *Social epidemiology.* 2nd ed. New York: Oxford University Press; 2014.
18. Smith KR, Woodward A, Campbell-Lendrum D, et al. Human health: impacts, adaptation, and co-benefits. In Field CB, Barros VR, Dokken DK, et al., eds. *Climate change 2014: impacts,*

adaptation, and vulnerability. Part A: global and sectoral aspects. Contribution of Working Group II to the Fifth Assessment Report of the Intergovernmental Panel on Climate Change. Cambridge: Cambridge University Press; 2014:709–754.

19. Klinenberg E. Denaturalizing disaster: a social autopsy of the 1995 Chicago heat wave. *Theory Soc.* 1999; 28(2):239–295.

20. *Obesity: preventing and managing the global epidemic: report of a WHO Consultation.* Geneva, Switzerland: World Health Organization; 2000.

21. Arroyo-Johnson C, Mincey KD. Obesity epidemiology trends by race/ethnicity, gender, and education: National Health Interview Survey, 1997–2012. *Gastroenterol Clin North Am.* 2016; 45(4):571–579.

22. Ogden CL. Prevalence of obesity among adults, by household income and education—United States, 2011–2014. *MMWR Morb Mortal Wkly Rep.* 2017; 66(50):1369–1373.

23. Freudenberg N, Galea S. Cities of consumption: the impact of corporate practices on the health of urban populations. *J Urban Health.* 2008; 85(4):462–471.

24. Wisman JD, Capehart KW. Creative destruction, economic insecurity, stress, and epidemic obesity. *Am J Econ Sociol.* 2010; 69(3):936–982.

25. Scott KA, Melhorn SJ, Sakai RR. Effects of chronic social stress on obesity. *Curr Obes Rep.* 2012; 1(1):16–25.

26. Chernomas R, Hudson I. To live and die in America: labor in the time of cholera and cancer. *Int J Health Serv.* 2014; 44(2):273–284.

27. Sparke M. Health and the embodiment of neoliberalism: pathologies of political economy from climate change and austerity to personal responsibility. In Springer S, Birch K, MacLeavy J, eds. *The handbook of neoliberalism.* New York: Routledge; 2016:237–251.

28. Kletzer L. Globalization and job loss, from manufacturing to services. *J Econ Perspect.* 2005; 29(2):38–46.

29. Moore AA. Decentralized decision-making and urban planning: a case study of density for benefit agreements in Toronto and Vancouver. *Can Public Adm.* 2016; 59(3):425–447.

30. Luft RE. Beyond disaster exceptionalism: social movement developments in New Orleans after Hurricane Katrina. *Am Q.* 2009; 61(3):499–527.

31. Poor people's campaign. A national call for moral revival. Poor People's Campaign website. Available at https://www.poorpeoplescampaign.org/. Accessed July 11, 2018.

32. Patel R. What does food sovereignty look like? *J Peasant Stud.* 2009; 36(3):663–673.

10

Migration

SABRINA HERMOSILLA AND TAHILIA J. REBELLO

1 Overview

This chapter examines the impact of the movement of individuals to cities, within or across borders, on urban health. It discusses the challenges and opportunities that this human movement has on the health of both those who move and those who reside in the urban centers facing this movement.

1.1 Migration Defined

Freedom of movement is a fundamental human right.[1] The movement of a person or group of persons from their initial area of residence, their home community, or community of origin to a new geographical location known as the "destination" (sometimes referred to as the "receiving" or "host") community is termed "migration."[2-4] Migration is not a novel process and has been occurring since early human history; modern migration to cities, in particular, has its roots in the Industrial Revolution.[2] Migration can occur both internally (within a political state) or externally (movement across political borders).[2,3] The flow of migrants within and across countries is dynamic.[2] Internal migration, most notably rural to urban migration, has accelerated over the past 20 years, specifically in populous countries such as China and India.[5] Urban areas house more than half of the global population, and both internal and external migrants often settle here; with more than 3 million people moving to cities weekly, migration is becoming synonymous with urbanization.[2,3,6] Global cities, such as Dubai (83%) and Brussels (62%) have the highest percentage of foreign-born populations and are central to global financial and economic systems.[3] Across North American and Europe, internal or regional migration has increased in the past two decades to smaller urban centers (500,000–3 million residents), driven by the search for improved employment, education, and quality of life, often taxing existing infrastructure and governance structures.[7] Urban centers have also begun to depopulate (e.g., Detroit's population decreased by one-quarter in 10 years), leading local governments to encourage international immigration to stabilize their cities, spur economic development, and shore up labor shortages.[3,8]

Migration is a multiphased process that may occur over diverging periods of time. It includes the pre-migration or pre-departure phase; the migration phase, which involves transit between the community of origin and the destination community; and the post-migration phase when individuals arrive at and resettle in their destination community.[3,4] In some cases, there may be a fourth return phase in which individuals may repatriate or move back to their communities of origin (circular migration). An individual who is moving or has moved is referred to as a "migrant," regardless of their reasons, where they move from or to, their legal status, or the length of their (intended) stay.[2–4]

1.2   Reasons for Urban Migration and Types of Migrants

There are a multitude of diverse motivations that drive migration. The push–pull model is used to define the interplay between those factors that push individuals away from their home communities and those that pull or attract individuals to their intended destinations.[2,4] These factors can be broadly categorized into four groups.

First, there are economic factors: economic migrants and migrant workers constitute approximately two of every three international migrants, with more than 98% in high- and middle-income countries.[2] In 2013, economic migrants worked primarily in the service industry (71%), manufacturing and construction (18%), and agriculture (11%).[2]

Second, political factors: this includes forcibly displaced individuals such as refugees, internally displaced persons (IDPs), and asylum seekers. According to the United Nations High Commissioner for Refugees (UNHCR), in 2016, 65.6 million individuals had been forcibly displaced from their homes globally (22.5 million considered refugees, 40.3 million internally displaced, and 2.8 million asylum-seekers), with 10.3 million displaced in 2016 alone.[9] Among refugees, most are children (51% under 18 years old), and 75,000 in 2016 were unaccompanied or separated from their primary caregivers. Per capita, Lebanon hosts the most refugees (one in six within Lebanon are refugees), with more than half of the global refugee population originating from the Syrian Arab Republic (5.5 million), Afghanistan (2.5 million), and South Sudan (1.4 million).[9] A common misconception is that forced migrants reside in refugee or organized camps; in Turkey, for example, only 8% of refugees reside in camps, while Istanbul alone has at least 539,000 Syrian refugees.[10] Human trafficking, forced labor, and modern-day slavery estimates are harder to obtain due to their illicit nature. In 2014, 17,752 victims were detected across 85 nations.[11] Detected trafficked victims are often women and girls (71%) and are either sexually exploited (women and girls) or subjected to forced labor (men); more than half reside in Bangladesh, China, India, Pakistan, and Uzbekistan.[11,12]

Third, social factors: this includes migration for the purposes of family reunification and improved living conditions.

Finally, there are environmental factors: migration in response to environmental triggers and natural disasters.[2–4] Of those internally displaced by disasters, climate-related incidents (e.g., droughts and flooding, which can lead to the destruction of habitable land and food insufficiency) were responsible for almost all (97%) displacements.[13] The preceding four groups are not mutually exclusive, and an individual's push–pull factors for migrating may fall into more than one category.

1.3 Migrant Demographics in Urban Centers

A basic understanding of the existing demographic profile of migrants is essential to understanding the urban health implications of migration. In 2015, an estimated 984 million migrants—one in every seven people—moved across international borders (244 million) or within their country of birth (740 million).[2,11,14] While the majority of citizens remain within their country of birth for their lifetime, the proportion of international migrants to the global population has remained stable over the past 40 years (2.3% in 1970 to 3.3% in 2015).[2] Migrants are primarily working aged (72% aged 20–64 years), with slightly more males (52%) migrating than females.[14] Europe, Asia, and North America hosted 84% of the total international migrant stock in 2015; however, based on per capita estimates, Oceania hosted the highest at 21% of the total population, and Asia saw the largest amount of growth from 2000 to 2015 (a greater than 50% increase).[14] The United States (46.6 million) and Germany (12 million) were the top two destinations for international migrants in 2015, while India and Mexico were the top two countries of emigrants.[14] Of note, 10 of the top 20 destination countries for international migrants were also top emigrant countries, evidence of the complexity of international migration flows.[14] There are limited data available on dynamic international migrant flows.[15]

2 Relevance of Migration to Urban Health

Migration is a major contributor to urban population growth, and migrants compose a substantial proportion of urban residents globally.[2,16] Figure 10.1 presents the 15 countries with the largest percentage of foreign-born residents and the respective percentage of urbanicity within each country.[14] Thus, addressing the health impact of the migration process is an integral component of urban health.

Migration is associated with significant transitions and disruptions that may occur in the various phases of migration.[3,4,16] This includes the disruption of social structures, transitions to new socioeconomic and/or cultural environments, and potential exposure to extreme conditions, violence, and malnutrition.[2,4] All of these can impact the health status of migrants, and, as such, migration can be considered a social determinant of health.[2,4] Certain subsets of migrants, such as children, women, the elderly, refugees, asylum seekers, victims of human trafficking, IDPs, low-skilled laborers, undocumented or irregular migrants, and those with preexisting health conditions, may be especially vulnerable to the health impacts of migration.[2,4,16] Factors in the receiving community, such as the experience of social inclusion or exclusion (e.g., due to discrimination, xenophobia), human rights violations, and the availability of housing, employment and education opportunities, and health services, can all impact migrant health.[2,4,16] Moreover, urban migrants impact the demographic and epidemiological profile of their destination communities, thereby potentially impacting health outcomes for nonmigrant urban residents as well.[2,4,16] Migration can result in rapid and dynamic growth of cities, posing new challenges and opportunities to address inequities and inefficiencies in health systems and to develop effective services, structures, and policies that accommodate the needs of a more pluralistic urban demographic.[2,16]

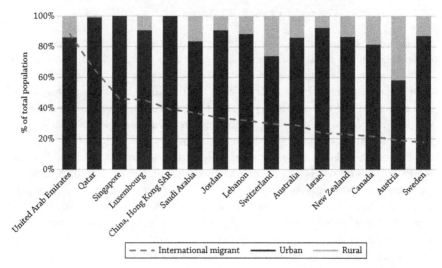

Figure 10.1 **Urban residence by countries hosting the largest percentage of international migrants, 2017.** Countries selected based on percentage of international migrants (out of total population) estimated within each country. Urban/rural distinction is based on country-specific criteria. Data combining both international and domestic migrant counts with urbanicity are not available on a global scale. Percentage of international migrants by country: 88.4% United Arab Emirates, 65.2% Qatar, 46.0% Singapore, 45.3% Luxembourg, 39.0% Hong Kong, 37.0% Jordan, 33.3% Lebanon, 32.0% Saudi Arabia, 29.6% Switzerland, 29.0% Australia, 24.0% Israel, 23.0% New Zealand, 21.5% Canada, 19.0% Austria, 18.0% Sweden, and 16.0% Cyprus. Source: International migrant stock: the 2017 revision. United Nations website; 2017. Available at http://www.un.org/en/development/desa/population/migration/data/estimates2/estimates17.shtml. Accessed May 1, 2018.

3 Migration Journeys' Influence on Health

Pre-departure, migrants tend to be healthier and more mobile than those who choose not to or are unable to migrate. Migrants suffer deleterious health outcomes during the migration journey related to exposure, exploitation and violence, unsafe transportation, and lack of basic needs and illnesses.[2] The International Organization for Migration (IOM) started collecting information in the Missing Migrants Project (MMP) in 2013 to quantify the scope of migrant deaths globally.[2] Data collection is significantly limited by many factors, including inaccessibility of migrant routes, lack of official reporting, and inaccurate or incomplete testimonies from fellow migrants.[2] Yet, given these severe underestimations, in 2016, the MMP reported 7,927 missing or dead migrants globally, primarily in the Mediterranean Sea and North Africa.[2] In recognition of migrants' plight, the United Nations General Assembly adopted the New York Declaration for Refugees and Migrants in 2016 to set a roadmap for a global compact to improve the safety of migrants throughout their journeys.[2,17] Migrant journeys also deleteriously influence a migrant's family and social network, including the health of those left behind.[5,18]

4 Challenges and Opportunities Motivated by Migration to Urban Centers

4.1 Health Services and Systems

Urban migrants present unique challenges to existing health services and systems, but, if these challenges are addressed, they may provide a unique opportunity to address and improve the very systems they challenge. In identifying and accommodating the health service needs of migrants and their impact on urban health, we consider health-care access, vulnerable subpopulations, health service effectiveness, health outcomes monitoring, and a multisectoral approach to improving health for all.

4.1.1 Barriers to Accessing Care

Urban migrants may experience logistical, language, and legal barriers that limit their ability to access and receive quality healthcare. These include a lack of familiarity with the health system, which may prevent them from efficiently navigating bottlenecks, administrative procedures, or clinical processes; lack or high cost of transportation to physically access services; prohibitive costs of health and diagnostic services; inability to speak the language(s) of the destination community; limited health literacy and the influence of the home culture on help-seeking behavior; experience of real or perceived discrimination and social exclusion, xenophobia, and stigma; lack of insurance coverage and/or legal immigration status; and legal and regulatory frameworks that prevent or exclude migrants from services.[3,4]

4.1.2 Vulnerable Subsets and Urban Spaces

Certain migrant subsets, such as women, children, and the elderly; those with preexisting health conditions prior to migration; refugees and asylum seekers who may have experienced extreme conditions, violence, and trauma; and immigrants who lack legal status may have enhanced and specific service needs. Moreover, those individuals living in vulnerable contexts within urban centers—such as in slums, informal, or low-income housing—may find it particularly hard to access services as health structures may be limited or nonexistent in their spaces.[3,4,16,19] They may also be more likely to experience overcrowding, lack of sanitation, and violence, and they are less likely to be able to afford or access services, which can substantially impact health.[3,16]

4.1.3 Effective Services

Migrants require services that are culturally, linguistically, and logistically sensitive to the migrant experience. This may require training and support for health professionals to implement culturally appropriate care and to strengthen their understanding of how migration serves as a social determinant of health. This also warrants engagement of community members/groups; inclusion of migrants in service and system design; presence of translators, interpreters, and cultural brokers to overcome communication barriers; and promotion of regulations and/or policies that make services more accessible to migrants.[3,4,20]

4.1.4 Migrant Health Outcome Tracking

There is a dearth of data on migrant status. Definitions for relevant variables are not standardized, and the quality of data collected is limited.[3] This makes it difficult to track migrant flow, subsequently impeding the ability to enhance continuity of care and provide longitudinal services to migrants and impeding efforts to monitor and evaluate their health outcomes. This lack of robust and effective data collection structures hinders the assessment of the impact of migrant health services, programs, and policies for the purposes of service planning and strengthening.

4.1.5 Multisectoral Approaches

Beyond health services, the barriers just listed affect the ability of migrants to access services in other relevant sectors including education, housing, employment, and social services—all of which can, in turn, impact health outcomes.[3,4,20] Thus, services for migrants in multiple sectors warrant strengthening, and a cohesive, collaborative approach is recommended. Addressing the health needs of urban migrants may require specialized health services and financial and human resources, but the injection of capital and resources into the health system can potentially benefit all urban dwellers.

The Johannesburg Migrant Health Forum (JHB-MHF) provides a unique example of a multisectoral, integrated, local response to migration in urban settings. Domestic (more than 30% in 2011) and international (13% in 2011) migrants have long been drawn to Johannesburg, South Africa, in search of economic opportunity and security.[21] In 2008, the JHB-MHF was established by the African Centre for Migration and Society at the University of Witwatersrand, the IOM South Africa, and the Wits Reproductive Health and HIV Institute to address critical unmet needs in the densely migrant-populated Hillbrow inner-city region.[21] To date, this purposively informal forum has fostered local migration and health responses by (1) actively monitoring discrimination against migrants in the public sector, (2) linking community members with policymakers, and (3) facilitating collaboration between service providers and nongovernmental organizations to improve migrant health.[21]

4.2 Urban Context Matters

Linguistic, cultural, and religious diversity—hallmarks of urban settings—are both a byproduct of migration and a draw for migrants. However, the specific urban context within which migrants reside influences their experience, challenging the creation of global frameworks and supporting a case-based approach to tackling their unique health needs.[19] For example, migration is central to both the megacity and the shrinking city phenomena.

In *megacities*, urban planners struggle to keep up with housing stock and infrastructure demand, resulting in more than one-third of migrants residing in informal settlements.[2] The hazardous conditions here—poor health resulting from poor water and sanitation, poverty, crime, and lack of education and economic opportunity—are well documented.[2,12,16] Historic efforts to improve economic conditions have often relied on policies of low-wage labor, exploitation, and other factors detrimental to health outcomes.[22] Current efforts to create inclusive urban development, whereby residents of slums are empowered to actively participate in development projects (e.g., clean community cook stove initiative in Nairobi, the public water and sewage system in Caracas, and the Johannesburg Migrant Health Forum) have been met with some success in poverty reduction and gains in education and health, and they are potentially applicable outside of the informal settlements where they were developed.[21–24] Similarly, context-specific planning practices that operate within global frameworks of inclusion and ethical treatment could be adapted beyond urban settings.

Shrinking cities (almost 10% of cities in the United States), where outmigration and low fertility levels have resulted in smaller populations and tax bases, have found increased international immigration beneficial to their existing population and future stability, translating a potential challenge into an opportunity for growth.[2,8]

Understanding the unique challenges faced by migrants and their health needs across settings, IOM has begun supporting health screening and vaccination campaigns targeted at migrants both before, during, and after arriving at their host communities.[2] From 2012 to 2016, the IOM and the US Refugee Admissions Program, for example, vaccinated more than 215,000 refugees across 21 countries.[2] While the estimated unmet need for vaccines and other health services remains significant, this serves as an example of supranational partnerships with local bodies to improve health outcomes for all.

4.3 Governance and Policy Fragmentation

Urban migration can present new challenges and opportunities to existing government structures and policymakers. Modern governance systems, whose origins stem from a predominantly rural era when urban centers were the minority, must adapt to the changing needs and balance of power that an urbanized society requires. While nations create international migration policy (and are thus often the unit of analysis for documenting migration), the importance of global cities in guiding and developing local and national policy and governance rules should be respected.[25] Migrant health policy fragmentation between the national and local levels—reflecting the tension between national migration policy and urban service provision and inclusivity—can be addressed through empowering local urban governments to respond to and guide migration patterns, as exemplified by the US, UK, and Canadian sanctuary city initiatives and supported by the international community in the Sutherland Report.[2,17,26] City governments must work with multicultural urban planners to realize plans that allow for economic, health, and religious sites for migrants. Jurisdictional change may be required to ensure that urban centers can address the needs of their changed migrant population, such as revenue and tax generation, land use, and infrastructure, which can then be leveraged to improve the lives of all urban residents.

5 Maximizing Opportunities of Migration for Urban Health

We are living in the most mobile era in history. Substantial migration to cities has been accompanied by stress on existing population, governance, and health systems.

The influx of migrants provides an opportunity for citizens and policymakers to reflect on and improve existing societal structures and processes to better serve not only the newly arrived but also the underserved in all communities. Failure to respond coherently to the increased needs in urban settings threatens to destabilize local and regional governments. Cities urgently need to develop, adopt, and implement inclusive, sustainable, multicultural urban plans that leverage migrant populations' inherent perseverance, social connections, and ingenuity.

Acknowledgments

The authors would like to thank Natalie Tikhonovsky for her invaluable assistance providing background research and copyediting for this chapter.

References

1. Assembly UNG. Universal declaration of human rights. In: Assembly UNG, ed1948. http://www.un.org/en/universal-declaration-human-rights/
2. Migration IOF. World Migration Report 2018. 2017. https://www.iom.int/wmr/world-migration-report-2018
3. Migration IOF. World Migration Report 2015. Migrants and Cities: New Partnerships to Manage Mobility. 2015. https://www.iom.int/world-migration-report-2015
4. Shultz C. Migration, Health and Urbanization: Interrelated Challenges. 2014. https://www.iom.int/sites/default/files/our_work/ICP/MPR/WMR-2015-Background-Paper-CSchultz.pdf
5. Mou J, Griffiths SM, Fong H, Dawes MG. Health of China's rural–urban migrants and their families: a review of literature from 2000 to 2012. *Br Med Bull.* 2013; 106(1):19–43.
6. Habitat UN. *State of the world's cities 2008/2009: harmonious cities.* London: *Earthscan,* 2008.
7. Esipova N, Pugliese A, Ray J. The demographics of global internal migration. *Migration Policy Pract.* 2013; 3(2):3–5.
8. Tacoli C, McGranahan G, Satterthwaite D. *Urbanisation, rural-urban migration and urban poverty.* Human Settlements Group, International Institute for Environment and Development; 2015. London, UK; http://pubs.iied.org/pdfs/10725IIED.pdf
9. UNHCR GT. Forced Displacement in 2016. 2017. Available at http://www.unhcr.org/globaltrends2016/. Accessed April 10, 2018.
10. Erdoğan M. Urban refugees from "detachment" to "harmonization" Syrian refugees and process management of municipalities: the case of Istanbul. *Marmara Belediyeler Birliği Kültür Yayınları.* 2017. https://mmuraterdogan.files.wordpress.com/2016/06/mmu-urban-refugees-report-2017_en.pdf
11. Barriers O. Human mobility and development. *Human Dev Rep.* 2009. http://hdr.undp.org/sites/default/files/reports/269/hdr_2009_en_complete.pdf
12. Foundation WF. The Global Slavery Index 2016. 2016. Available at https://www.globalslaveryindex.org/findings/. Accessed April 18, 2018.
13. Center IDMC. Global Report on Internal Displacement, 2017. http://www.internal-displacement.org/global-report/grid2017/
14. United Nations. International Migrant Stock: The 2017 Revision. Available at http://www.un.org/en/development/desa/population/migration/data/estimates2/estimates17.shtml. Accessed May 1, 2018.

15. United Nations. International Migration Flows to and from Selected Countries: The 2015 Revision. 2015. Available at http://www.un.org/en/development/desa/population/migration/data/empirical2/migrationflows.shtml.

16. Alirol E, Getaz L, Stoll B, Chappuis F, Loutan L. Urbanisation and infectious diseases in a globalised world. *Lancet Infect Dis.* 2011; 11(2):131–141.

17. Assembly UNG. Report of the Special Representative of the Secretary-General on Migration. In: Assembly UNG, ed2017. http://www.un.org/en/development/desa/population/migration/events/coordination/15/documents/Report%20of%20SRSG%20on%20Migration%20-%20A.71.728_ADVANCE.pdf

18. Murphy R, Zhou M, Tao R. Parents' migration and children's subjective well-being and health: evidence from rural China. *Population, Space Place.* 2016; 22(8):766–780.

19. Wild V, Dawson A. Migration: a core public health ethics issue. *Public Health.* 2018; 158:66–70.

20. Pottie K, Greenaway C, Feightner J, et al. Evidence-based clinical guidelines for immigrants and refugees. *CMAJ.* 2011; 183(12):E824–E925.

21. Vearey J, Thomson K, Sommers T, Sprague C. Analysing local-level responses to migration and urban health in Hillbrow: the Johannesburg Migrant Health Forum. *BMC Public Health.* 2017; 17(3):427.

22. Roy M, Cawood S, Hordijk M, Hulme D. *Urban poverty and climate change: life in the slums of Asia, Africa and Latin America.* New York: Routledge; 2016.

23. Lesirma S. Energy access among the urban poor in Kenya: a case study of Kibera slums. *Intl J Environ Sci.* 2016; 1(1):17–28.

24. Smith CE. Design with the other 90%: Cities. *Places Journal.* 2011. https://placesjournal.org/article/design-with-the-other-90-cities/

25. Sassen S. *The global city: New York, London, Tokyo.* Princeton, NJ: Princeton University Press; 1991.

26. Bauder H. Sanctuary cities: policies and practices in international perspective. *International Migration.* 2017; 55(2):174–187.

11

Education

JENNIFER KARAS MONTEZ AND AMY ELLEN SCHWARTZ

1 Challenges and Opportunities in Delivering Education in Urban Areas

The importance of educational attainment for an individual's health and the importance of mass education for population health has been documented in numerous countries.[1] Education is so crucial, in fact, that ensuring inclusive and quality education for all by the year 2030 is one of the United Nation's 17 Sustainable Development Goals.

The importance of education to health differs in magnitude across geographic contexts, however.[1] In the United States, which is the focus of this chapter, education is one of strongest predictors of how healthy an individual will be and how long an individual will live.[2] Graduating from high school with a diploma is crucial, especially in urban areas.[3] At the same time, high school graduation rates are lower in urban than rural areas, in part due to the unique challenges in delivering education in city school districts. This chapter reviews those challenges, explains the importance of schooling (especially receiving a high school diploma) for adult health and longevity, and illustrates the extent to which the health of urban residents suffers from their lower average level of education.

1.1 Urban School Districts Are Large and Complex

Almost one-third of America's school children—roughly 15 million students—are educated in city school districts, and more than 8 million of these children are educated in the 190 largest city school districts.[4] These large city school districts serve an average of 42,000 students across roughly 75 schools that differ in numerous and significant ways from the typical suburban, rural, and smaller city districts, which educate a few thousand students across a handful of schools. The largest city school district in the country, New York City, enrolls more than 1.1 million students in more than 1,800 schools, with a current operating budget of $24 billion.[5] Staffing, monitoring, coordinating, and managing such a large set of schools presents greater complexity than typically arises in smaller districts. The scale of assessment and accountability requires layered administrative structures and engenders a web of rules and regulations designed to foster equity and fairness; however, it too often creates rigidities that hinder innovation and efficiency.

The politics of large city education is often particularly fraught. School district decisions often involve large, professional union locals and advocacy organizations (from all sides of the political spectrum), national media markets, as well as city leaders hoping to use their particular school district stage to pursue national ambitions. The combined complexities make it difficult to enact beneficial changes in policy and practice.

The large size of urban school districts does, however, offer several key opportunities. In particular, it allows for a diversity of schools differentiated by curriculum, mission, or pedagogical style; by size or facilities; by grade span or admissions criteria; and by programs and services for students with disabilities or in need of special services, among others. This offers the opportunity to match students to more effective programs, to take advantage of economies of scale in delivering specialized services, and to experiment with alternatives methods. Indeed, some of the country's *best* public schools are city schools, including high schools and specialized programs of many kinds.[6] Finally, the professionalism and size of the staff in city schools can foster the development of best practices, and some of the best new evidence about "what works" in education comes from urban schools.

1.2   Urban Students Are Diverse and Disadvantaged

Large city school districts differ markedly from other districts in the demographic characteristics of their students. Roughly one-quarter of city students are black and one-third are Hispanic, with a significantly lower share of white students (less than a third) than the national average and a significantly larger share of Asian students.[4] Thus, city schools must contend with the consequences of discrimination and racial inequality. Many cities serve as gateways for immigrants to the United States, and thus city schools enroll new students from a wide array of countries, speaking many different languages, and bringing widely varying prior educational experiences. Mirroring these, the students are disproportionately English language learners and economically poor (as measured by eligibility for free or reduced-price lunch programs).[4] Thus, students' educational and support needs are particularly high. At the same time, their parents are less likely to be able to provide assistance in navigating school. Urban school parents are less likely to have completed high school, attended college, or have the resources and flexibility that suburban parents leverage to support their children's academic success. Taken together, the features of urban schools and the students they serve mean that the cost of educating urban school children is higher than elsewhere.

That said, the rich diversity of urban school children offers opportunities for students to engage with other cultures, thus preparing students for a diverse world. Dual-language schools, for example, offer unique educational opportunities for native English speakers to learn alongside students for whom English is a second language. Furthermore, immigrant students are often among the best performing students and highly engaged in their schooling, making them good classmates.

1.3 School Funding Disadvantages Cities

Although there is significant variation across US states, school finance places much of the responsibility for funding schools on local districts, which rely heavily on property taxation. In fact, local sources of revenues typically account for 40–50% of school budgets. Revenues from property taxation alone typically represent two-thirds of this sum. Thus, school funding depends critically on the income and wealth of district residents. This is particularly problematic for city schools given the comparatively high proportion of economically disadvantaged residents within city school districts versus, for example, suburban districts. At the same time, cities often face higher operating costs: wages are higher, making it more expensive to hire teachers, principals, and support staff; land and construction are more expensive; and so on. While state and federal aid are also often higher in these districts (designed to compensate for both higher costs and lower ability to pay), the assistance is rarely sufficient to close the gaps in funding with wealthier districts. These inequalities persist, in part, because households can easily move to adjacent non–city districts when family economic circumstances improve, where school spending is higher, property values lower, and the costs of education are lower.

1.4 Implications for Educational Attainment

The challenges facing urban education just discussed are easily seen reflected in the lower performance of urban students on standardized tests. On the 2015 National Assessment for Educational Progress among fourth- and eighth-grade students, the percentage of students scoring "Below Basic" on reading and mathematics was highest in the large city school districts.[7] For instance, among fourth graders, 41% in large city districts scored "Below Basic" compared to 28% of their peers in suburban districts. Among eighth graders, these percentages were 33% and 22%, respectively. For many urban students, the inadequacy of their primary and secondary education translates into relatively low levels of attainment. For example, an analysis of data from 2009–2010 found that the high school graduation rate for public high school students was roughly 68% in city districts, compared to more than 80% in suburban and rural districts.[8] The lower likelihood of graduating from high school with a diploma in urban school districts may be one of the most crucial consequences for these students, one that will reverberate throughout their lifetimes. For instance, a study spanning the latter part of the twentieth century found that graduating from high school lowers a person's risk of death more than any other single year of education.[3]

In the next section, we describe the importance of educational attainment on a host of outcomes including economic well-being and social ties, but we focus on its implications for health and longevity in adulthood. We explain key theories about why education matters and why it matters especially so in urban environments. We also show how much the health of adults in urban environments might improve by raising high school and college graduation rates.

2 Importance of Educational Attainment for the Health of Urban Residents

Schooling influences numerous experiences and outcomes in life. It influences work, marriage, family size, income, home ownership, friendship networks, hobbies, and lifestyles, to name a few. Schooling is especially important for health and longevity. In fact, in high-income countries such as the United States, the amount of schooling individuals obtain is one of the strongest determinants of how healthy they will be and how long they will live.[2] The more education an individual has obtained, the less likely he or she is to develop chronic conditions such as diabetes, metabolic syndrome, cardiovascular disease, hypertension, disability, depression, and many types of cancer.[9]

2.1 Educational Attainment Is a Fundamental Cause of Adult Health

The association between educational attainment and adult health is so robust and strong that education is often referred to as a "fundamental cause" of health.[10] Education teaches critical skills such as how to read, write, synthesize information, communicate, persevere through challenges, and reconcile conflicting information and points of view.[11] Individuals can then draw on these human capital skills to navigate all domains of contemporary life, such as employment and social relationships. Education is unlike other types of socioeconomic resources such as income, employment, or occupational prestige. Education provides human capital skills that are intrinsic; they inhere within the individual. In contrast, other socioeconomic resources such as income and employment are extrinsic and fluctuate greatly across the life span and across macroeconomic cycles.

Explanations for why education strongly predicts health in adulthood are numerous and complex. Even so, they are often consolidated into three main groups.[11] The first explanation points to economic well-being. Adults with more years of education tend to be stably employed, to have jobs that are safe and satisfying, to make higher incomes, and to own homes in safe, clean, and healthy neighborhoods. All of these factors, in turn, enhance health. A second explanation is lifestyles. Adults with more schooling tend to engage in physical exercise, maintain a healthy body weight, and avoid smoking and heavy consumption of alcohol. A third explanation points to social relationships. Adults with more years of education tend to marry, stay married, and maintain beneficial social networks. In addition to these explanations, medical care is sometimes proposed as a fourth explanation, although the evidence is quite mixed. The importance of education for garnering all of these economic, social, and lifestyle resources for health has increased over the last half century.[12]

2.2 The Importance of Education for Health Depends on Geography

Education may be more critical for health in some environments than others. In fact, a small but growing number of US studies have found that the health benefits of education strongly depend on which region or state an individual resides in and whether he or she resides in an urban or rural area. For instance, a 2014 study of the four US Census regions found that the importance of education for reducing the risk of death was strongest in the South and weakest in the Northeast.[13] A 2017 study of US states found that the benefits of education for avoiding disability was strongest in states like Mississippi and West Virginia and weakest in states like Minnesota and New York.[14] A 1997 study of older US men found that the importance of education for reducing the risk of death was pronounced in urban areas but nonexistent in rural areas.[15] In urban areas, older men in that study with a primary school education had a 20% greater risk of death than did their peers with at least 1 year of college. Another key and consistent finding across these studies is that geography matters more for the health of low-educated adults than it does for high-educated adults. Having a low level of education is particularly bad for health in certain geographic locations.[14] Urban areas are one such location.

Why might having a low level of education elevate the risk of poor health and early death in urban areas more so than rural areas? The reasons seem to reflect the contextual characteristics of urban environments, net of any personal characteristics of urban residents.[15] For instance, compared to rural environments, urban environments are more often characterized by higher crime rates, ambient hazards such as noise and air pollution, greater social disorder, wider income inequality, greater variability in the quality of the physical environment due to residential segregation, and higher prevalence of unhealthy behaviors, including smoking, heavy alcohol consumption, and sedentary lifestyles.[15,16] Consequently, in urban areas, a higher socioeconomic status (e.g., higher education, higher income) may be necessary to avoid, or at least mitigate, these major risks to health by, for instance, moving to a more desirable part of the urban area.

2.3   Documenting the Importance of Education for Health in Urban and Rural Areas

This section documents the association between educational attainment and adult health within urban and rural areas of the United States. To estimate the association, we used data from the 2017 Annual Social and Economic Supplement to the Current Population Survey (the data are made available by the Minnesota Population Center).[17] It is one of the largest nationally representative surveys of the noninstitutionalized population, including roughly 70,000 households. We include 73,951 adults in the survey who were US-born and 30–70 years of age.

The survey contains information on health, education, and urban–rural residence, in addition to other demographic and economic factors. Respondents were asked whether they considered their health to be excellent, very good, good, fair, or poor. We defined "favorable" health as excellent, very good, or good, and unfavorable as fair or poor. The survey also asks respondents' their highest level of education, which we collapse into four groups. It also identifies whether respondents resided in a metropolitan statistical area; we considered these areas to approximate urban areas. Using a regression model, we estimated the percentage of adults in favorable health by education level within urban and rural areas and accounted for differences between urban and rural areas in adults' age, sex, and race.

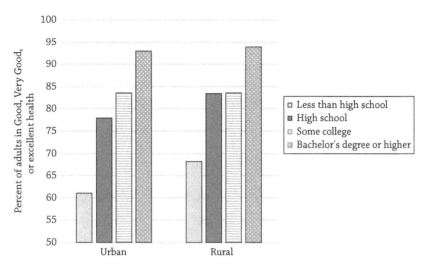

Figure 11.1 **Percentage of adults in favorable health by level of educational attainment, within urban and rural areas of the United States.** Data are from 73,951 US-born individuals aged 30-70 years in the 2017 Annual Social and Economic Supplement of the Current Population Survey. Using a logit model, probabilities are estimated from four categories of education, urban-rural status, cross-product terms between education and urban-rural status, age, sex, and race. Probabilities shown for average-aged adults.

In both urban and rural areas, the percentage of adults who report favorable health is positively associated with education level. For instance, Figure 11.1 shows these percentages for adults 50 years of age. In urban areas, just 61% of them without a high school credential were in favorable health, compared to 78% of those with a high school credential, 84% of those with some college, and 93% of them with a bachelor's degree or higher. In rural areas, the percentages of adults in favorable health were 68%, 83%, 86%, and 94%, respectively. As expected, having a low level of education—especially lacking a high school credential—is more problematic for health within urban than rural areas. The health disadvantage of urban residents becomes increasingly smaller with each successive level of education; the urban health disadvantage effectively vanishes among adults with a bachelor's degree or higher.

2.4 Topics for Future Research

More work is needed to understand why having low education, particularly lacking a high school credential, is so problematic for health in urban areas. While underlying differences in the characteristics of residents play some role, substantial evidence points to certain features of the environment.[15] Our data provide some support for this. In our analyses, even if we had accounted for several additional characteristics of the survey respondents (employment status, occupation, poverty status, marital status), the health gap between low-educated urban and rural residents persists. There is some evidence from prior studies, however, that lifestyle behaviors such as smoking play a small role, at least for older cohorts of men.[15] The question is then: What environmental factors account for the gap in health between low-educated urban and rural residents? Is it due to the content and quality of K–12 schooling in urban areas? Is it due to the greater concentration of poverty, crime, substandard housing, and pollution in precisely those sections of urban areas where low-educated adults tend to reside? Addressing these questions is imperative for developing strategies to mitigate the health risks of having low education in urban areas.

3 Conclusion

Urban school districts face many unique challenges which often manifest in lower achievement scores and lower graduation rates compared to other school districts. Given the importance of schooling for adult health and longevity, these challenges also manifest in poor health for urban residents, particularly for those without a high school diploma. These challenges are not limited to the United States, however. As the proportion of the world's population living in urban areas continues to grow, improving access and quality of urban education will be essential for human capital and economic development, human health, and perhaps even the sustainability of cities. In sum, investment in urban schooling districts is a global public health imperative.

Acknowledgments

This research was supported in part by grant R01AG055481-01, "Educational Attainment, Geography, and US Adult Mortality Risk," awarded by the National Institute on Aging (Jennifer Karas Montez, Principal Investigator).

References

1. Smith WC, Anderson E, Salinas D, Horvatek R, Baker DP. A meta-analysis of education effects on chronic disease: the causal dynamics of the Population Education Transition Curve. *Soc Sci Med.* 2015; 127:29–40.
2. Galea S, Tracy M, Hoggatt KJ, DiMaggio C, Karpati A. Estimated deaths attributable to social factors in the United States. *Am J Public Health.* 2011; 101:1456–1465.
3. Montez JK, Hummer RA, Hayward MD. Educational attainment and adult mortality in the United States: a systematic assessment of functional form. *Demography.* 2012; 49:315–336.
4. Urban education in America. National Center for Education Statistics website. Available at https://nces.ed.gov/surveys/ruraled/tables/a.1.a.-1.asp?refer=urban2013. Accessed May 18, 2018.
5. NYC Department of Education website. Available at https://www.schools.nyc.gov/about-us/reports/doe-data-at-a-glance. Accessed September 5, 2018.
6. Best public high schools in America. Niche website. Available at https://www.niche.com/k12/search/best-public-high-schools/. Accessed May 18, 2018.
7. The nation's report card. National Assessment of Educational Progress website. Available at https://www.nationsreportcard.gov/. Accessed May 18, 2018.
8. The status of rural education. National Center for Education Statistics website. Available at https://nces.ed.gov/programs/coe/indicator_tla.asp. Accessed May 18, 2018.

9. Zajacova A, Lawrence EM. The relationship between education and health: reducing disparities through a contextual approach. *Annu Rev Public Health.* 2018; 39: 271–289. doi:10.1146/annurev-publhealth-031816-044628

10. Link BG. Epidemiological sociology and the social shaping of population health. *J Health Soc Behav.* 2008; 49:367–384.

11. Mirowsky J, Ross CE. *Education, social status, and health.* New York: Aldine de Gruyter; 2003.

12. Goesling B. The rising significance of education for health. *Soc Forces.* 2007; 85:1621–1644.

13. Montez JK, Berkman LF. Trends in the educational gradient of mortality: bringing regional context into the explanation. *Am J Public Health.* 2014; 104:e82–e90. doi:10.2105/AJPH.2013.301526

14. Montez JK, Zajacova A, Hayward MD. Disparities in disability by educational attainment across U.S. states. *Am J Public Health.* 2017; 107:1101–1108.

15. Hayward MD, Pienta AM, McLaughlin DK. Inequality in men's mortality: the socioeconomic status gradient and geographic context. *J Health Soc Behav.* 1997; 38:313–330.

16. House JS, Lepkowski JM, Williams DR, et al. Excess mortality among urban residents: how much, for whom, and why? *Am J Public Health.* 2000; 90:1898–1904.

17. Flood S, King M, Ruggles S, Warren JR. *Integrated Public Use Microdata Series, Current Population Survey: Version 5.0. [dataset].* Minneapolis: University of Minnesota. 2017. doi:10.18128/D030.V5.0.

12

Healthy Places to Play, Learn, and Develop

RENÉE BOYNTON-JARRETT

> The requisite for any of these varieties of incidental play is not preten-
> tious equipment of any sort, but rather space at an immediately conven-
> ient and interesting place. The play gets crowded out if sidewalks are too
> narrow relative to the total demands put on them.
>
> —Jane Jacobs

1 Introduction

Global trends in urbanization have a disproportionate impact on children, adolescents, and young adults. By 2025, 6 out of 10 children will be living in cities.[1] By 2030, the majority of urban residents will be under the age of 18.[2] Low-income regions of the world account for 90% of urban growth globally, yet a third of these urban residents live in slums—characterized by inadequate sanitation and housing and overcrowding.[2] Children are also uniquely vulnerable given that, typically, they cannot change or choose their residential environments.

Throughout history, periods of rapid urbanization have posed challenges to the health and well-being of populations.[3] As urbanization expanded, a growing recognition of the need for health-promoting urban planning and city design that reduces environmental impacts sharpened. As a result, there is a growing interest in the design of "livable" and "healthy" cities. Entering the fray is a more precise agenda to design "child-friendly" and "child-centered" cities.

This chapter reviews the history of urban planning with respect to the health and developmental needs of children, outlines the impact of urbanization on child health and development, and highlights emerging strategies to improve outcomes.

2 Urban Planning and Child Health and Development

Traditionally, urban planning has focused on efficiency and minimizing environmental impacts. A now well-established body of research on the impact of place on health, well-being, and health behaviors converges on and has expanded the role of urban planning and its responsiveness to population health, public health, and health promotion efforts.

Historically, children were conceptualized as complications rather than beneficiaries in urban planning.[4] A primary focus of urban planning was on safety, with urban design models for children that required adult supervision and a focus on modifying child behavior. It is not surprising that a central paradox faced with growing urbanization is that of how to keep children safe and active.[4] Most urban policies have undervalued the importance of play and opportunities for exploration and independent mobility for healthy child development and the emergence of life skills, and, as a result, there has been an erosion of spaces for free and independent play.[5] Public spaces for play are often in direct competition with more financially lucrative land uses.

There is a growing movement to develop "child-friendly" and "child-centered" urban communities that engage children in the design and implementation process.[6] The United Nations 2016 Habitat III conference included a commitment to vulnerable populations, including children, to promote "a safe, healthy, inclusive, and secure environment in cities and human settlements enabling all to live, work, and participate in urban life without fear of violence and intimidation," as well as a commitment to children's right to participation in key decision-making processes.[7] This builds on the precedent set by Article 31 of the United Nations Convention on the Rights of the Child (UNCRC) that protects and promotes the right of the child to engage in play and recreational activities. It is also supported by the now well-established body of research that embraces the importance of early childhood experiences as life course social determinants of health and wellness. Efforts to transform and redesign cities to be child friendly have considered the impact of green spaces, traffic control, and opportunities for safe recreational activity on the right to play.[1]

3 Urban Environments and Child Health

Place is a central and enduring determinant of child health, development, and well-being over the life course. Attributes of urban areas, including features of the built and social environment and associated neighborhood infrastructure and opportunities, are associated with child health and developmental outcomes. Urbanization is associated with trends in population health and well-being. Key factors in urban environments that influence child health and development include green space, crime and safety, traffic, air pollution, blight, crowding and housing conditions. Pollution, environmental toxins, and housing are not reviewed in this chapter because they are covered elsewhere in this collection.

3.1 Urban Green Space and Health

Urban green space and usage of green space in urban settings is consistently associated with health and well-being.[3] Exposure to a green environment has been associated with lower socioeconomic inequities in health and positive health outcomes.[8,9] Exposure to urban green space is positively associated with cognitive function and development including attention and memory, improved mood or emotion, and physical activity, and it is negatively linked to mortality, heart rate, and violence or urban crime.[10] There is a more concerted effort to proactively consider how ecosystem services within urban environments (vegetation to purify the air, playgrounds for activity, trees to provide cooling) may be leveraged as nature-based solutions to the potentially health-harming effects of urbanization.[9]

3.1.1 Green Space and Cognition and Mental Health

A series of classic studies exploring the effects of vegetation surrounding Chicago public housing found that greener views from apartment windows were associated with concentration, self-control, and attention.[11] A citywide cluster randomized trial found that remediation of dilapidated and vacant physical environments demonstrated a significant decrease in depression and worthlessness.[12] Exposure to urban natural environments is associated with reduced cardiovascular disease–related mortality, likely mediated by the influence of urban natural environments on affect, mood, and ecosystems (heat).[13]

3.1.2 Green Space and Play

Green space in urban public housing has been associated with imaginative play, creativity, and socially cooperative play, which is critical for the development of capacities and psychological well-being.[14] Opportunities to play and to access play spaces are associated with child development, socioemotional regulation, and well-being. Attachment to place and cultural access play a role in the development of personal identity and sense of the right to use the space; mastery of the environment is associated with social and cognitive development, and place-based memories and experiences impact self-regulation.[15]

3.1.3 Recreational Space and Childhood Obesity

Urban and minority youth are disproportionately at greater risk for access to fewer and less safe recreational facilities. Lower access to recreational areas and green space is associated with overweight and reduced physical activity in youth.[16] Children who live in areas with a higher density of recreational spaces and in closer proximity to supermarkets are more likely to maintain a healthy body mass index (BMI), perhaps through greater opportunities for healthy activity and nutrition.[17] Racial/ethnic disparities in childhood obesity risk are associated with neighborhood socioeconomic status and, to a lesser degree, with built environment features and resources that may mediate differences in energy intake, physical activity, stress, and weight trajectory.[18] Inequitable distribution of resources, such as recreational facilities, is associated with activity levels and overweight, suggesting that policies to improve accessibility would be beneficial. Unfavorable social and built environment conditions appear to have a greater impact on risk for obesity among girls and younger children.[19]

Rapid urbanization, with inadequate urban planning for recreational areas, walkability, and safety, has been associated with negative shifts in dietary behaviors and physical activity patterns.[20] The impact of built environment features on play and walking appears to be strongest among adolescents.[21]

3.2 Crime and Safety

Neighborhood safety is a product of the social and built environment.

3.2.1 Crime and Asthma

Neighborhood violent crime has been associated with childhood asthma prevalence, as has perceived neighborhood safety.[22] Family stress and maternal stress have been associated with wheezing and asthma morbidity.[22]

3.2.2 Crime and Mental Health

Depression and depressive symptoms have been more consistently associated with neighborhood social processes such as crime and social disorder.[23] Built environment features are associated with depression and are believed to interact with dimensions of the social environment.

Children residing in distressed communities experience elevated psychiatric morbidity.[23,24] Exposure to community violence has been associated with cognitive performance on standardized exams and concentration.[25] While mental health problems are associated with neighborhood factors, such as concentrated disadvantage, the presence of collective efficacy, or informal social control and social cohesion among residents, seemed to buffer this effect.[24] Moreover relocating from high-poverty urban environments to low-poverty communities is associated in changes in adolescent depressive symptom profiles and perceived stress, although results vary by gender.[26]

3.2.3 Crime and Obesity Risk

Neighborhood violence may contribute to obesity risk through impacts on mental health and/or health-related behaviors. Neighborhood physical and social disorder is a direct stressor and also limits physical activity.[27] Although the majority of existing studies are observational, a social experiment that randomly assigned variation in neighborhood conditions by allowing women with children to move from high-poverty to low-poverty communities, was associated with reduced prevalence of morbid obesity and diabetes among adults.[28]

Childhood obesity is a multifactorial phenomenon. Neighborhood socioeconomic disadvantage, high crime and social disorder, and low perceived safety, collective efficacy, and recreational areas are positively associated with obesity in childhood.

3.3 Built Environment

The built environment is defined as all buildings, spaces, and products that are created by people.

3.3.1 Traffic, Walking, and Injury

Features of the built environment that slow traffic (traffic calming) and create recreational areas that separate children from traffic (playgrounds) are associated with increased walking and reduced pedestrian injury.[29] Pedestrian safety declines in areas with higher population and road density. Walking increases in areas with more crosswalks and closer proximity to facilities; however, these attributes are also associated with higher rates pedestrian injury.[29] Whereas high-speed traffic and busy major roads are associated with both more injury and less walking. Although traffic safety educational programs are a common public health strategy, there is no evidence of their effect on traffic injuries, whereas traffic calming measures are associated with a 15% reduction in injury accidents.[30] Interventions to change the built environment support evidence that improving road traffic safety can reduce injury and mortality for children, and improving street connectivity and pavements facilitate an increase in active travel (physical active transportation including walking, cycling).[31]

3.3.2 Blight

Neighborhood physical conditions—vacant lots, dilapidated spaces, trash, and deteriorating buildings and the lack of quality infrastructure, such as sidewalks, parks, and playgrounds—are associated with depression.[23] Neighborhood blight is a daily source of stress for residents in these areas.[32] Attributes of the urban social environment in cities, including noise level, violent crime, residential segregation, concentrated poverty, underemployment, and unemployment, may heighten levels of stress and associated stress-related disorders.[33] Research suggests that community residents' perceptions of poor conditions are as important to influencing health as the actual physical conditions.[34]

Urban sprawl has been associated with decreased physical activity, decreased overall health, higher BMI, and higher motor vehicle collisions and pedestrian fatalities.[35] Neighborhood design can create geographic isolation, diminish opportunities for social contact, and wither social networks, thus leading to a parallel social isolation.

3.3.3 Physical Disorder

Physical disorder is believed to influence health through its impact on the perception of social control over neighborhood conditions. Physical structures may influence social trust and relationships, may directly create opportunities for crime, or may limit informal social controls. Physical deterioration of neighborhood buildings, as measured by boarded-up vacant housing, has been associated with premature mortality risk and sexually transmitted infections in ecological studies.[36] Physical conditions, social connections, and social controls are connected; environmental conditions provide opportunities for health-promoting and health-undermining practices.[37]

The association between neighborhood disorder and the breakdown of social cohesion and networks has been well researched, and social contact, social capital, and fear of crime mediate the association between deterioration and depression symptoms.[38] Social connections have also been noted to buffer the impact of neighborhood disorder, and individual perception of disorder mediates the impact on well-being.[39] Child maltreatment risk has been associated with community social disorder.[40]

3.4 Slums

The proportion of city-dwellers around the world who reside in urban slums is growing. Urban slums are characterized by poverty, overcrowding, and substandard housing, water quality, and sanitation. Children living in slums are at increased risk for infection, injury, malnutrition, poor cognitive development, lack of economic and educational opportunity, and limited enrichment and developmental stimulation.[41] Risk differs based on developmental stage and gender: infant mortality rates are notably elevated in slums, and girls are at greater risk for limited educational opportunities.[41] Gender differences in developmental outcomes are also observed in urban slums in that girls are at greater risk for illiteracy, malnutrition, early marriage, and pregnancy.[41]

4 Strategies to Mitigate Negative Health Effects and Promote Healthy Development

4.1 Multidisciplinary Approaches

Although urban planning and public health emerged with similar interests in preventing the spread of infectious disease, these fields are largely disconnected, arguably to the detriment of efforts to address health inequities disproportionately experienced by the urban poor and minority communities.[42] Interdisciplinary approaches may best illuminate how place and the use of land impacts population health.[42] Intentionally highlighting the impact of the political economy on "place-making" is an important first step. Creating opportunities to align research agendas, metrics, and frameworks may further facilitate collaboration. Green space, traffic volume, residential density, land use mix, walkability, and traffic speed are all intersecting variables of the built environment that also interact with social factors such as crime, safety, and social cohesion. Ultimately, an urban agenda for healthy cities for children will also require collaboration with educators, child development specialists, caregivers, and children themselves. Past work has demonstrated the importance and resourcefulness of children as active agents in shaping their environments to promote healthy development.[14]

4.2 Research Directions

A systems-oriented, multilevel research agenda is needed to understand how macro-level systems influence urban community settings and how they ultimately interact with interpersonal and biological processes to influence health and health behaviors.[43] *Ecological systems theory* is a model that has been used to guide interdisciplinary research and interventions to address multifactorial health outcomes, such as obesity, by carefully considering individual, community-level, and policy- and social norms–level factors, thereby expanding an understanding of the influencers of the neighborhood built and social environments. But examining the contributions of the social and built environments to child health is insufficient. It is important to also consider the influence of macro-environments—agricultural and food policy, food marketing, social norms and cultural values, and socioeconomic status—on opportunities to promote an optimal health trajectory.[43]

Important future research directions to inform policy and practice include (1) developing a comprehensive theoretical framework that specifically considers the unique features of urban communities and pathways through which health may be impacted; (2) improving and standardizing metrics of the built and social environments and indicators of child-friendly cities; (3) developing stronger research methods, including studies using longitudinal, quasi-experimental, or experimental designs; and (4) identifying and addressing bias in reporting and confounding variables.[23] Research on the health benefits of sustainable communities is needed to balance the predominance of research on negative health impacts. Multidisciplinary research training opportunities and community participation in research are essential to achieving meaningful outcomes.

4.3 Community Engagement

Community-generated solutions may address features of the built and social environments that impact health.[44] Addressing the priorities of local residents is a basic step in incorporating community stakeholders. Engaging residents in design, implementation, and leadership is a deeper commitment to community-generated solutions.

Urban residents may support policies that not only address the built environment but also address the social environment and encourage community engagement and cohesion.[44] Since one pathway through which the built environment undermines health is through fear and erosion of social trust, urban residents may be able to improve health through the ability to exert social control through informal surveillance.[45]

Engagement of community resident perspectives and community-generated solutions is essential to ensuring the health benefit and uptake of neighborhood interventions. Collective revitalization processes also build social cohesion and empowerment and thereby influence health. Increasing transparency and the participatory nature of budgeting processes can lead to more child-inclusive governance and has been associated with more equitable resource distribution and reduced infant mortality rates.[1]

Child participation is widely considered a core strategy for child-friendly city initiatives. The engagement of children and youth in decision-making on policies and design encourages civic engagement and the exercise of rights and citizenship from a young age.[1] Involvement of children in community planning acknowledges their participation in the local economy and ways in which the local economy directly impacts their development and health.[15]

4.4 Policy Implications

In order to develop a systematic approach to addressing health inequities for urban children, policymakers should consider a child-focused approach to evaluating marginalization based on social, developmental, or spatial processes related to childhood.[46] Cities can be designed to protect the rights of children (e.g., through prevention of child labor, holistic approaches to child protection, policies to care for homeless youth and those at risk for sex work and trafficking).[1] With supportive research evidence, municipal leadership can consider the health impact of vacant land when developing and selecting policies than may influence the presence of green space and the safety and renewal of these properties.[44]

Importantly, disadvantaged urban communities are produced by socioeconomic processes that concentrate wealth or resources in other areas (i.e., suburbs); therefore, ultimately, improvements in urban environments must consider the interdependence of these respective environments and address those sociopolitical processes.[47] Policies that focus exclusively on addressing a "problem" within the urban environment fail to engage a major fulcrum of change associated with the policies, practices, and historical processes of adjacent environments.

Neighborhood improvement policies may improve infrastructure (playgrounds, sidewalks, traffic) but may simultaneously impact affordability and ultimately neighborhood composition, disproportionately negatively impact poor families, and widen social inequities experienced by low-income children. It is important to be mindful of the relative health implications of common housing policies to improve housing quality and neighborhood conditions which may ultimately elevate housing costs, and proactively work to reduce the potential housing insecurity and associated mobility that may arise.

Finally, nature-based solutions (NBS) is an emerging strategy to develop healthy cities and address challenges in the urban environment. NBS is based on actions that mimic nature.[13] A more explicit integration of population health into the NBS framework may support health-promoting urban landscapes.[13]

5 Conclusion

We are experiencing a renaissance in the understanding of the importance of places where children live, learn, and play as the ecosystem wherein health develops and emerges over the life course. This shared understanding is matched by a desire to translate research into practice with the design of child-friendly and child-centered cities. In this effort, we must go beyond the question, "What role does the urban environment play in contributing to inequities in population health?" and begin to ask "What role can urban planning play in promoting optimal health and well-being?"

A comprehensive agenda is needed to inform research, policy, and planning that may optimize the health and well-being of children who live in urban environments. To this end, an understanding of the impact of the built environment on child development, health, and play has to be strengthened by more rigorous studies and incorporated into policy and urban planning. Effective public health approaches to minimize risks to health associated with urbanization must consider the health implications of social policies that impact neighborhood characteristics and opportunity structures, as well as develop interventions to address modifiable elements of the social and physical environments.

Research has demonstrated that social and built environmental issues associated with urbanization impact physical activity, use of outdoor spaces, access to healthy foods, and mental health and wellness. A more comprehensive understanding of policy initiatives that impact land use planning and neighborhood safety, and thereby contribute to environmental conditions in cities, is needed. To proactively design urban environments that promote health, future research efforts should explore the impact of changes in policies on physical activity, diet, and mental health.

In order to design healthy places, multidisciplinary teams incorporating perspectives of traffic engineers, public health and child development practitioners, and urban planners are required. Resident-generated solutions to urban challenges and the inclusion of children in these processes are essential.

References

1. Riggio E. Child friendly cities: good governance in the best interests of the child. *Environ Urban.* 2002; 14(2):45–58.
2. Ragan D. *Cities of youth, cities of prosperity.* Nairobi: UN-Habitat; 2014.
3. Krefs A, Augustin M, Schlunzen KH, Obenbrugge J, Augustin J. How does the urban environment affect health and well-being? A systematic review. *Urban Science.* 2018; 2(21):2–21.
4. Davis A, Jones L. Whose neighbourhood? Whose quality of life? Developing a new agenda for children's health in urban settings. *Health Educ J.* 1997; 56(4):350–363.
5. Shackel R. *The impact of urbanization on the child's right to play.* University of Sydney Law School. Legal Studies Research Paper No. 11/103. 2011.
6. Wright H, Hargrave J, Williams S, zu Dohna F. Cities alive: designing for urban childhoods. ARUP website. 2017. Available at https://http://www.arup.com/perspectives/publications/research/section/cities-alive-designing-for-urban-childhoods. Accessed June 1, 2018.
7. *New urban agenda: with subject index.* Quito, Ecuador: UN-Habitat. 2017.
8. Mitchell R, Popham F. Effect of exposure to natural environment on health inequalities: an observational population study. *Lancet.* 2008; 372(9650):1655–1660.
9. Kabisch N, van den Bosch M, Lafortezza R. The health benefits of nature-based solutions to urbanization challenges for children and the elderly—a systematic review. *Environ Res.* 2017; 159:362–373.
10. Kondo MC, Fluehr JM, McKeon T, Branas CC. Urban green space and its impact on human health. *Int J Environ Res Public Health.* 2018; 15(3). doi:10.3390/ijerph15030445
11. Faber T, Kuo FE. Could exposure to everyday green spaces help treat ADHD? Evidence from children's play settings. *Appl Psychol Health Well-Being.* 2011; 3(3):281–303.
12. South EC, Hohl BC, Kondon, MC. Effect of greening vacant land on mental health of community-dwelling adults. *JAMA.* 2018; 1(3):e180298.
13. van den Bosch M, Sang, AO. Urban natural environments as nature-based solutions. *Environ Res.* 2017; 158:373–384.
14. Chawla L. Benefits of nature contact for children. *J Plan Lit.* 2015; 304(4):433–452.
15. Spencer C, Woolley H. Children and the city: a summary of recent environmental psychology research. *Child Care Health Dev.* 2000; 26(3):181–197.
16. Boone-Heinonen J, Casanova K, Richardson AS, Gordon-Larsen P. Where can they play? Outdoor spaces and physical activity among adolescents in U.S. urbanized areas. *Prev Med.* 2010; 51(3-4):295–298.
17. Fiechtner L, Cheng ER, Lopez G, Sharifi M, Taveras EM. Multilevel correlates of healthy BMI maintenance and return to a healthy BMI among children in Massachusetts. *Child Obes.* 2017; 13(2):146–153.
18. Sharifi M, Sequist TD, Rifas-Shiman SL, et al. The role of neighborhood characteristics and the built environment in understanding racial/ethnic disparities in childhood obesity. *Prev Med.* 2016; 91:103–109.
19. Singh GK, Siahpush M, Kogan MD. Neighborhood socioeconomic conditions, built environments, and childhood obesity. *Health Aff (Millwood).* 2010; 29(3):503–512.
20. Pirgon O, Aslan N. The role of urbanization in childhood obesity. *J Clin Res Pediatr Endocrinol.* 2015; 7(3):163–167.
21. McGrath LJ, Hopkins WG, Hinckson EA. Associations of objectively measured built-environment attributes with youth moderate-vigorous physical activity: a systematic review and meta-analysis. *Sports Med.* 2015; 45(6):841–865.

22. DePriest K, Butz A. Neighborhood-level factors related to asthma in children living in urban areas. *J Sch Nurs.* 2017; 33(1):8–17.

23. Mair CF, Roux AVD, Galea S. Are neighborhood characteristics associated with depressive symptoms? A review of evidence. *J Epidemiol Community Health.* 2008; 62(11):940–946, 948.

24. Xue Y, Leventhal T, Brooks-Gunn J, Earls FJ. Neighborhood residence and mental health problems of 5- to 11-year-olds. *Arch Gen Psychiatry.* 2005; 62(5):554–563.

25. McCoy DC, Raver CC, Sharkey P. Children's cognitive performance and selective attention following recent community violence. *J Health Soc Behav.* 2015; 56(1):19–36.

26. Osypuk TL, Tchetgen EJ, Acevedo-Garcia D, et al. Differential mental health effects of neighborhood relocation among youth in vulnerable families: results from a randomized trial. *Arch Gen Psychiatry.* 2012; 69(12):1284–1294.

27. Miles R. Neighborhood disorder, perceived safety, and readiness to encourage use of local playgrounds. *Am J Prev Med.* 2008; 34(4):275–281.

28. Ludwig J, Sanbonmatsu L, Gennetian L, et al. Neighborhoods, obesity, and diabetes: a randomized social experiment. *N Engl J Med.* 2011; 365(16):1509–1519.

29. Rothman L, Buliung R, Macarthur C, To T, Howard A. Walking and child pedestrian injury: a systematic review of built environment correlates of safe walking. *Inj Prev.* 2014; 20(1):41–49.

30. Liabo K, Lucas P, Roberts H. Can traffic calming measures achieve the Children's Fund objective of reducing inequalities in child health? *Arch Dis Child.* 2003; 88(3):235–236.

31. Audrey S, Batista-Ferrer H. Healthy urban environments for children and young people: a systematic review of intervention studies. *Health Place.* 2015; 36:97–117.

32. South EC, Kondo MC, Cheney RA, Branas CC. Neighborhood blight, stress, and health: a walking trial of urban greening and ambulatory heart rate. *Am J Public Health.* 2015; 105(5):909–913.

33. Evans GW. Child development and the physical environment. *Annu Rev Psychol.* 2006; 57:423–451.

34. Warr D, Tacticos T, Kelaher M, Klein H. "Money, stress, jobs": residents' perceptions of health-impairing factors in "poor" neighbourhoods. *Health Place.* 2007; 13:743–756.

35. Lopez RP, Hynes HP. Obesity, physical activity, and the urban environment: public health research needs. *Environ Health.* 2006; 5:25.

36. Cohen DA, Mason K, Bedimo A, Scribner R, Basolo V, Farley TA. Neighborhood physical conditions and health. *Am J Public Health.* 2003; 93(3):467–471.

37. Kawachi I, Kennedy BP, Wilkinson RG. Crime: social disorganization and relative deprivation. *Soc Sci Med.* 1999; 48(6):719–731.

38. Kruger DJ, Reischl TM, Gee GC. Neighborhood social conditions mediate the association between physical deterioration and mental health. *Am J Community Psychol.* 2007; 40(3-4):261–271.

39. Ross CE, Jang SJ. Neighborhood disorder, fear, and mistrust: the buffering role of social ties with neighbors. *Am J Community Psychol.* 2000; 28(4):401–420.

40. Coulton CJ, Korbin JE, Su M, Chow J. Community level factors and child maltreatment rates. *Child Dev.* 1995; 66(5):1262–1276.

41. Nair MK, Radhakrishnan SR. Early childhood development in deprived urban settlements. *Indian Pediatr.* 2004; 41(3):227–237.

42. Corburn J. Confronting the challenges in reconnecting urban planning and public health. *Am J Public Health.* 2004; 94(4):541–546.

43. Larson N, Story M. A review of environmental influences on food choices. *Ann Behav Med.* 2009; 38(S1):S56–S73.

44. Garvin EBC, Keddem S, Sellman J, Cannuscio C. More than just an eyesore: local insights and solutions on vacant land and urban health. *J Urban Health.* 2013; 90(3):412–426.

45. Jacobs J. *The death and life of great American cities.* New York: Random House; 1961.

46. Stephens C. Urban inequities; urban rights: a conceptual analysis and review of impacts on children, and policies to address them. *J Urban Health.* Jun 2012; 89(3):464–485.

47. Loyd J, Bonds A. Where do Black lives matter? Race, stigma and place in Milwaukee, Wisconsin. *Sociol Rev.* 2018; 66(4):898–918.

13

Pollution

JONATHAN M. SAMET

1 Introduction

1.1 Overview

This chapter addresses pollution in urban environments. Pollution can be variably defined, but, for this chapter, pollution is considered as comprising agents exogenous to the body and including both those resulting from man's activities and those having natural origins. The pollution problems discussed here are not unique to urban environments, but some (e.g., air pollution) reach a degree of severity far greater than in typical suburban and rural environments. Consider air pollution, for example; some of the same pollutants that are problematic in urban environments because of vehicles, power generation, and industry, such as airborne particulate matter (PM), also have regional reach, reflecting spread from urban locales and local sources. However, across urban environments, PM levels, typically indexed by $PM_{2.5}$ (PM less than 2.5 microns in aerodynamic diameter), may vary widely, reaching higher concentrations alongside heavily trafficked roadways and adjacent to polluting facilities. Furthermore, there is a wide range of PM sources across urban areas by the area's socioeconomic level, tending to be amassed in poorer neighborhoods. In lower income countries, biomass burning for space heating and cooking remains prevalent as does open refuse burning in urban environments, and these may be critical sources of urban air pollution.

An additional consideration is the multiplicity of exposures sustained in urban environments: air pollution, high noise levels, sustained light exposure, contaminated water and food, and the psychological stress associated with high-density living (Box 13.1). Research and management tend to focus on the risks of the individual agents (e.g., PM) or linked groups of agents but not on overall consequences that reflect the effects of the agents themselves and the potential synergisms among them. Studies addressing such synergisms call for complex designs and assessment of multiple exposures, and, consequently, relevant research remains limited.

Two other concepts are also relevant: vulnerability and susceptibility. These represent differing but complementary concepts: *vulnerability* refers to an increased risk either for being exposed or for being exposed at higher levels, and *susceptibility* refers to an increased risk for an outcome at a given level of exposure. For example, in many urban

Box 13.1 **Sources of Exposure in Urban Environments**

Air pollution
Motor vehicles
Power generation
Trash/refuse burning
Biomass burning
Windblown dust
Industrial activities

Water pollution
Contaminated water from central systems, river and lakes, wells, piping
Industrial pumping

Noise pollution
Motor vehicles
Industrial activities
Aviation

environments, those who are poorer live in more polluted environments and in poorer quality housing than do the more affluent, thus making the poor vulnerable. Research has now identified a broad array of factors that determine susceptibility across the life course from gestation to late adulthood, when age itself and the associated high prevalence of noncommunicable diseases (NCDs) enhance susceptibility. Across the life course, other NCDs also increase susceptibility to environmental agents: asthma and other chronic lung diseases, obesity, diabetes, and cardiovascular diseases. With the tools of genomics, much research is now directed at genetic determinants of susceptibility to environmental agents.

The disease burden from environmental pollution is substantial, particularly given the substantial burden estimated for air pollution (Table 13.1). Although the air pollution burden from ambient PM has not been estimated for urban areas specifically, the bulk of the premature deaths from environmental pollution occur among urban dwellers. The problem of household air pollution spans both urban and rural dwellers.

1.2 Exposures and Sources of Exposure

The concept of *exposure* underlies consideration of the risks associated with urban pollution and its management.[1] Figure 13.1 presents a general schema that is integrative in setting out sources and their drivers, time-activity patterns of people, and the resulting exposures. The left-most side sets out sources, including the upstream drivers of exposures (i.e., factors determining the types of sources, their locations, the intensity of exposures, and the control measures used). Construed broadly, the upstream drivers reach across the range of social determinants of health; in many urban locales, industrial sources are located more densely in poorer neighborhoods, as are heavily trafficked roadways.

Table 13.1 **Global estimated deaths (millions) due to pollution risk factors from the Global Burden of Disease study (GBD; 2015) versus World Health Organization data (WHO; 2012)**

	GBD study best estimate (95% Confidence Interval)	WHO best estimate (95% Confidence Interval)
Air (total)	6.5 (5.7–7.3)	6.5 (5.4–7.4)
Household air	2.9 (2.2–3.6)	4.3 (3.7–4.8)
Ambient particulate	4.2 (3.7–4.8)	3.0 (3.7–4.8)
Ambient ozone	0.3 (0.1–0.4)	--
Water (total)	1.8 (1.4–2.2)	0.8 (0.7–1.0)
Unsafe sanitation	0.8 (0.7–0.9)	0.3 (0.1–0.4)
Unsafe source	1.3 (1.0–1.4)	0.5 (0.2–0.7)
Occupational	0.8 (0.8–0.9)	0.4 (0.3–0.4)
Carcinogens	0.5 (0.5–0.5)	0.1 (0.1–0.1)
Particulates	0.4 (0.3–0.4)	0.2 (0.2–0.3)
Soil, heavy metals, and chemicals	0.5 (0.2–0.8)	0.7 (0.2–0.8)
Lead	0.5 (0.2–0.8)	0.7 (0.2–0.8)
Total	9.0	8.4

Note that the totals for air pollution, water pollution, and all pollution are less than the arithmetic sum of the individual risk factors within each of these categories because these have overlapping contribution (e.g., household air pollution also contributes to ambient air pollution and vice versa).

From Landrigan PJ, Fuller R, Acosta NJR, et al. The Lancet Commission on pollution and health. 2018; 391(10119):462–512.

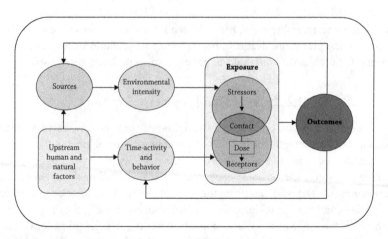

Figure 13.1 **Conceptual framework showing the core elements of exposure science as related to humans and ecosystems.** Source: Taken from National Research Council. *Exposure science in the 21st century: a vision and a strategy.* Washington, DC: National Academies Press; 2012.

Moving to the right, contact with exposure and the intensity of exposure are driven by what is released into the environment and how people interact with the environment, as determined by time-activity patterns (i.e., the places where people spend time and the amount of time spent in these locations). The term "microenvironment" refers to locations where exposures are consistent during the time of exposure, including, for example, the air pollution within a home or office. Pollution concentrations in some locations may be temporally and spatially dynamic, such as on the sidewalks of busy streets where stalled traffic may result in "hot spots."

The concept of exposure (the diagram's middle) has been broadened to encompass contact of people with agents, whether external or internally incorporated. As captured by the diagram, environmental agents enter the body and may interact with critical receptors that drive processes leading to injury, ill health, and disease. Here, the *dose* refers to the materials reaching the targeted receptors. Some stressors act more generally, such as psychological stress, which may affect health through the multiple mechanisms underlying the stress response. At the far right, *outcomes* refers to the consequences of pollution exposures, comprising a broad array of adverse effects, some transitory (e.g., exacerbation of asthma or increased coughing) and some long-term and irreversible (e.g., development of lung cancer).

1.3 Adverse Outcomes

The range of adverse health outcomes relevant to urban environments is extensive but reflective of the broad array of exposures and the multiplicity of processes by which they cause adverse effects: carcinogenicity, inflammation and irritation, immune mechanisms including allergic sensitization, and stress.[2] The outcomes include incremental risk for various diseases, such as lung cancer, and exacerbation of underlying disease, such as asthma. Air pollution also broadly affects quality of life, particularly at the extremely high levels now present in many countries.

2 Ambient (Outdoor) Air Pollution

2.1 Overview

Air pollution in cities has long been known to harm the health of urban dwellers. The density of combustion sources in urban environments produces pollution that is typically visible and readily evident, and, in the past, levels were high enough in many places to have posed a visible public health threat. The air pollution experience in London, long one of the world's largest cities, has been well documented and its historical course over centuries exemplifies the path from dramatic episodes of high pollution to control.[3] During the twentieth century, excess mortality was documented in London and elsewhere at times when "fogs"—episodes of atmospheric stagnation—occurred and air pollution levels were high. The most dramatic, the London Fog of 1952, caused thousands of excess deaths (Figure 13.2).[4] The high levels of smoke (an index of airborne particles) and sulfur dioxide during the fog—approximately two orders of magnitude higher than values permitted under World Health Organization (WHO) guidelines—reflected coal combustion for space heating, industrial emissions, and vehicle exhaust.[5] This and other

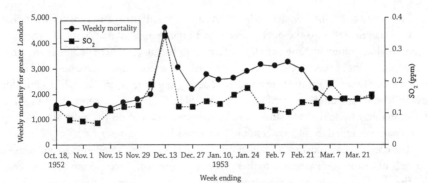

Figure 13.2 **Approximate weekly mortality and sulfur dioxide (SO$_2$) concentrations for Greater London, 1952–1953.** Source: Taken from Bell ML and Davis DL. Reassessment of the lethal London Fog of 1952: novel indicators of acute and chronic consequences of acute exposure to air pollution. *Env Health Persp.* 2001; 109(3):389–394.

disasters during the twentieth century motivated research, including epidemiological studies, on the health effects of air pollution and the development of effective evidence-based approaches to air quality management.

Now, air quality has improved in most large cities in higher income countries consequent to regulation, reduced emissions from vehicles, and a sharp decline in smokestack industries. However, air pollution remains a threat to public health in many large cities in lower income countries, reflecting industry and power generation, high-emitting vehicles, burning of biomass fuels for space heating and cooking, and dust suspended by wind and traffic. The problems are particularly severe in the ever-increasing megacities, such as Bangkok, Beijing, Jakarta, and Delhi, although the challenge of air pollution has been met in some to a substantial extent (e.g., Mexico City). Megacities—urban agglomerations with populations of at least 10 million—now number 19 and pose major challenges for assuring environmental quality.

Global estimates of concentrations of small or "fine" particles in the air reflect a bi-modal distribution; the high-income countries are to the left side of the distribution, while low- and middle-income countries are to the right (Figure 13.3). Given the large population size of some of these countries, the majority of the world's population sustains exposures to airborne particles well above the WHO guidelines, driving the high disease burden attributable to air pollution.

2.2 Overview of Health Risks

Table 13.2 provides a listing of major regulated pollutants and associated health effects, as well as some of the current standards and guidelines for controlling their concentrations. Diverse health effects have been linked to ambient air pollution, including increased risk for respiratory infections, exacerbation of asthma and chronic obstructive pulmonary disease (COPD—a disease involving destruction of the lung structure) and cardiac (heart) events, contributions to development of major chronic diseases (coronary heart disease, COPD, and cancer), and impaired lung growth and

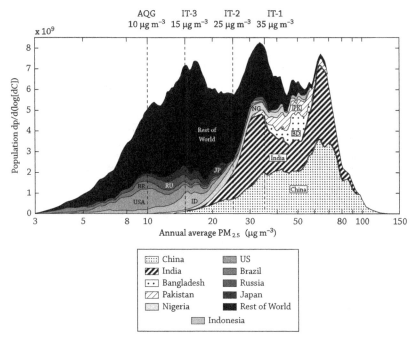

Figure 13.3 **Global and regional distributions of population as a function of annual average ambient particulate matter (PM$_{2.5}$) concentration for the 10 most populous countries in 2013.** Plotted data reflect local smoothing of bin-width normalized distributions computed over 400 logarithmically spaced bins; equal sized plotted areas would reflect equal populations. Dashed vertical lines indicate World Health Organization Interim Targets (IT) and the Air Quality Guideline (AQG). Source: Brauer M, Freedman G, Frostad J, et al. Ambient air pollution exposure estimation for the global burden of disease 2013. *Environ Sci Technol.* 2016; 50(1):79–88, figure 3.

respiratory symptoms during childhood. Additional adverse health outcomes are under investigation: autism and other neurodevelopmental disorders, adverse reproductive outcomes, obesity and metabolic syndrome, and more rapid "brain aging." There are general mechanisms underlying these health effects, particularly oxidant stress, an excess of reactive molecules, and a heightened inflammatory state, given the oxidative nature of ambient air pollution. The increased risk for cancer causally linked to air pollution likely comes primarily from the presence of specific cancer-causing agents in ambient air pollution (e.g., polycyclic aromatic hydrocarbons) and inflammation; particles collected in outdoor air are *mutagenic*, meaning they can damage DNA.

Multiple investigational approaches have been used to characterize the health effects of ambient air pollution. Initially, simple counts of events associated with dramatic pollution episodes made clear that high levels of air pollution caused excess mortality, particularly in elderly people with chronic diseases and in infants and young children. As air pollution levels declined with regulation, increasing emphasis was placed on understanding the quantitative risks of air pollution so that air quality standards could be set to be protective of public health. In other words, researchers did studies to understand by how much risk changes as air pollution increases or decreases. Observational

Table 13.2 **Major ambient air pollutions: sources, health effects, and regulations**

	Source types and major sources	Health effects	Regulations and guidelines
Lead	Primary Anthropogenic: Leaded fuel (phased out in some locations such as the US), lead batteries, metal processing	Accumulates in organs and tissues. Learning disabilities, cancer, damage to the nervous system	US NAAQS: Quarterly average: 1.5 μg/m^3 WHO Guidelines: Annual: 0.50 μg/m^3
Sulfur dioxide	Primary Anthropogenic: Combustion of fossil fuel (power plants), industrial boilers, household coal use, oil refineries Biogenic: Decomposition of organic matter, sea spray, volcanic eruptions	Lung impairment, respiratory symptoms. Precursor to PM. Contributes to acid precipitation	US NAAQS: Annual arithmetic mean: 0.03 ppm (80 μg/m^3) 24-hour average: 0.14 ppm (365 μg/m^3) WHO Guidelines: 10-minute average: 500 μg/m^3 Annual: 20 μg/m^3
Carbon monoxide	Primary Anthropogenic: Combustion of fossil fuels (motor vehicles, boilers, furnaces) Biogenic: Forest fires	Interferes with delivery of oxygen. Fatigue, headache, neurological damage, dizziness	US NAAQS: 1-hour average: 35 ppm (40 mg/m^3) 8-hour average: 9 ppm (10 mg/m^3) WHO Guidelines: 15-minute average: 100 mg/m^3 30-minute average: 60 mg/m^3 1-hour average: 30 mg/m^3
Particulate matter[a]	Primary and secondary Anthropogenic: Burning of fossil fuel, wood burning, natural sources (e.g., pollen), conversion of precursors (NO$_x$, SO$_x$, VOCs) Biogenic: Dust storms, forest fires, dirt roads	Respiratory symptoms, decline in lung function, exacerbation of respiratory and cardiovascular disease (e.g., asthma), mortality	US NAAQS: PM$_{10}$ 24-hour average 150 μg/m^3 PM$_{2.5}$ Annual arithmetic mean: 15 μg/m^3 24-Hour average: 35 μg/m^3

			WHO Guidelines: PM_{10} Annual: 20 µg/m³ 24-hour average: 50 µg/m³ $PM_{2.5}$: Annual: 10 µg/m³ 24-hour average: 25 µg/m³
Nitrogen oxides	Primary and secondary Anthropogenic: Fossil fuel combustion (vehicles, electric utilities, industry), kerosene heaters Biogenic: Biological processes in soil, lightning	Decreased lung function, increased respiratory infection Precursor to ozone. Contributes to PM and acid precipitation	*US NAAQS for NO_2:* Annual arithmetic mean: 0.053 ppm (100 µg/m³) Related to compliance with NAAQS for ozone. *WHO Guidelines for NO_2:* 1-hour average: 200 µg/m³ Annual: 40 µg/m³
Tropospheric ozone	Secondary Formed through chemical reactions of anthropogenic and biogenic precursors (VOCs and NO_x) in the presence of sunlight	Decreased lung function, increased respiratory symptoms, eye irritation, bronchoconstriction	*US NAAQS:* 1-hour average: 0.12 ppm (235 µg/m³). Applies in limited areas. 8-hour average: 0.075 ppm (147 µg/m³) *WHO Guidelines:* 8-hour average: 100 µg/m³

(continued)

Table 13.2 Continued

	Source types and major sources	Health effects	Regulations and guidelines
"Toxic" pollutants ("hazardous" pollutants) (e.g., *asbestos, mercury, dioxin, some VOCs*)	Primary and secondary Anthropogenic: Industrial processes, solvents, paint thinners, fuel	Cancer, reproductive effects, neurological damage, respiratory effects	EPA rules on emissions for more than 80 industrial source categories (e.g., dry cleaners, oil refineries, chemical plants) EPA and state rules on vehicle emissions
Volatile organic compounds (e.g, benzene, terpenes, toluene)	Primary and secondary Anthropogenic: Solvents, glues, smoking, fuel combustion Biogenic: Vegetation, forest fires	Range of effects, depending on the compound. Irritation of respiratory tract, nausea, cancer Precursor to ozone. Contributes to PM.	EPA limits on emissions EPA toxic air pollutant rules Related to compliance with NAAQS for ozone.
Biological pollutants (e.g., pollen, mold, mildew)	Primary Biogenic: Trees, grasses, ragweed, animals, debris Anthropogenic systems, such as central air conditioning, can create conditions that encourage production of biological pollutants.	Allergic reactions, respiratory symptoms, fatigue, asthma	

ᵃSources and effects of PM can differ by size. From Bell ML, Samet JM. Air pollution. In Frumkin H, ed. *Environmental health: from local to global*. San Francisco, CA: John Wiley & Sons: 2010; 387–415 (fig. 12.1).

This table lists only a sample of the sources and health effects associated with each pollutant. Additionally, health effects may be the result of characteristics of the pollutant mixture rather than the independent effects of a pollutant. Additional legal requirements often apply, such as state regulations.

epidemiological studies (i.e., research based in populations) were critical to that purpose. Cohort or longitudinal studies were informative; such studies involve following participants over time, estimating pollution exposures, and tracking health events; analyses focused on quantifying the risks associated with air pollution exposure during follow-up. For example, the Children's Health Study in Southern California tracked lung growth and respiratory health in school children from communities having a range of pollution concentrations.[6] Now in progress for more than two decades, the study has shown that higher levels of air pollution slow lung growth and that reduction of pollution enhances it.

These epidemiological approaches are complemented by toxicological studies that provide insights into the mechanisms by which air pollution causes adverse health effects. Such evidence is critical in reaching causal conclusions on the adverse health effects of air pollution. In the past, toxicological studies often involved exposure of animals to a single pollutant, such as ozone, to isolate the pollutant's effect from those of other pollutants present in the air pollution mixture. For studying some pollutants, human volunteers inhaled the pollutants in an exposure chamber over a short interval and their responses were closely monitored. Additionally, pollutants are also studied in cell systems; these systems are likely to gain increasing prominence as new, sophisticated systems probe gene expression of different kinds of cells following exposure.

There are national bodies that periodically assess the evidence on adverse effects of air pollution and provide guidance to the setting of standards and guidelines. In the United States, the Environmental Protection Agency carries out evidence reviews as the basis for establishing major air quality standards (the National Ambient Air Quality Standards or NAAQS) on a 5-year cycle. Reviews are conducted by the United Kingdom, the European Commission, and other nations. The WHO regularly releases air quality guidelines (last issued in 2005).

While air pollution research and regulation generally focuses on specific pollutants, outdoor air pollution comprises a complex mixture. Effects attributed to a single pollutant, particularly when studied in the "real-world" context, may reflect the toxicity of the mixture as indexed by a particular pollutant. Ambient PM, for example, comes from many sources, is emitted as a primary pollutant from combustion and other sources, and is also formed by chemical transformations of gaseous pollutants (e.g., formation of particulate nitrates from gaseous nitrogen oxides). The mixture of pollutants formed from vehicle emissions, generally referred to as *traffic-related air pollution* (TRAP), may have specific toxicity beyond that of its individual components.

2.3 Particulate Matter

The literature on health effects of particles is enormous, comprising many epidemiological and toxicological studies carried out for a half-century. The risks of PM have assumed worldwide prominence because particles are widely monitored and used as the principal indicator for estimating the worldwide burden of morbidity and premature mortality attributable to air pollution. Particles are a robust indicator of ambient air pollution because of the myriad sources of primary particles and the contributions of sulfur and nitrogen oxides and organic compounds to secondary particle formation. Particles in outdoor air have both natural and man-made sources. The man-made sources include power plants, industry, and motor vehicles; the last category includes diesel-powered vehicles that emit small particles capable of penetrating into the lung. In areas where biomass fuels are used, the contributions of indoor combustion to outdoor air pollution may be substantial.

Particles in outdoor air span a range of sizes and are highly diverse in composition and physical characteristics, including size (as indicated by *aerodynamic diameter*). Thus, $PM_{2.5}$ includes those particles less than 2.5 μm in aerodynamic diameter, a size band that contains most man-made particles in outdoor air and of a size that can reach the smaller airways and air sacs of the lungs. The very small *ultrafine particles*, which include freshly generated combustion particles, are another concerning set. These particles are emitted by vehicles, and exposure to them may occur alongside roadways. Those living near roadways, walking along streets with heavy traffic, or driving in heavy traffic may experience substantial exposures to ultrafine particles.

There has been extensive epidemiological and toxicological investigation of the effects of particles on health since the air pollution disasters of mid-century. The extensive body of toxicological evidence shows that particles are injurious and also indicates the mechanisms by which particles could cause adverse effects on the respiratory and cardiovascular systems. The epidemiological studies have grown in their size and geographic scope and in the sophistication of their methodology. Recent studies involve large, national-level populations (all people in the United States who are 65 years and older) and the estimation of exposures at all household locations using models that incorporate available monitoring data, satellite information, and land-use data (such as that available on roadways and manufacturing). In a recent study utilizing the Medicare data for persons 65 years of age and older—more than 60 million people—Di and colleagues showed increased mortality at annual averages below 12 μg/m, the current annual standard in the United States.[7]

One analysis has suggested that reductions in particulate air pollution during the 1980s and 1990s led to measurable improvements in life expectancy in the United States.[8] The researchers estimated that for each 10 μg/m³ reduction in air pollution over this period, the average gain in life expectancy was 0.61 years (about 7.3 months). The authors concluded that as much as 15% of the total life expectancy increase seen during this time in the United States was attributable to air pollution reductions.

This strong evidence on the adverse health effects of PM has led to increasingly tighter ambient air quality standards. Nonetheless, adverse health effects are still observed, and much of the world's population is exposed at high concentrations at which adverse effects are certain (Figure 13.3).

2.4 Ozone

Ozone is a gas that has been studied for its toxicity using laboratory and epidemiological approaches. It is also used as the indicator for photochemical pollution, or "smog," the complex oxidant mixture produced by the action of sunlight on hydrocarbons and nitrogen oxides. From its original identification in Los Angeles in the 1940s, smog has become a worldwide problem as vehicle fleets and sources of other ozone precursors have grown.

Ozone, a highly reactive molecule, has been extensively investigated using toxicological approaches that have included exposures of human volunteers and short- and long-term exposures of animals.[9] The human studies have involved exposures of volunteers, generally young and healthy, to concentrations of ozone found in urban areas in the United States and elsewhere. Collectively, the studies show that exposures of up to 6–8 hours with intermittent exercise result in temporary drops in lung function and that some individuals have greater susceptibility to ozone. While the effects are transient, they are of sufficient magnitude in some people (loss of around 10% of function) to be considered adverse. In experimental animals, sustained low-level exposure damages the small airways and leads to early changes of COPD; thus, there is concern about permanent structural alteration in ozone-exposed populations. In the human studies, those with asthma have not been shown to have increased susceptibility to ozone compared with those who do not have asthma.

Epidemiological studies provide coherent evidence on the short-term effects of ozone on respiratory health. There is also evidence from daily time-series studies (studies examining day-to-day variation in death counts in relationship to variation in pollution levels) that ozone increases risk for mortality. There is inconsistent evidence for cardiovascular effects, and a just-completed exposure study of older persons with cardiovascular disease did not find adverse effects.

Reflecting the evidence on short-term effects on lung function, standards for ozone concentrations are directed at brief time spans (Table 13.1). Given the range of susceptibility of the population and the ubiquity of ozone, it is likely that feasibly achieved standards will not protect the full population from adverse respiratory effects.

2.5 Nitrogen Oxides

Gaseous nitrogen oxides are produced by combustion processes and also contribute to the formation of aerosols. Nitrogen dioxide (NO_2), an oxidant gas, is the indicator that is generally monitored. The principal source of NO_2 in outdoor air is motor vehicle emissions, and NO_2 is considered to be a useful marker of TRAP in urban environments. NO_2 has emerged as a key pollutant in urban environments, reflecting both rising vehicle numbers and choking congestion. Power plants and industrial sources may also contribute.

The health effects of NO_2 emitted into outdoor air probably come mainly from the formation of secondary pollutants, including ozone and particles, but NO_2 itself has adverse effects. NO_2, along with hydrocarbons, is an essential precursor of ozone, and the nitrogen oxides also form acidic nitrate particles. Consequently, disentangling the effects of NO_2 alone from those of the secondary pollutants to which it contributes is problematic in epidemiological research.

NO_2 itself has been studied in animal models and in clinical studies. It can reach the small airways and air sacs of the lung because of its low solubility. The toxicological evidence at high exposures has raised concern that NO_2 exposure can impair lung defenses against infectious agents like viruses and cause airway inflammation and thereby increase the risk for respiratory infections. Human exposure studies have been performed to investigate the immediate effects of NO_2 on persons with asthma but with inconsistent findings.

2.6 Carbon Monoxide

Carbon monoxide (CO), an invisible gas formed by incomplete combustion, is a prominent indoor pollutant with sources including biomass fuel combustion and space heating with fossil fuels. At high levels indoors, fatal CO poisoning may result. Outdoors, vehicle exhaust is the major source, and concentrations are highly variable, reflecting vehicle density and traffic patterns. Urban locations with high traffic density (i.e., "hot spots") tend to have the highest concentrations. The toxicity of CO comes from its tight binding to hemoglobin, which carries oxygen in the blood, and the resulting reduction of oxygen delivery to tissues.

Because of the reduction of oxygen delivery, persons with cardiovascular disease are considered at greatest risk from CO exposure, and research has focused on CO and adverse effects in this susceptible group. The evidence from studies of CO-exposed individuals with cardiovascular disease has produced some coherent epidemiological evidence indicating that CO exposure leads to earlier evidence of myocardial ischemia (inadequate oxygenation of the heart). There are other potential susceptible groups: fetuses, as well as persons with COPD, may also be harmed by CO, and healthy persons may have reduced oxygen uptake during exercise.

The exposure studies have provided robust evidence for standards for CO, which are based on brief time windows, reflective of the handling of CO in the body. In higher-income countries, outdoor levels of CO have fallen greatly over recent decades as controls have greatly reduced emissions. Nonetheless, CO may be a concern in some high-traffic locations.

2.7 Sulfur Oxides

Sulfur oxides are generated by combustion of fuels containing sulfur, such as coal, crude petroleum, and diesel, and by smelting operations. The water-soluble gas, sulfur dioxide or SO_2, is the indicator that is generally monitored. However, other sulfur oxides are emitted, and the sulfur oxides undergo transformation to form particulate sulphate compounds. SO_2 is a reactive gas that is effectively scrubbed or cleaned from inhaled air in the upper airway. With exercise and a switch to oral breathing as ventilation increases, the inhaled dose of SO_2 increases and more reaches the lung.

Much of the evidence that has driven regulation comes from studies of people with asthma showing adverse effects of SO_2 without exposures to other pollutants. Those with asthma are particularly sensitive; with exercise and hyperventilation, some people with asthma respond to SO_2 with a drop in lung function and respiratory symptoms. Such effects have been demonstrated at concentrations that might be reached in the United States in high-exposure situations and that may be common in some heavily industrialized countries.

2.8 Lead

Although lead in gasoline is now phased out in almost all nations, exposure continues from industrial activities, such as smelting, and sometimes results in dangerous exposures for children. Exposure to lead may occur through inhalation and also ingestion of lead in food, house dust, and water, routes of exposure that have become the most important in high-income countries. Lead is of particular concern for fetuses and young children who may have unacceptable exposures from ingestion of lead paint and contamination of water systems. A substantial body of epidemiological evidence links lead exposure of children to adverse neurodevelopmental effects, such as lower intelligence levels, and, as a result of that evidence, recommendations have progressively lowered the acceptable levels of lead exposure for children.[10] Lead has also been linked to higher blood pressure and cardiovascular disease and to low bone mineral density and osteoporosis.

2.9   Traffic-Related Air Pollution

Epidemiological studies have provided evidence that the pollution mixture associated with motor vehicle emissions may have toxicity beyond that anticipated from the single pollutants in the mixture. This emerging literature is significant for the large groups of people who live and work near roadways and as a consideration in urban design. The pollution from traffic is distinguished by being composed of fresh emissions, which include high concentrations of ultrafine particles and various gaseous pollutants, such as carbonyl compounds.

The evidence on TRAP was systematically reviewed by a panel convened by the Health Effects Institute in 2010.[11] For that review, the zone comprising TRAP was considered to be up to 300–500 meters from a major roadway. A wide range of respiratory, cardiovascular, allergic, reproductive, and other outcomes was considered. For many outcomes, the evidence was limited, and clear causal conclusions could not be draw, but the evidence was sufficiently suggestive to indicate an issue of public health concern. Asthma has been an outcome of particular concern, given the potential for inhaled pollutants to possibly contribute to the causation of the disease and of acute exacerbations. A meta-analysis of 41 studies found statistically significant associations of multiple TRAP pollutants with asthma onset.[12]

Given increasing urbanization and greater density of urban areas, the emerging evidence on TRAP must be considered in guiding the placement of major roadways and dwellings. In some cities, multiunit housing is still being built in close proximity to major roadways with dense and slow-moving traffic (e.g., Los Angeles). Some potential solutions have been implemented, such as the congestion charging scheme and low-emission zone in London, but such approaches are insufficient in the context of rapidly increasing numbers of vehicles in many cities such as Beijing.[13]

3   Noise

3.1   Overview

Noise has been defined as "unwanted sound."[14] It is generally measured as sound pressure level in decibels (dB) on a logarithmic scale in relation to a reference value corresponding to the human hearing threshold.

Urban environments have numerous sources of noise, including industrial activity, motor vehicles, and airports, which may be within cities or become surrounded by residences and businesses because their presence fosters growth. The problem of noise in cities has long been recognized and managed with anti-noise ordinances.[15]

3.2 Health Risks

Evidence indicates that noise may adversely affect health, with both auditory and nonauditory consequences. The auditory consequences are well studied and include noise-induced hearing loss resulting from direct damage to the auditory sensory cells in the inner ear. An emerging literature links noise exposure to cardiovascular disease risk, cognitive performance, disturbed sleep, and annoyance, as noise is by definition unwanted.

In urban environments, noise and air pollution are co-occurring, and, consequently, research has been directed at the joint consequences of these two exposures, reflecting their ubiquity as stressors in urban environments. For example, Tzivian and colleagues investigated long-term exposure to air pollution and road traffic noise in a cross-sectional study of cognitive function in adults in the Ruhr region of Germany.[16] The findings were indicative of possible synergy. A review by the same team identified 15 studies of air pollution and mental health in adults and eight on noise, but no studies considered both exposures.[17] The studies of noise exposure by itself provided some evidence on possible adverse cognitive and psychological effects. A growing body of literature, much directed at airports, links noise exposure to increased risk for cardiovascular events.

4 Water

4.1 Overview

The public health problems of water supply in urban areas are diverse, including lack of a safe water supply for drinking and hygiene, aged infrastructure with the potential for lead and copper contamination of drinking water, and pollution of water with chemicals coming from man's activities—antibiotics and other pharmaceuticals, hormones, pesticides, and other compounds. While issues related to water in urban areas vary widely, there are some commonalities: increasing scarcity as urban areas grow, increasing need for recycling of water, and increasing contamination with bioactive molecules.

Across the urban water cycle, water can be contaminated with chemicals through direct run-off from surfaces, incomplete treatment of wastewater, and discharge of effluent into surface water, from which it may eventually return to aquifers and be recycled for human use. The discharges that introduce contaminants into the urban water cycle are many and include human wastes and discharges from sewage systems, industrial sites and medical care facilities, landfills, and streets.[18] Urbanization increases the density of sources and the number of people contributing waste, particularly as density grows.

4.2 Health Risks

Studies that have assessed concentrations of contaminants in urban water have documented the presence of numerous agents that may affect human health, including plasticizers, perfluorinated surfactants, pesticides, surfactants, antibiotics, pharmaceuticals, hormones, x-ray contrast media, artificial sweeteners, fragrances, UV-filters (sunscreens), antimicrobial preservatives, and other products.[18] Some of these compounds are not particularly biodegradable (e.g., perfluorinated surfactants) and have biological activity that raises broad concerns for human and ecosystem health. Promotion of antibiotic resistance is a rising concern given the sustained exposure of microbial organisms to antibiotics across the urban water cycle.[19]

5 Conclusion

The urban environment poses multiple stressors to human health, most notably—across history and to the present—air pollution coming from outdoor and indoor sources. Air pollution illustrates the challenge of maintaining a healthy urban environment as increasing population size and density increases emissions into the atmosphere. And, even though the risks of air pollution are now well known, air quality worsened over recent decades in many of the mega-cities of Asia. Other critical elements of the environment (e.g., water) are similarly affected by population growth. These manmade exposures are overlaid by the possibly synergistic stresses of urban living. Approaches to improving the health of urban dwellers need to be holistic in their scope.

References

1. National Research Council. *Exposure science in the 21st century: a vision and a strategy.* Washington, DC: National Academies Press; 2012.
2. Thurston GD, Kipen H, Annesi-Maesano I, et al. A joint ERS/ATS policy statement: what constitutes an adverse health effect of air pollution? An analytical framework. *Eur Respir J.* 2017; 49(1).
3. Brimblecombe P. *The big smoke: a history of air pollution in London since medieval times.* Abingdon, UK: Routledge; 1987.
4. Bell ML, Davis DL. Reassessment of the lethal London Fog of 1952: novel indicators of acute and chronic consequences of acute exposure to air pollution. *Environ Health Perspect.* 2001; 109(3):389–394.
5. *Air quality guidelines: global update 2005-particulate matter, ozone, nitrogen dioxide and sulfur dioxide.* Copenhagen, Denmark: World Health Organization; 2006.
6. Gauderman WJ, Urman R, Avol E, et al. Association of improved air quality with lung development in children. *N Engl J Med.* 2015; 372(10):905–913.
7. Di Q, Wang Y, Zanobetti A, et al. Air pollution and mortality in the Medicare population. *N Engl J Med.* 2017; 376(26):2513–2522.
8. Pope CA III, Ezzati M, Dockery DW. Fine-particulate air pollution and life expectancy in the United States. *N Engl J Med.* 2009; 360(4):376–386.
9. *Integrated science assessment for ozone and related photochemical oxidants.* Research Triangle Park, NC: US Environmental Protection Agency; 2013.
10. Dapul H, Laraque D. Lead poisoning in children. *Adv Pedr.* 2014; 61:313–333.
11. *Special report 17: traffic-related air pollutions: a critical review of the literature on emissions, exposure, and health effects.* Boston, MA: Health Effects Institute; 2010.
12. Khreis H, Kelly C, Tate J, Parslow R, Lucas K, Nieuwenhuijsen M. Exposure to traffic-related air pollution and risk of development of childhood asthma: A systematic review and meta-analysis. *Environ Int.* 2017; 100:1–31.

13. Kelly FJ, Zhu T. Transport solutions for cleaner air. *Science*. 2016; 352(6288):934–936.

14. Basner M, Babisch W, Davis A, et al. Auditory and non-auditory effects of noise on health. *Lancet*. 2014; 383(9925):1325–1332.

15. Wagner K. City noise might be making you sick. *Atlantic*. February 20, 2018. Available at https://www.theatlantic.com/technology/archive/2018/02/city-noise-might-be-making-you-sick/553385/. Accessed August 7, 2018.

16. Tzivian L, Dlugaj M, Winkler A, et al. Long-term air pollution and traffic noise exposures and mild cognitive impairment in older adults: a cross-sectional analysis of the Heinz Nixdorf Recall Study. *Environ Health Perspect*. 2016; 124:1361–1368.

17. Tzivian L, Winkler A, Dlugaj M, et al. Effect of long-term outdoor air pollution and noise on cognitive and psychological functions in adults. *Int J Hyg Environ Health*. 2015; 18(1):1–11.

18. Pal A, He Y, Jekel M, Reinhard M, Gin KYH. Emerging contaminants of public health significance as water quality indicator compounds in the urban water cycle. *Environ Int*. 2014; 71:46–62.

19. Manaia CM, Macedo G, Fatta-Kassinos D, Nunes OC. Antibiotic resistance in urban aquatic environments: can it be controlled? *Appl Microbiol Biotechnol*. 2016; 100(4):1543–1557.

14

Climate Change and the Health of Urban Populations

PATRICK L. KINNEY

1 Introduction

Climate change has been called the greatest threat to global health of the twenty-first century.[1] Cities are central to both the impacts of climate change and to solutions to the climate crisis. As home to a growing proportion of the world's population, including the urban poor, cities are increasingly bearing the impacts of climate extremes, including extreme flood and heat events and unhealthy air pollution concentrations. Urban areas, while producing 70% of global carbon emissions, generate fewer emissions per capita than do less dense living arrangements.[2] Thus cities can play a central role in achieving global sustainability goals. Cities are engines of economic growth and policy innovation, and cities around the world are taking a leadership role in climate change planning, both from the perspective of building resilience to climate risks as well as in setting aggressive targets for carbon emission reductions.[3,4] What happens in cities over the next few decades will determine how severely our future world is shaped by climate change.

That our climate is changing due to human interference with the chemistry and physics of our atmosphere is now unequivocal.[5] Over the past century, average global temperatures rose by about 1 degree Celsius (C), and the pace of change is accelerating, with a current warming rate of about 0.2 degrees C per decade. Due to the inertia in the earth system, temperatures will continue to rise for several more decades regardless of carbon emission policies we enact. However, substantial global climate benefits of carbon emission controls we enact now will begin to be realized starting around 2050 and will be hugely important for the world we leave to our children and grandchildren in the latter half of this century and beyond (Figure 14.1). Furthermore, most climate friendly actions taken at the city level can bring immediate and substantial health benefits for local populations.[6,7]

Global average temperature is a convenient way to measure the health of the planet, just as our body temperature gives us insight into whether we are sick. But, like the body, the earth system is highly complex, and the damage we are doing to the climate extends to fundamental determinants of life on the planet, including how much rain falls where and when in the world, and thus affecting agricultural productivity, mental

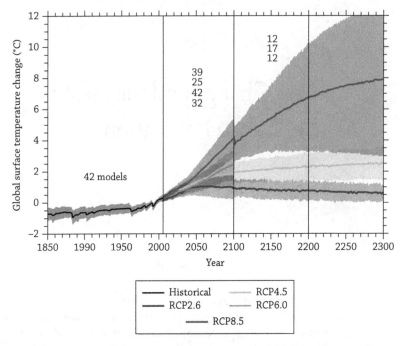

Figure 14.1 **Change in global mean temperature.** Time series of global annual mean surface air temperature anomalies (relative to 1986–2005) from the fifth coupled model intercomparison project (CMIP5) concentration-driven experiments. Projections are shown for each representative concentration pathway (RCP) for the multimodel mean (solid lines) and the 5–95% range (±1.64 standard deviation) across the distribution of individual models (shading). Discontinuities at 2100 are due to different numbers of models performing the extension runs beyond the twenty-first century and have no physical meaning. Only one ensemble member is used from each model, and numbers in the figure indicate the number of different models contributing to the different time periods. No ranges are given for the RCP6.0 projections beyond 2100 as only two models are available. Source: Intergovernmental Panel on Climate Change. *Climate change 2013: the physical science basis.* Cambridge: Cambridge University Press; 2014, figure 12.5.

health, conflict, migration, and other complex downstream impacts. Along with rising temperatures, changing patterns of extreme storms, droughts, wildfires, and sea level rise will introduce complex challenges to populations throughout the world, with impacts felt especially strongly in cities.

The term "climate" refers to long-term average conditions over a period of several decades. "Weather: is what we experience each day, week, and year, and, at these temporal scales, conditions vary widely around the climate average. Many though not all of the most severe societal impacts of climate change are caused by the wide swings in those shorter term temporal variations (e.g., too much rain in too short a time, several weeks with no rain, prolonged heat waves). But it is important to note that extreme values are directly linked to averages, as shown in Figure 14.2. For example, a small shift in the average of the temperature distribution can lead to enormous increases in the number of days above thresholds for impacts such as heat-related mortality risk.

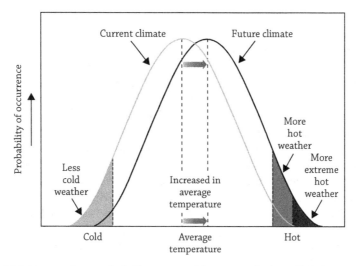

Figure 14.2 **Future climate shift.** Illustration of the way in which small shifts in the mean of a distribution can lead to manifold increases in the proportion of days above high thresholds. For example, how the areas under the curve grow in the future climate.

While extremes of temperature, precipitation, winds, and/or tidal surges can lead to immediate deaths and injuries, medium- to long-term health impacts may also follow after a climate disaster. Also, gradual changes in climate can be harmful as well, for example, by shifting patterns of risks related to air pollution, vector-borne disease, and aeroallergen exposures. In the next three sections, I review current knowledge regarding health risks of climate change with a focus on cities.

2 Storms and Floods

Many cities experience severe storms and flooding events due to their proximity to the coastline and/or situation in river valleys. Climate change compounds those risks as sea level rises and storms become more intense.[8] Health risks from severe storms and floods include direct trauma and secondary risks related to evacuation, utility outages, damage to transportation systems, exposures to contaminated air and water, and disruption of healthcare infrastructure.

Direct impacts from storms include deaths and injuries from drowning, electrocution, exposure to falling or windblown debris, and acute deaths related to preexisting chronic conditions such as heart disease. Impacts vary greatly depending on financial and institutional capacity.[9] Hurricane Katrina was estimated to have caused almost 1,000 deaths in Louisiana, with 40% due to drowning, 25% due to trauma and injury, and 11% due to cardiovascular causes.[10] Hurricane Sandy killed 44 people in New York City and dozens more in New Jersey.[11] In the Philippines in 2013, Typhoon Haiyan killed more than 6,300.[9] Inland flooding due to severe rains in Pakistan in 2010 resulted in an estimated 2,000 deaths.[12] While the urban proportion of these latter statistics has not been quantified, it is likely to have been large.

Evacuation in advance of or during weather events carries risks, including traffic accidents. Living in shelters can increase risks of communicable diseases and lead to interruption of routine treatment for chronic conditions.[13] Power outages triggered by storms can disrupt interior climate control, cold storage of food, water supplies reliant on pumping to upper floors of high-rise buildings, elevator operation, and medical support equipment.[14] Exposure to excessive indoor heat or cold in the absence of climate control may exacerbate underlying chronic conditions. Carbon monoxide and particulates emitted from backup generators or cooking equipment present poisoning and acute respiratory risks. After Hurricane Sandy made landfall, hundreds of thousands of New York City residents initially lost power. However, even after the electric grid had been largely restored, many residential buildings in storm-inundated areas still lacked electric power, heat, or running water, often because of saltwater flood damage to buildings' electrical and heating systems. Many people who did not evacuate in advance of the storm sheltered in place in housing conditions that lacked one or more services.

Flooding can compromise water and air quality by mobilizing pathogens and/or toxins from sewage and toxic waste reservoirs.[15] Flooding often leads to interior mold growth and subsequent respiratory problems, including childhood asthma.[16,17]

Healthcare institutions such as hospitals and nursing homes can be damaged by extreme storms. New York City health facilities affected by Sandy included a psychiatric hospital, nursing homes, long-term care facilities, outpatient and ambulatory care facilities, community-based providers, and pharmacies.[11] Five acute care hospitals shut down, three of which required evacuation of patients after the storm due to flooding in lower floors.[11] Four weeks following the storm, there was still a 5% reduction in hospital beds city wide.

Diverse direct and ongoing stresses associated with storm events, including displacement, can adversely affect mental health, including exacerbation of existing disease and contributing to new cases.[18,19] Posttraumatic stress disorder (PTSD) is commonly observed following natural disasters. Mental health impacts can linger or intensify long after storm events, as emergency support services wind down.

3 Heat

High temperatures have been shown to be an important risk factor for premature mortality throughout the world.[20] Excessive heat exposure has also been associated with morbidity outcomes including hospital admissions and preterm birth.[21,22] Low temperatures are also associated with higher mortality, but it is not yet clear to what extent temperature, as opposed to other seasonal factors, is causally related to excess winter mortality.[23] A typical "exposure-response" function, relating mortality to temperature in Manhattan, New York, is shown in Figure 14.3.

Workers exposed to high temperatures can experience dehydration, heat stroke, fatigue, nausea, and loss of coordination, as well as chronic effects such as chronic kidney disease, cardiovascular and respiratory diseases, and mental health problems.[24,25]

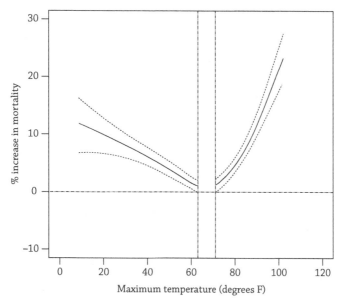

Figure 14.3 **Exposure-response function for temperature-related mortality in Manhattan, NY, based on daily data from 1982–1999.** While both cold and warm temperatures are associated with mortality risk, warming is associated with a rapid increase in risk at high temperatures and a more gradual decrease in risk at low temperatures. The dashed lines indicate the 95% confidence bounds around the curve. Source: Li T, Horton RM, Kinney PL. Projections of seasonal patterns in temperature-related deaths for Manhattan, New York. *Nat Clim Chang.* 2013; 3:717–721.

Since air conditioning confers protection from heat, health effects may be especially severe if a blackout occurs during an extreme heat event. In August 2003, the largest blackout in US history occurred in the Northeast. Weather was moderately warm during the blackout, and researchers estimated there were 90 excess deaths and an increase in respiratory hospitalizations as a result.[26]

Projecting potential future health impacts that could result from higher temperatures is challenging, in part because it is impossible to predict future changes in adaptive capacity. Assuming no change in adaption, a study by Li and colleagues projected heat-related mortality in Manhattan over the twenty-first century in the face of climate change.[27] Results are summarized in Figure 14.4 and suggest that increasing impacts may occur.

4 Other Climate Hazards

While storms and heat are two ubiquitous and important climate-related health drivers, climate change can influence the health of urban populations via other pathways as well; these include worsening air quality, exposure to pollen and mold, and changing patterns of vector-borne, water-borne, and food-borne infectious diseases.[28]

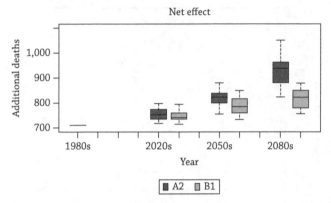

Figure 14.4 **Projection of temperature-related deaths in the 1980s, 2020s, 2050s, and 2080s for 16 global climate models and two greenhouse gas emission scenarios.** The A2 scenario assumes relatively high and the B1 assumes relatively low greenhouse gas emissions over the twenty-first century. This depicts the net effect of warming, taking into account both warm season increases and cold season decreases in future deaths. Source: Li T, Horton RM, Kinney PL. Projections of seasonal patterns in temperature-related deaths for Manhattan, New York. *Nat Clim Chang.* 2013; 3:717–721.

Health damaging air pollution is closely linked with climate change because many of the same pollution sources are responsible for both problems, especially sources where fossil fuels are burned without adequate controls on emissions. Also, pollution concentrations are strongly influenced by the weather through wind, rain, temperature, humidity, and by temperature inversions that hold pollution near the ground.[29] Changes in the climate will affect air quality, and control of pollution sources will bring benefits both for human health and for avoiding dangerous climate change. Ground-level ozone pollution, also commonly referred to as *smog*, is the pollutant most strongly influenced by climate change. Studies suggest that climate change could lead to increases in ozone concentrations in areas already impacted by ozone in the absence of more aggressive efforts to control emissions of the pollutants that are responsible for ozone pollution.[30] Ozone is formed through reactions in the atmosphere from other pollutants that are emitted in and around urban areas, including nitrogen oxides and volatile organic compounds from motor vehicles. In a future, warmer climate, ozone-forming reactions will happen faster, leading to higher concentrations and potential health impacts that include premature deaths and asthma exacerbations.[31,32] In addition to air pollutants, there is evidence that pollen seasons are lengthening, with potential impacts on allergic asthma.[33,34] Also, wildfire smoke is expected to be an increasing problem as the climate changes.[35]

Since people spend most of their time indoors, climatic influences on indoor air quality also are important for health.[36] Clearance of pollutants produced indoors, such as gas stove emissions and cigarette smoke, is affected by air exchange rates, which are in turn affected by indoor/outdoor temperature differences, wind speed and direction, and occupant behaviors related to window opening.

Climate change may affect the seasonal cycle and/or spatial distribution of some vector-borne diseases such as malaria, dengue fever, and zika virus, although climate is only one of many drivers of vector-borne disease distribution.[37] Also, some pathogens that cause water- and food-borne illnesses in humans are sensitive to climate change, including increased temperature, changing precipitation patterns, more frequent extreme precipitation events, and associated changes in seasonal patterns in the hydrological cycle.[38,39]

5 Health Vulnerability and Adaptive Capacity

Because of carbon emissions by rich countries over the past 150 years, there will be unavoidable further changes in climate over the next several decades regardless of global emission control policies. Thus, cities will need to adapt to ongoing changes in temperature, storm intensity, sea level rise, and the many downstream impacts these have for human health. After mid-century, much more devastating climate changes will be faced in the absence of immediate and effective global action to curb carbon emissions starting now.

The pathways linking climate change to adverse health outcomes are numerous and complex, and the resulting health impacts will be highly variable by region and across different groups within regions. Climate change can be viewed as a striking case of global environmental justice, in which the rich countries, those most responsible for the problem, will generally be most resilient to the adverse impacts of climate change. Poor countries, which have contributed little to climate change so far, will bear the major brunt of climate change impacts. Within countries, similar inequities exist. At the individual and population level, vulnerability tends to be greatest where multiple risk factors are present, including young and old age; preexisting physical, mental, or substance-abuse diseases; low income; and outdoor jobs, and for homebound persons with minimal social connections and those dependent on critical infrastructure including electric power.

Inversely related to vulnerability is the concept of adaptive capacity, which refers to the capacity of society to respond in ways that reduce the vulnerability of social and biological systems to actual or anticipated effects of climate change. Cities are well positioned to lead in climate adaptation planning, though technical and economic capacity is often lacking. The 100 Resilient Cities initiative of the Rockefeller Foundation is one prominent effort to address those capacity needs. Global funding mechanisms for adaptation planning and investment in low-income countries have been developed as part of the United Nations Framework Convention on Climate Change; however, funding commitments remain largely unfulfilled. Urban climate adaptation measures include infrastructure projects to limit flooding, planting of vegetation to absorb excess rainfall, and providing localized cooling, such as white roofs. Also, they can include warning and response systems for severe storms and heat events. Prioritizing adaptation investments based on their projected benefits for human health should be a core urban policy priority this century.

6 Health Dividends of Carbon Mitigation

While building capacity to reduce the health impacts of ongoing climate change–related hazards, cities are also assuming an increasingly active leadership role in carbon mitigation, the goal of which is to reduce carbon emissions to levels that would put the world on a pathway toward minimizing future climate change. New York City was one of the first cities to set carbon mitigation goals as part of Mayor Michael Bloomberg's PlaNYC initiative of 2007. Other cities have jumped on board with 80% or even 100% carbon emission reduction goals for 2050, roughly consistent with the Paris Climate Accord's global warming target of 1.5–2°C. Interestingly, Mayor Bloomberg was among the first urban leaders to highlight the health benefits for local residents that would accrue in the near term from adopting carbon mitigation targets.[40] This concept has found a growing focus in the public health and sustainable development literature.[6,7,41]

One of the biggest benefits of carbon mitigation is clean air. Most steps that cities can take to eliminate greenhouse gas emissions, such as clean vehicles and renewable energy for buildings, lead directly to far fresher, healthier air. That means fewer sick days and less medication for children who suffer from asthma. It also means longer lives for adults by reversing gradual but insidious pollution-caused changes in our bodies that can result in early death from heart disease or lung cancer. These benefits begin immediately following emission reduction and can be large. For example, the Clean Power Plan proposed under the Obama administration would have prevented thousands of premature deaths each year from particle pollution.[42]

In addition to clean air, low-carbon transportation policies can provide increased opportunities for routine physical activity. Inactivity is a major risk factor for obesity, heart disease, and diabetes. Cities can address these health problems by designing cities that weave walking and biking opportunities into the fabric of everyday life. According to recent studies, even small mode shifts away from commuting by car can have profound benefits for population health. Many other opportunities for healthier living come with low-carbon solutions, from healthier foods to greater access to green space.

7 Conclusion

Climate change is emerging as one of the most significant health challenges of our time, and cities have a crucial role to play both in adapting to the impacts and in leadership to reduce future global change. Extreme heat and storm events will increasingly expose urban residents to hazardous conditions, with both immediate and long-term risks for health. Gradual changes in temperature and precipitation will affect other pathways that affect human health, including through changes in air and water quality; vector-, food-, and water-borne infections; food security; competition for resources; and conflict. The extent to which cities of the twenty-first century are able to harness their economic and creative advantages to address the many challenges that climate change will create for urban health will be a defining question of our time.

References

1. Costello A, Abbas M, Allen A, et al. Managing the health effects of climate change. *Lancet.* 2009; 373:1693–1733.

2. Seto KC, Dhakal S, Bigio A, et al. *Human settlements, infrastructure, and spatial planning.* Cambridge: Cambridge University Press; 2014.
3. 100 Resilient Cities Program website. 2018. Available at http://www.100resilientcities.org. Accessed May 11, 2018.
4. C40 Cities website. 2018. Available at http://www.c40.org/. Accessed May 11, 2018.
5. Intergovernmental Panel on Climate Change. *Climate change 2013: the physical science basis.* Cambridge: Cambridge University Press; 2014.
6. Watts N, Adger WN, Agnolucci P, et al. Health and climate change: policy responses to protect public health. *Lancet.* 2015; 386:1861–1914.
7. Haines A, McMichael AJ, Smith KR, et al. Public health benefits of strategies to reduce greenhouse-gas emissions: overview and implications for policy makers. *Lancet.* 2009; 374:2104–2114.
8. Lane K, Charles-Guzman K, Wheeler K, Abid Z, Graber N, Matte T. Health effects of coastal storms and flooding in urban areas: a review and vulnerability assessment. *J Environ Public Health.* 2013; 15:1–13.
9. *Final report: effects of Typhoon "Yolanda" (Haiyan).* Quenzon City, Philipphines: The Philippine National Disaster Risk Reduction and Management Council; 2015.
10. Brunkard J, Namulanda G, Ratard R. Hurricane Katrina Deaths, Louisiana, 2005. *Disaster Med Public Health Prep.* 2008; 2:215–223.
11. *A stronger, more resilient New York: NYC special initiative for rebuilding and resiliency.* New York: City of New York; 2013.
12. *Pakistan floods: the deluge of disaster: facts & figures as of 15 September 2010.* Singapore: Singapore Red Cross; 2010.
13. Arrieta MI, Foreman RD, Crook ED, Icenogle ML. Providing continuity of care for chronic diseases in the aftermath of Katrina: from field experience to policy recommendations. *Disaster Med Public Health Prep.* 2009; 3:174–182.
14. Beatty ME, Phelps S, Rohner C, Weisfuse I. Blackout of 2003: public health effects and emergency response. *Public Health Rep.* 2006; 121:36–44.
15. Ruckart PZ, Orr MF, Lanier K, Koehler A. Hazardous substances releases associated with Hurricanes Katrina and Rita in industrial settings, Louisiana and Texas. *J Hazard Mater.* 2008; 159:53–57.
16. Barbeau DN, Grimsley LF, White LE, El-Dahr JM, Lichtveld M. Mold exposure and health effects following Hurricanes Katrina and Rita. *Annu Rev Public Health.* 2010; 3:165–178.
17. Jaakkola JJK, Hwang BF, Jaakkola N. Home dampness and molds, parental atopy, and asthma in childhood: a six-year population-based cohort study. *Environ Health Perspect.* 2005; 113:357–361.
18. Pietrzak RH, Tracy M, Galea S, et al. Resilience in the face of disaster: prevalence and longitudinal course of mental disorders following Hurricane Ike. *PLoS One.* 2012; 7. doi:10.1371/journal.pone.0038964
19. Galea S, Brewin CR, Gruber M, et al. Exposure to hurricane-related stressors and mental illness after Hurricane Katrina. *Arch Gen Psychiatry.* 2007; 64:1427–1434.
20. Gasparrini A, Guo Y, Hashizume M, et al. Mortality risk attributable to high and low ambient temperature: a multicountry study observational study. *Lancet.* 2015; 386(9991): 369–375.
21. Basu R, Malig B, Ostro B. High ambient temperature and the risk of preterm delivery. *Am J Epidemiol.* 2010; 172:1108–1117.
22. Knowlton K, Rotkin-Ellman M, King G, et al. The 2006 California Heat Wave: impacts on hospitalizations and emergency department visits. *Environ Health Perspect.* 2009; 117:61–67.
23. Kinney PL, Schwartz J, Pascal M, et al. Winter season mortality: will climate warming bring benefits? *Environ Res Lett.* 2015; 10:8.
24. Roncal-Jimenez CA, Garcia-Trabanino R, Wesseling C, Johnson RJ. Mesoamerican nephropathy or global warming nephropathy? *Blood Purif.* 2016; 41:135–138.
25. Xiang J, Bi P, Pisaniello D, Hansen A. Health impacts of workplace heat exposure: an epidemiological review. *Ind Health.* 2014; 52(2): 91–101.

26. Anderson GB, Bell ML. Lights out: impact of the August 2003 power outage on mortality in New York, NY. *Epidemiology*. 2012; 23(2):189–193.

27. Li T, Horton RM, Kinney PL. Projections of seasonal patterns in temperature-related deaths for Manhattan, New York. *Nat Clim Chang*. 2013; 3:717–721.

28. Crimmins A, Balbus J, Gamble JL, et al. *The impacts of climate change on human health in the United States: a scientific assessment*. Washington, DC: US Global Change Research Program. 2016. doi:10.7930/J0R49NQX

29. Kinney PL. Climate change, air quality, and human health. *Am J Prev Med*. 2008; 35:459–467.

30. Kinney PL. Interactions of climate change, air pollution, and human health. *Curr Environ Health Rep*. 2018; 5(1):179–186.

31. Knowlton K, Rosenthal J, Hogrefe C, et al. Assessing ozone-related health impacts under a changing climate. *Environ Health Perspect*. 2004; 112:1557–1563.

32. Sheffield PE, Knowlton K, Carr JL, Kinney PL. Modeling of regional climate change effects on ground-level ozone and childhood asthma. *Am J Prev Med*. 2011; 41:251–257.

33. Anenberg S, Weinberger KR, Roman H, et al. Impacts of oak pollen on allergic asthma in the USA and potential effect of future climate change: a modelling analysis. *Lancet*. 2017; 389:S2.

34. Ziska L, Knowlton K, Rogers C, et al. Recent warming by latitude associated with increased length of ragweed pollen season in central North America. *Proc Natl Acad Sci U S A*. 2011; 108(10):4248–4251.

35. Jolly WM, Cochrane MA, Freeborn PH, et al. Climate-induced variations in global wildfire danger from 1979 to 2013. *Nat Commun*. 2015; 6:11.

36. Spengler JD. Climate change, indoor environments, and health. *Indoor Air*. 2012; 22:89–95.

37. Lafferty KD. The ecology of climate change and infectious diseases. *Ecology*. 2009; 90:888–900.

38. Curriero FC, Patz JA, Rose JB, Lele S. The association between extreme precipitation and waterborne disease outbreaks in the United States, 1948–1994. *Am J Public Health*. 2001; 91:1194–1199.

39. Semenza JC, Suk JE, Estevez V, Ebi KL, Lindgren E. Mapping climate change vulnerabilities to infectious diseases in Europe. *Environ Health Perspect*. 2012; 120:385–392.

40. Bloomberg MR, Aggarwala RT. Think locally, act globally: how curbing global warming emissions can improve local public health. *Am J Prev Med*. 2008; 35:414–423.

41. Jack DW, Kinney PL. Health co-benefits of climate mitigation in urban areas. *Curr Opin Environ Sustain*. 2010; 2:172–177.

42. Buonocore JJ, Lambert KF, Burtraw D, Sekar S, Driscoll CT. An analysis of costs and health co-benefits for a US power plant carbon standard. *PLoS One*. 2016; 11(6). doi:10.1371/journal.pone.0156308

15

Crime and Criminal Justice in Cities

MATT VOGEL AND STEVEN F. MESSNER

1 Introduction

Writing nearly 80 years ago, Ernst Burgess summarized the state of existing knowledge on crime in urban areas by noting that "the distribution of juvenile delinquents in space and time follows the pattern of the physical structure and social organization of the American city."[1] Seven decades later, this general observation still holds true. Crime rates vary in predictable ways across the urban landscape, and although the socioeconomic composition and features of the built environment of cities are constantly changing, rates of crime and delinquency remain intricately linked to the structural characteristics of neighborhoods and the shared experiences of the people residing within them. This chapter provides a broad overview of contemporary research on urban crime in the United States. We begin by describing temporal and spatial patterns in urban crime rates, placing recent trends within a broader historical context. We then focus on prominent theoretical perspectives that help illuminate the processes underlying these trends. We end with a discussion of contemporary criminal justice practices that have been enacted to lessen the burden of crime on urban areas and draw some general inferences about crime in cities that apply to countries beyond the United States.

2 Trends in Urban Crime

Contemporary research on urban crime is often oriented around one of three general "facts." First, crime rates in urban areas are declining and have been for some time. Second, despite these declines, crime rates are much higher in cities than in suburban or rural communities. Third, crime is not evenly distributed within cities. Instead, crime rates vary substantially from neighborhood to neighborhood, with a handful of places responsible for the vast majority of criminal activity.

Figure 15.1 presents the homicide rates in 17 major urban centers in the United States between 1960 and 2017. We focus on homicide because the definition has remained relatively consistent over time and the official statistics are unlikely to be influenced by reporting bias. As demonstrated here, homicide increased markedly throughout the 1970s and 1980s, peaked around 1991, and has declined dramatically since. Despite

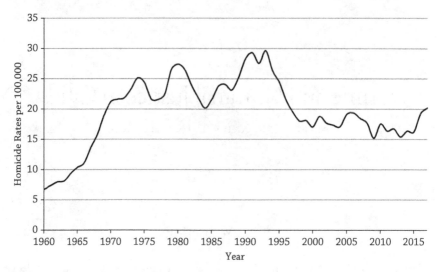

Figure 15.1 **Homicide rates in 17 major cities, 1960–2017.** Cities include Atlanta, GA; Boston, MA; Chicago, IL; Cincinnati, OH; Cleveland, OH; Detroit, MI; Houston, TX; Kansas City, MO; Los Angeles, CA; Milwaukee, WI; New York; Philadelphia, PA; Pittsburgh, PA; Portland, OR; San Francisco, CA; Seattle, WA; and St. Louis, MO.

some recent fluctuations (discussed in greater detail later), recent crime rates parallel those experienced in the late 1960s. On the whole, US cities are much safer today than they were 30 years ago.

Despite the crime decline, the concentration of violence and property crime remains a salient feature of urban life in the twenty-first century. Table 15.1 presents levels of seven types of offending across different types of communities. Rates of robbery and motor vehicle theft are more than twice as high in urban areas relative to the suburbs and rural communities, a fact likely attributed to greater population density and a higher concentration of vehicles. Yet urban areas also have considerably higher rates of homicides, assaults, burglaries, and thefts. Even after adjusting for population size, crime is much more heavily concentrated in cities than in other community types.

Finally, crime and violence are not evenly distributed across urban space; instead, crime rates tend to cluster around other indicators of social and economic well-being. Figure 15.2 presents the spatial distribution of violent crime, socioeconomic disadvantage, and race in the city of St. Louis in 2016. These figures use block groups, the smallest geographical unit for which the US Census Bureau publishes sample data. Panel 1 presents the spatial distribution of violent crime (homicide, assault, robbery). Panel 2 presents the distribution of African Americans, and Panel 3, the distribution of poverty, measured as the proportion of families at or below the federal poverty line. For each panel, the variables are split into quartiles, with the darkest shaded region corresponding to the highest concentration of each indicator. As illustrated in this figure, crime, race, and economic disadvantage all cluster together in space. The highest levels of crime are found in neighborhoods characterized by the highest levels of socioeconomic deprivation and the largest concentrations of minority residents. These general trends

Table 15.1 **Uniform Crime Reporting Part I crime rates (per 100,000) by urbanicity, 2016**

	Homicide	Rape	Robbery	Aggravated assault	Burglary	Larceny theft	Motor vehicle theft
Cities	8.1	46.7	185.5	344.0	556.5	2207.2	372.4
Suburban areas	3.2	31.5	52.1	170.5	370.5	1406.7	156.5
Rural counties	3.6	39.1	11.6	149.5	378.7	736.2	99.4

Source: Crime in the United States, 2016, Table 11. United States Department of Justice Federal Bureau of Investigation website. Available at: https://ucr.fbi.gov/crime-in-the-u.s/2016/crime-in-the-u.s.-2016/topic-pages/tables/table-10. Published 2016. Accessed April 14, 2018.

Urban rates are calculated from agencies within cities having populations greater than 50,000. Suburban rates are calculated from agencies that exist within metropolitan statistical areas but excluding reporting agencies from principal cities (those with populations 50,000 or greater). Rural crime rates consist of agencies reporting from nonmetropolitan counties. Due to the inability to disaggregate FBI Crime in the US cities by their metropolitan statistical area distinction, the rural county measure excludes agencies reporting regularly from the city level.

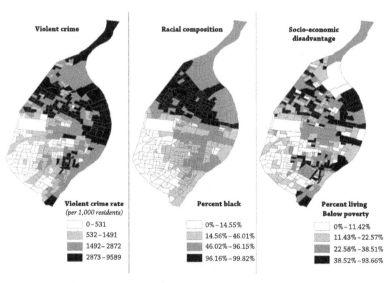

Figure 15.2 **Spatial distribution of violent crime, percent black, and percent at or below federal poverty line by block-group, St. Louis, MO, 2016.**

are characteristic of most major American cities: crime flourishes in areas characterized by the highest concentration of socioeconomic disadvantages.[2]

3 Explanations of Urban Crime

Several factors may help to explain patterns of urban crime. In the following sections, we discuss trends in urban crime over time and spatial distribution of crime in cities.

3.1 Trends in Urban Crime Over Time

Much contemporary research has centered on the trends and spatial patterns described in Figures 15.1 and 15.2. Explanations of temporal fluctuations in crime rates often point to the role of changing economic conditions. For example, rapid deindustrialization in the latter half of the twentieth century had profound consequences for the structure of urban neighborhoods. Tectonic shifts in the US economy led to the migration of manufacturing jobs away from core urban centers.[3] Working and middle-class whites followed the jobs out of cities, leaving behind communities characterized by relatively high levels of socioeconomic disadvantage, fewer resources to combat impending social problems, and limited prospects for outward mobility.[4] As a result, crime rates began a long, upward crawl from the 1960s through the early 1990s.

Other explanations of long-term crime trends have focused on more proximate economic correlates of crime, such as shifts in consumer sentiment, unemployment, and inflation. For example, ebbs and flows in the crime rates from 1960 through the present map closely onto year-over-year changes in inflation. Some have argued that consumers are especially attuned to changes in price levels. As inflation increases, so, too, does the demand for cheap, stolen goods (and the people who supply underground markets), thus driving up rates of acquisitive crime.[5]

Moving beyond economic indicators, a sizeable body of research has accumulated alternative explanations for the abrupt decline in urban crime beginning in the early 1990s. Much of this literature points to innovations in policing that targeted low-level offenders, reduced signs of physical disorder, and helped eradicate inner-city drug markets.[6] Others have highlighted the growth of "tough on crime" policies that incapacitated large numbers offenders for longer periods of time. While the changes in criminal justice practices undoubtedly contributed to the crime decline, recent scholarship points to a subtler culprit—the growth of nonprofit organizations. Throughout the 1990s and early 2000s, a large number of nonprofit organizations were established across the United States. Many of these organizations were explicitly focused on reducing youth violence, reinvigorating neighborhoods, and making communities safer places. Emerging research suggests that, on the whole, these programs achieved their goal—the more funding these organizations received within cities over time, the more crime declined.[7]

3.2 Spatial Distribution of Urban Crime

The uneven distribution of crime within cities has been a central puzzle in criminological research for more than a century. Studying rates of juvenile delinquency in Chicago
in the first half of the twentieth century, Clifford Shaw and Henry McKay observed
that neighborhoods characterized by high levels of residential turnover, ethnic heterogeneity, and socioeconomic disadvantage displayed the highest levels of offending.[8]
These trends remained relatively stable over time, suggesting that characteristics of
neighborhoods, above and beyond the shared characteristics of the people living there,
were consequential for understanding the concentration of crime within cities. Their
conceptual framework, referred to as "Social Disorganization Theory," provided the
scaffolding for decades of research examining how characteristics of residential places
affect criminal conduct.

Early studies of social disorganization focused on how structural disadvantage
influences interpersonal relationships among neighborhood residents and, in turn, how
these relationships affect efforts at crime control. Drawing from Coleman's theory of
social capital, relationships among neighbors can be viewed as producing intangible
resources that are mutually beneficial for all neighborhood residents (e.g., the joint
supervision of youth).[9] Social organization can be viewed as the extent to which a neighborhood utilizes interactional networks among residents to effectively control group
behavior (referred to as the "systemic model of crime").[10] In socially organized areas,
neighbors are more likely to be acquaintances or friends and as such are more willing
to watch out for others' property and intervene in others' affairs should trouble arise.
Socially disorganized neighborhoods, then, are characterized by deficient friendship,
kinship, and acquaintanceship networks that diminish the capacity to regulate criminal
behavior.[11]

Of course, not all neighborhoods are organized around the goal of crime reduction. Cohesive social networks can also impede the facilitation of social control.[12] In
disadvantaged communities, dense connections among residents sometimes insulate
the criminal element (such as drug dealers and gang members) from law enforcement.
Moving beyond the systemic approach, the prevalence of social networks and participation in community organizations have been hypothesized to facilitate the development
of "collective efficacy," or a mutual sense of trust among neighbors and a willingness
to intervene on behalf of the common good. Insofar as community residents desire
to live in crime-free environments, their collective capacity to control group behavior should be negatively associated with crime rates. From this vantage point, dense
social networks alone are not sufficient to prevent crime, but rather crime rates are a
function of the community's capacity for collective action. And, indeed, collective efficacy has been consistently associated with lower levels of violence and homicide, often
mediating the effects of neighborhood disadvantage on violence.[13]

More recent scholarship has recognized that neighborhoods themselves tend to be
heterogeneous; for instance, crime rates often vary significantly from one street to the
next within the same census tract. This growing body of research highlights the ways in
which *microplaces*—often conceptualized as street segments or addresses—affect the
geographic concentration of crime. A common observation is that approximately 5%

of all addresses in a city account for 50% of all crime, and these "hot-spots" are the key drivers of crime in urban areas.[14]

The recognition that some places are more (or less) likely to experience crime has also led scholars to explore how elements of the built environment can enable or constrain criminal conduct. The earliest of these theories, commonly referred to as Routine Activities Theory (RAT), argues that the key elements of a criminal event are the presence of motivated offender, a suitable target, and the absence of capable guardianship.[15] From this general observation sprang an entire subdiscipline, referred to as *environmental criminology*, dedicated to understanding the ways in which offenders and victims come together in space and time.[16] A sizeable portion of this research focuses on how communities can reduce crime by altering features of the physical environment, for instance, by creating barriers to limit through-traffic, installing street lights, and placing CCTV cameras on local businesses.

4   Controlling Crime in Urban Areas Through Law Enforcement

The trends described in Section 2 have given rise to a number of innovative policing strategies. For example, the observation that criminal behavior is unevenly clustered at small spatial scales has led many police departments to focus their efforts at crime "hot spots." By targeting resources at high-crime areas, law enforcement can effectively utilize limited resources to maximize crime reduction. There have been numerous evaluations of hot spots policing, including several randomized control trials. The majority of these studies find a significant effect: when police focus their efforts on hot spots, crime goes down.[17]

However, not all attempts at crime control have been as effective. Many urban police departments are facing criticism for controversial practices that have disproportionately affected low-income communities of color. Take New York City's stop, question, and frisk policy (SQF). Officers have the right to stop suspects who they believe have committed or are in the process of committing a crime. If the officer feels there is a reasonable threat to his safety, he may pat down the exterior clothing of a suspect for weapons. Between 2003 and 2011, the number of such stops quadrupled in New York City. Opponents to the policy pointed out that these stops had disproportionately targeted young, minority males in predominantly low-income communities of color. In 2012, the New York State Supreme Court, in *Floyd v. City of New York,* declared this practice to be unconstitutional as it violated the Fourth Amendment. The presiding judge concluded that the policy was one of "indirect racial profiling" that overwhelmingly affected young black and Hispanic males.

This general pattern is not confined to New York City. Many have argued that aggressive policing and mass incarceration have disproportionately affected low-income, minority communities.[18] This differential contact with the criminal justice system can erode public trust in law enforcement, leading neighborhood residents to cast law enforcement in a negative light. As a result, minority communities are often characterized by high levels of legal cynicism—defined as the belief that law enforcement is illegitimate, unresponsive, and ill-equipped to ensure public safety.[19] In these places, residents are more willing to resolve disputes with violence than to seek police intervention. This phenomenon has been amplified in recent years due to the highly publicized and often politicized cases involving officer use of deadly force. Recent research suggests that calls for service decline in the wake of the highly publicized officer-involved shootings, which, in turn, places upward pressure on rates of criminal violence in minority communities.[20] And some have even argued that the increasing media coverage and ensuing social unrest are at least partially responsible for the increased urban crime rates observed since 2014.[21]

5 Conclusion

There are several important take-away points from the empirical literature on crime and criminal justice in urban areas. For one, despite some very recent upticks, crime rates in the United States today are significantly lower than they were 30 years ago. That being said, crime rates remain much higher in cities than in suburban and rural areas, and the uneven spatial distribution of crime *within* urban areas remains a defining feature of modern cities. Given the legacy of socioeconomic and racial segregation in the United States, it is not surprising that levels of crime, as well as the criminal justice response to criminal behavior, vary significantly across neighborhoods of differing sociodemographic compositions. While there are a number of explanations for these trends, most coalesce around structural barriers that inhibit the formation of collective efficacy and limit the ability of local residents to work together for their own common good.

From a criminal justice standpoint, the spatial concentration of crime in urban areas has had several profound implications for policing in recent decades. The observation that crime tends to be concentrated in small geographic areas suggests that targeted policing can go a long way toward reducing crime. However, such policing needs to be implemented judiciously, given the evidence that overly aggressive practices have strained police–community relationships, especially in communities of color, which has the potential to increase rates of crime in the future.

Although this chapter has focused on research findings from the United States, it is important to note in closing that many of these general patterns characterize crime in other urban contexts. For example, the geographic concentration of crime at small spatial scales has been documented in places as diverse as Venezuela, the Netherlands, Australia, Colombia, and China.[22,23] Similarly, the relationship between structural neighborhood characteristics and crime also appears to be generalizable to a much broader range of urban centers in a variety of countries.[24-26] To be sure, the ways in which neighborhood characteristics influence rates of crime invariably reflect features of the sociocultural context.[27] Nevertheless, on the whole, criminological research continues to reaffirm Ernest Burgess's basic insight that, despite marked differences in the socioeconomic composition, cultures, and unique historical developments of cities across the globe, the disproportionate concentration of crime within urban areas can be attributed to identifiable features of the structure and social organization of the city.

References

1. Burgess R. Forward. In Shaw CR, McKay HD, eds. *Juvenile delinquency and urban areas.* Chicago, IL: University of Chicago Press; 1942.
2. Peterson RD, Krivo LJ. *Divergent social worlds: neighborhood crime and the racial-spatial divide.* New York, NY: Russell Sage Foundation; 2010.
3. Wilson WJ. *The truly disadvantaged: the inner city, the underclass, and public policy.* Chicago, IL: University of Chicago Press; 2012.
4. Sharkey P. *Stuck in place: urban neighborhoods and the end of progress toward racial equality.* Chicago, IL: University of Chicago Press; 2013.
5. Rosenfeld R, Vogel M, McCuddy T. Crime and inflation in US cities. *J Quant Criminol.* 2017; 1–16.
6. Blumstein A, Wallman J, eds. *The crime drop in America.* Cambridge: Cambridge University Press; 2006.
7. Sharkey P, Torrats-Espinosa G, Takyar D. Community and the crime decline: the causal effect of local nonprofits on violent crime. *Am Sociol Rev.* 2017; 82(6):1214–1240.
8. Shaw CR, McKay HD. *Juvenile delinquency and urban areas.* Chicago, IL: University of Chicago Press; 1942.
9. Coleman JS. Social capital in the creation of human capital. In Lesser E, ed. *Knowledge and social capital: foundations and applications.* Wobum, MA: Butterworth-Heinemann; 2000: 17–41.
10. Bursik Jr RJ, Grasmick HG. *Neighborhoods and crime: the dimensions of effective community control.* New York: Lexington Books; 1993.
11. Sampson RJ, Morenoff JD, Gannon-Rowley T. Assessing "neighborhood effects": social processes and new directions in research. *Annu Rev Sociol.* 2002; 28(1):443–478.
12. Pattillo-McCoy M. *Black picket fences.* Chicago, IL: University of Chicago Press; 1999.
13. Sampson RJ, Raudenbush SW, Earls F. Neighborhoods and violent crime: a multilevel study of collective efficacy. *Science.* 1997; 277(5328):918–924.
14. Weisburd D, Groff ER, Yang SM. *The criminology of place: street segments and our understanding of the crime problem.* Oxford: Oxford University Press; 2012.
15. Cohen LE, Felson M. Social change and crime rate trends: a routine activity approach. *Am Sociol Rev.* 1979; 588–608.
16. Brantingham PJ, Brantingham PL. Environmental criminology: from theory to urban planning practice. *Studies on Crime and Crime Prevention.* 1998; 7(1):31–60.
17. Braga A, Papachristos A, Hureau D. Hot spots policing effects on crime. *Campbell Systematic Reviews.* 2012; 8(8):1–96.
18. Alexander M. *The new Jim Crow: mass incarceration in the age of colorblindness.* New York: The New Press; 2012.
19. Kirk DS, Papachristos AV. Cultural mechanisms and the persistence of neighborhood violence. *Am J Sociol.* 2011; 116(4):1190–1233.
20. Desmond M, Papachristos AV, Kirk DS. Police violence and citizen crime reporting in the black community. *Am Sociol Rev.* 2016. 81(5):857–876.
21. Rosenfeld R. Studying crime trends: normal science and exogenous shocks. *Criminology.* 2018; 56(1):5–26.
22. Feng J, Dong Y, Song L. A spatio-temporal analysis of urban crime in Beijing: based on data for property crime. *Urban Stud.* 2016; 53(15):3223–3245.
23. Sanguinetti P, Ortega D, Berniell L, et al. *Toward a safer Latin America. A new perspective to prevent and control crime.* Bogotá, Colombia: CAF Development Bank of Latin America; 2015.
24. Liu D, Song W, Xiu C. Spatial patterns of violent crimes and neighborhood characteristics in Changchun, China. *Aust NZ J Criminol.* 2016; 49(1):53–72.

25. Bruinsma GJ, Pauwels LJ, Weerman FM, Bernasco W. Social disorganization, social capital, collective efficacy and the spatial distribution of crime and offenders: an empirical test of six neighbourhood models for a Dutch city. *Br J Criminol.* 2013; 53(5):942–963.
26. Mazerolle L, Wickes R, McBroom J. Community variations in violence: the role of social ties and collective efficacy in comparative context. *J Res Crime Delinq.* 2010; 47(1):3–30.
27. Messner SF, Zhang L, Zhang S, Gruner CP. Neighborhood crime control in a changing China: Tiao-jie, Bang-jiao, and neighborhood watches. *J Res Crime Delinq.* 2017; 54(4):544–577.

16

Improving Access to Healthy Food in Cities

MONICA L. WANG AND MARISA OTIS

1 Introduction

Substantial evidence now exists that the food environment is associated with health.[1-3] This makes healthy food environments in urban settings a priority nationally and globally. Healthy food access is a key characteristic of healthy food environments. Living in unhealthy food environments such as *food deserts* (geographic areas with limited access to affordable, healthy foods) is associated with poor diet and elevated risk for obesity, diabetes, hypertension, heart disease, diet-related cancers, and premature mortality among youth and adults.[3-11] More recent research indicates that *food swamps* (geographic areas saturated with fast food outlets) better predict obesity rates than food deserts.[11,12] In contrast, living in healthy food environments, characterized by accessibility, availability, affordability, and acceptability of healthy foods, is associated with healthy eating (e.g., increased fruit and vegetable intake) and decreased risk of diet-related chronic conditions.[1,2,8,13] These associations remain significant after adjusting for a variety of individual- and neighborhood-level factors.

1.1 Assessing Food Environments

The availability and placement of supermarkets are commonly used as proxy measures of healthy food environments.[14] Using that measure, an estimated 4 million urban US households have inadequate access to a supermarket (reside over half a mile away with no vehicle access), and approximately 19 million Americans (6.2% of the population) live in food deserts.[15] Food environments, however, systematically differ depending on the socioeconomic and racial/ethnic composition of neighborhoods in the United States. Neighborhoods with higher proportions of low-income or racial/ethnic minority residents are characterized by fewer supermarkets, smaller grocery stores, and higher densities of convenience and fast food stores than are higher income, predominately white communities.[16]

1.2 Food Environment and Health Disparities

Disparities in exposure to poor-quality food environments translate into health disparities. The excessive exposure to nutrient-poor, energy-dense foods and limited access to healthy foods among poor, urban communities and communities of color may partially contribute to disproportionately higher rates of obesity and diabetes among these communities than their counterparts.[17-19] It is important to note that the proliferation of poor urban "foodscapes" is largely the result of institutionalized discriminatory policies, such as redlining and restrictive covenants, that systematically promoted economic opportunity for white families over racial/ethnic minority families.[17,20] Such policies encouraged white flight from inner cities to suburban neighborhoods, resulting in disinvested urban communities of color that continue to struggle in attracting businesses—including supermarkets—today.[17]

Providing equitable access to healthy food across urban settings therefore is a critical priority that has yet to be sufficiently addressed. The following sections describe key opportunities and challenges for targeting disparities in healthy food access and improving the food environment for urban populations using several examples from the US context. While these examples are domestically focused, they provide perspectives that we suggest can inform the global effort to provide healthy food universally for all.

2 Opportunities

The creation of healthy food environments has the potential to yield multiple opportunities that benefit urban communities.

2.1 Cross-Sector Collaboration

Targeting healthy food access can bridge efforts and leverage resources among government, business, academia, industry, and community. Improving healthy food access in urban settings provides multiple avenues for interdisciplinary, cross-sector collaborations. Such efforts are often led by nonprofit or community organizations and/or state and local departments.[21,22] However, engaging critical players (e.g., food producers and distributors, policymakers) in the process is not yet common practice in food environment interventions.[23] More recently, an increasing number of cities and states in the United States are pursuing healthy food financing initiatives that are dedicated to the development or renovation of healthy food retail (e.g., grocery stores, corner stores, mobile markets, farmers markets), particularly in underserved communities and food deserts.[24] Such initiatives include leaders and representatives from a wide range of sectors, including local government, business, academia, community, nonprofit, and philanthropy.

For example, Mandela MarketPlace, a nonprofit organization, initiated a cross-sector partnership to inform the development of a cooperative grocery store in a historically disinvested community in Oakland, California. Resources leveraged included community outreach from trained residents, food assessment expertise from local academic researchers, agricultural skills of family farmers, assets from small businesses, expertise of a retail consultant, political support of a city council member, and financial support from government programs and private lenders. Their collective efforts led to the opening of Mandela Foods Cooperative, a community-owned cooperative grocery store in 2009.[25] Such cross-cutting partnerships facilitate the identification and implementation of strategies to improve healthy food access that are tailored for each setting.

2.2   Urban Revitalization

Increasing healthy food access can provide opportunities for urban revitalization; such effects need to be systematically evaluated in order to generate interest and sustained investment in food environment interventions. The opening of new sources of healthy, affordable foods, such as full-service supermarkets and grocery stores, can provide opportunities for economic and social revitalization for urban communities. According to The Food Trust, every 10,000 square feet of added retail grocery space generates approximately 24 jobs in the United States.[24] Pennsylvania's Fresh Food Financing Initiative led to the development of 88 grocery stores and the creation of 5,000 jobs over a 6-year period.[26] Establishing healthy food retailers can increase community tax revenue and overall economic activity (thus catalyzing further commercial revitalization) and is also linked with increased neighborhood livability. Results from a time-series analysis indicated that the development of new supermarkets in Philadelphia was associated with subsequent increases in the city's residential real estate values.[27] Improving healthy food access can be a catalyst for urban revitalization that strengthens the community's economic, social, and cultural fabric.[28] However, efforts to document and evaluate urban revitalization as an outcome of healthy food access interventions are sparse. Expanding the types of outcomes assessed beyond sales, store environment, and consumer perceptions and health behaviors is needed to generate findings that are not only useful to researchers, but also to policymakers, business owners, and community members who are key stakeholders in influencing the spread and adoption of healthy food access interventions.[23]

2.3   Private Sector Engagement

Improving access to healthy food opens the possibility for collaborations with industry for population health promotion. Efforts to prevent obesity and related conditions through strategies such as increasing healthy food access often conflict with the business interests of powerful economic operators, such as the food and beverage industry.[29] Kickbusch and colleagues coined the term "commercial determinants of health" to describe strategies used by the private sector to "promote products and choices that are detrimental to health."[30] However, commercial determinants need not be health-undermining by default. Pursuing proactive partnerships with industry can lead to a more systematic integration of science in shaping the food and beverage industry and subsequent food environment (e.g., product reformulation to meet evidence-based dietary recommendations) that contribute to improved dietary changes and health outcomes in the long term.

For example, several US cities and countries around the world have passed legislation on sugar-sweetened beverage taxation as a food environment policy approach to curb the obesity epidemic.[31] Such legislative actions have sparked national and international

Improving Access to Healthy Food in Cities 151

conversations on the health impact of sugar-sweetened beverages, leading to beverage industry executives convening to discuss ways to reformulate recipes to meet growing consumer demand for lower sugar products.[32] This serves as an excellent opportunity to engage with industry through approaches such as product reformulation, marketing, and partnerships to promote population health.[33] A partnership between the Clinton Foundation and the beverage industry led to a voluntary industry agreement to remove full-calorie beverages from schools and adhere to school beverage guidelines.[34] As a result, calories from beverages shipped to US schools decreased by 90%. Another partnership between the Healthy Weight Commitment Foundation and 16 major food and beverage companies, including General Mills and PepsiCo, led to an industry pledge to reduce calories in the marketplace by introducing new, lower calorie products or reformulating existing products.[35] Collectively, industry members removed 6.4 trillion calories from the US marketplace over a 5-year period (the equivalent of 78 calories/ person per day).[35] However, opportunities to build healthy food environments in urban settings must be considered within the context of key challenges.

3 Challenges

While creating healthy food environments can yield benefits to communities, there are also challenges and costs.

3.1 Targeted Access and Demand

Improving the built urban food environment and ultimately urban health requires targeting access and demand. While several studies indicate that limited access to healthy food (e.g., full-service supermarket) is associated with poor diet and obesity, other studies demonstrate that saturated access to unhealthy foods (e.g., high density of fast food outlets and convenience stores) matters more for obesity risk.[1,2,10,36–39] These findings suggest that placing supermarkets in food deserts may not be enough to drive utilization and subsequent improvements in diet and related health outcomes. Several US cities have limited the presence of fast food establishments through zoning mechanisms such as total or partial bans, distance or density requirements, quotas, and use restrictions as a strategy to restructure food swamps.[40]

However, to be successful in promoting healthy eating and overall urban health, reshaping local food environments must also be accompanied by a community demand for such changes. A study of residents living in urban food deserts indicated that the majority conducted their grocery shopping further than the nearest supermarket, underscoring the importance of involving residents in urban planning to increase the likelihood that any new food market meets residents' needs and preference and thus utilization.[41] Though South Los Angeles, California, implemented a 1-year ban on new fast food restaurants, no changes were observed in residents' fast food consumption or obesity rates over a 5-year period.[42] A possible explanation for this finding is a lack of change in community diet norms and preferences, given a long-standing culture of a fast food diet. Food environment interventions must target both supply and demand for healthy foods, though how to achieve this efficiently and effectively remains a key challenge.[43]

3.2 Investment from Multiple Sectors

The creation of healthy urban food environments requires substantial time, resources, and investment from multiple sectors, particularly government through policy-making. Improving the built food environment is costly and requires multisector investment. A 1977 landmark study analyzing supermarket operating costs found that nearly every expense was higher for urban stores than for their suburban counterparts.[44] Costs such as training, inventory loss, taxes, and maintenance are substantially higher in urban locations. Although the grocery landscape has changed since then, contemporary comparisons have generated similar results.[45] Opening new food retailers, as opposed to transforming existing ones, requires further time and resources. The Mandela Food Cooperative took a decade to come to fruition, with about half of that time dedicated to the food assessment and community planning process and the other half to business plan development and market build-out.[25]

Efforts to revitalize the urban food environment must be accompanied by political support and engagement. Using scientific evidence to appeal to policymakers is one method of garnering political support, particularly for healthy eating initiatives.[46–48] However, these evidence-based recommendations must often compete with policymakers' non–health priorities as well with the many influences affecting policymaker decisions, including budget, policy compatibility, and stakeholder interests.[49] Understanding policymaker priorities and how to better target messages for this audience is critical for identifying leverage points in the policy process that facilitate the translation of evidence to policy.[50] Additional research and training on ways for public health professionals to strategically engage with policymakers to improve the urban food environment are needed.

3.3 Exacerbating Health Disparities

Improving urban food environments may lead to the displacement of low-income, racial/ethnic minority populations and exacerbate health disparities. Revitalizing urban communities through changes such as improving healthy food access can result in relatively large increases in rents and home values in low- to moderate-income neighborhoods. This may in turn lead to the displacement of lower income residents who can no longer afford the rising cost of housing. Several cities have experienced this so-called *Whole Foods effect*, whereby the introduction of a healthy food retailer (like the Whole Foods chain) contributes to neighborhood gentrification.[51] Redevelopment projects accelerated and property values quadrupled after a Whole Foods store opened in the Logan Circle neighborhood of Washington, DC, in 2000.[51] Many low-income residents of color were displaced, and the black population decreased by 20% over a 5-year period. Such displacement ultimately widens socioeconomic and racial/ethnic health disparities in obesity, diabetes, heart disease, and other diet-related outcomes. Strategies that prevent marginalization and displacement of low-income, racial/ethnic minority populations, such as rent control, just-cause eviction policies, property tax breaks for longtime owner-occupants, and preservation and expansion of public and affordable housing, are needed to promote equitable and inclusionary urban healthy food environments.[52]

4 Conclusion

Improving access to healthy foods in urban settings remains a key priority for public health policy and population health promotion. To maximize impact, interventions and policies must also address area-level disparities in unhealthy food availability, strategically engage communities in driving demand to sustain long-term effects, and focus on revitalization efforts that minimize displacement of socioeconomically disadvantaged and racial/ethnic minority populations. Building healthy urban food environments and, ultimately, healthy urban living environments requires a commitment to health equity and can be achieved through proactive, interdisciplinary collaborations that span multiple sectors and levels of influence.

References

1. Morland K, Wing S, Roux AD. The contextual effect of the local food environment on residents' diets: the Atherosclerosis Risk in Communities Study. *Am J Public Health.* 2002; 92(11):1761–1768.
2. Morland K, Diez Roux A, Wing S. Supermarkets, other food stores, and obesity: the Atherosclerosis Risk in Communities Study. *Am J Prev Med.* 2006; 30(4):333–339.
3. Larson NI, Story MT, Nelson MC. Neighborhood environments: disparities in access to healthy foods in the U.S. *Am J Prev Med.* 2009; 36(1):74–81.
4. Budzynska K, West P, Savoy-Moore RT, Lindsey D, Winter M, Newby PK. A food desert in Detroit: associations with food shopping and eating behaviours, dietary intakes and obesity. *Public Health Nutr.* 2013; 16(12):2114–2123.
5. Rhone A, Ver Ploeg M, Dicken C, Williams R, Breneman V. *Low-income and low-supermarket-access census tracts, 2010–2015.* Washington, DC: United States Department of Agriculture Economic Research Service; 2017.
6. Black C, Moon G, Baird J. Dietary inequalities: what is the evidence for the effect of the neighbourhood food environment? *Health Place.* 2014; 27:229–242.
7. Liu GC, Wilson JS, Qi R, Ying J. Green neighborhoods, food retail and childhood overweight: differences by population density. *Am J Health Promot.* 2007; 21(4 Suppl):317–325.
8. Powell LM, Auld MC, Chaloupka FJ, O'Malley PM, Johnston LD. Associations between access to food stores and adolescent body mass index. *Am J Prev Med.* 2007; 33(4S):S301–S307.
9. Michimi A, Wimberly MC. Associations of supermarket accessibility with obesity and fruit and vegetable consumption in the conterminous United States. *Int J Health Geogr.* 2010; 9:49.
10. Bodor JN, Rice JC, Farley TA, Swalm CM, Rose D. The association between obesity and urban food environments. *J Urban Health.* 2010; 87(5):771–781.
11. Cooksey-Stowers K, Schwartz MB, Brownell KD. Food swamps predict obesity rates better than food deserts in the United States. *Int J Environ Res Public Health.* 2017; 14(11):1–20.
12. Rose D, Bodor NJ, Swalm CM, Rice JC, Farley TA, Hutchinson P. *Deserts in New Orleans? Illustrations of urban food access and implications for policy.* Ann Arbor, MI: National Poverty Center Working Paper; 2009.
13. Caspi CE, Sorensen G, Subramanian SV, Kawachi I. The local food environment and diet: a systematic review. *Health Place.* 2012; 18(5):1172–1187.
14. Treuhaft S, Karpyn A. *The grocery gap: who has access to healthy food and why it matters.* Philadelphia, PA: PolicyLink, The Food Trust; 2010.
15. Ver Ploeg M, Breneman V, Farrigan T, et al. *Access to affordable and nutritious food: measuring and understanding food deserts and their consequences.* Washington, DC: United States Department of Agriculture Economic Research Service; 2009.

16. Diez-Roux AV, Nieto FJ, Caulfield L, Tyroler HA, Watson RL, Szklo M. Neighbourhood differences in diet: the Atherosclerosis Risk in Communities (ARIC) Study. *J Epidemiol Community Health.* 1999; 53(1):55–63.

17. Bell J, Standish M. *Building healthy communities through equitable food access.* San Francisco, CA: Federal Research Bank of San Francisco Community Development Investment Review. 2009(3):75–87.

18. Hilmers A, Hilmers DC, Dave J. Neighborhood disparities in access to healthy foods and their effects on environmental justice. *Am J Public Health.* 2012; 102(9):1644–1654.

19. Powell LM, Slater S, Mirtcheva D, Bao Y, Chaloupka FJ. Food store availability and neighborhood characteristics in the United States. *Prev Med.* 2007; 44(3):189–195.

20. Reel JJ, Badger BK. From food deserts to food swamps: health education strategies to improve food environments in urban areas. *J Obes Weight Loss Ther.* 2014; S4:1–2.

21. Gittelsohn J, Laska MN, Karpyn A, Klingler K, Ayala GX. Lessons learned from small store programs to increase healthy food access. *Am J Health Behav.* 2014; 38(2):307–315.

22. Gittelsohn J, Rowan M, Gadhoke P. Interventions in small food stores to change the food environment, improve diet, and reduce risk of chronic disease. *Prev Chronic Dis.* 2012; 9:E59.

23. Anderson Steeves E, Martins PA, Gittelsohn J. Changing the food environment for obesity prevention: key gaps and future directions. *Current Obesity Reports.* 2014; 3(4):451–458.

24. *HFFI impacts: the nationwide success of healthy food financing initiatives.* Philadelphia, PA: The Food Trust; 2017.

25. *Transforming West Oakland: a case study series on Mandela MarketPlace.* Oakland, CA: PolicyLink; 2015.

26. *A healthy food financing initiative: an innovative approach to improve health and spark economic development.* Philadelphia, PA: PolicyLink, The Food Trust, The Reinvestment Fund; 2012.

27. *The economic impacts of supermarkets on their surrounding communities.* Philadelphia, PA: The Reinvestment Fund; 2007.

28. *Cultivating equitable food-oriented development: lessons from West Oakland.* Oakland, CA: PolicyLink; 2017.

29. Chan M. WHO Director-General addresses health promotion conference. Paper presented at the 8th Global Conference on Health Promotion. Helsinki, Finland; 2013.

30. Kickbusch I, Allen L, Franz C. The commercial determinants of health. *Lancet Glob Health.* 2016; 4(12):e895–e896.

31. Mello MM, Pomeranz J, Moran P. The interplay of public health law and industry self-regulation: the case of sugar-sweetened beverage sales in schools. *Am J Public Health.* 2008; 98(4):595–604.

32. Welsh JA, Lundeen EA, Stein AD. The sugar-sweetened beverage wars: public health and the role of the beverage industry. *Curr Opin Endocrinol Diabetes Obes.* 2013; 20(5):401–406.

33. National Academies of Sciences, Engineering, and Medicine. *Strategies to limit sugar-sweetened beverage consumption in young children: proceedings of a workshop—in brief.* Washington, DC: The National Academies Press. doi:10.17226/24897

34. Wescott RF, Fitzpatrick BM, Phillips E. Industry self-regulation to improve student health: quantifying changes in beverage shipments to schools. *Am J Public Health.* 2012; 102(10):1928–1935.

35. Ng SW, Slining MM, Popkin BM. The healthy weight commitment foundation pledge: calories sold from U.S. consumer packaged goods, 2007–2012. *Am J Prev Med.* 2014; 47(4):508–519.

36. Powell LM, Han E, Chaloupka FJ. Economic contextual factors, food consumption, and obesity among U.S. adolescents. *J Nutr.* 2010; 140(6):1175–1180.

37. Dubowitz T, Ghosh-Dastidar M, Eibner C, et al. The Women's Health Initiative: the food environment, neighborhood socioeconomic status, BMI, and blood pressure. *Obesity.* 2012; 20(4):862–871.

38. Laska MN, Hearst MO, Forsyth A, Pasch KE. Neighbourhood food environments: are they associated with adolescent dietary intake, food purchases and weight status? *Public Health Nutr.* 2010;13(11):1757–1763.

39. Sallis JF, Floyd MF, Rodríguez DA, Saelens BE. Role of built environments in physical activity, obesity, and cardiovascular disease. *Circulation.* 2012; 125(5):729–737.

40. *The zoning diet: using zoning as a potential strategy for combating local obesity.* Boston, MA: Public Health Advocacy Institute at Northeastern University School of Law; 2008.

41. Dubowitz T, Zenk SN, Ghosh-Dastidar B, et al. Healthy food access for urban food desert residents: examination of the food environment, food purchasing practices, diet, and body mass index. *Public Health Nutr.* 2015; 18(12):2220–2230.

42. Sturm R, Hattori A. Diet and obesity in Los Angeles County 2007–2012: is there a measurable effect of the 2008 "Fast-Food Ban"? *Soc Sci Med.* 2015; 133:205–211.

43. Glanz K, Mullis RM. Environmental interventions to promote healthy eating: a review of models, programs, and evidence. *Health Educ Q.* 1988; 15(4):395–415.

44. Goldstein I, Loethen L, Kako E, Califano C. *CDFI financing of supermarkets in underserved communities: a case study.* Philadelphia, PA: Reinvestment Fund; 2008.

45. *Expanding New Jersey's supermarkets: a new day for the Garden State.* Philadelphia, PA: The Food Trust; 2012.

46. Murphy K, Fafard P. Taking power, politics, and policy problems seriously. *J Urban Health.* 2012; 89(4):723–732.

47. Brownson RC, Chriqui JF, Stamatakis KA. Understanding evidence-based public health policy. *Am J Public Health.* 2009; 99(9):1576–1583.

48. Finkelstein E, French S, Variyam JN, Haines PS. Pros and cons of proposed interventions to promote healthy eating. *Am J Prev Med.* 2004; 27(3S):163–171.

49. Wang ML, Goins KV, Anatchkova M, et al. Priorities of municipal policymakers in relation to physical activity and the built environment: a latent class analysis. *J Public Health Manag Pract.* 2016; 22(3):221–230.

50. Bernier NF, Clavier C. Public health policy research: making the case for a political science approach. *Health Promot Int.* 2011; 26(1):109–116.

51. Newkirk VR. Irrigating the (food) desert: a tale of gentrification in DC. *Gawker.* August 11, 2014. Available at http://gawker.com/irrigating-the-food-desert-a-tale-of-gentrification-1617679708. Accessed September 3, 2018.

52. Douglas J. From disinvestment to displacement: gentrification and Jamaica Plain's Hyde-Jackson Squares. *Trotter Review.* 2016; 23(1):1–80.

17

Disasters

JAMES M. SHULTZ

1 Disaster Overview

A disaster is an encounter between forces of harm (hazards) and a vulnerable human population in harm's way, influenced by the ecological context, that creates demands that exceed the coping capacity of the affected community. When disasters occur in urban environments, this interplay of hazard and vulnerability creates complex patterns of risk and resilience (Figure 17.1).[1,2]

1.1 Disaster Frequency

On a worldwide basis, disasters are common. Extreme events are officially entered into the international disaster database maintained by the Centre for Research on the Epidemiology of Disasters (CRED) if they meet any of four threshold criteria: 10 or more people killed, 100 or more people affected, emergency declaration issued, or call for international assistance. CRED tallies more than 340 natural disasters annually, about one each day. During the 20-year period from 1994 to 2013, CRED recorded 6,873 natural disaster events worldwide that resulted in 1.35 million deaths and caused 4.3 billion instances where an individual was affected by a disaster, with many individuals exposed to multiple events.[3]

The number of people exposed to disasters each year is anticipated to increase. Escalating disaster risk to human populations is driven by three trends that operate interactively: population growth, urbanization, and global climate change.[4,5] Regarding population growth, the ongoing rise in numbers of human inhabitants is already straining Earth's carrying capacity. As populations grow and concentrate in urban centers, their collective activities contribute to the production of greenhouse gases and the accelerating pace with which the planet warms, the seas rise, and disasters strike with increasing frequency and ferocity.[4-6]

1.2 Disaster Classification

Disasters are classified based on the properties of hazards that produce disasters. CRED sorts disasters originating from forces of nature into six categories: meteorological

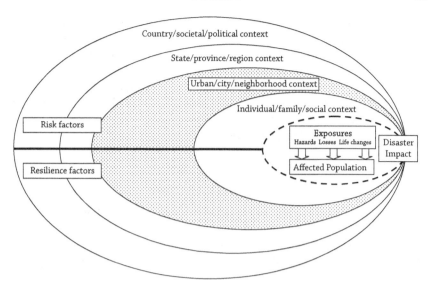

Figure 17.1 **An ecosocial model of disaster risk and resilience across contexts.**

(storms, extreme temperatures), hydrological (floods, waves, mudslides) climatological (wildfires, droughts), geophysical (earthquakes, volcanoes), biological (epidemics), and extraterrestrial (impacts) (Figure 17.2).[3] The term "natural" disaster is declining in usage with the recognition that human settlement patterns and behavior contribute instrumentally to the population impact of these events.

Nonintentional human-generated ("anthropogenic") disasters, numbering hundreds of incidents per year, usually result from a failure of technology. Anthropogenic disasters include structural collapses (buildings, bridges, tunnels), hazardous materials releases, fires and explosions, and transportation crashes. The catalog of human-caused events expands as new technologies are developed and accidents happen. The advent of

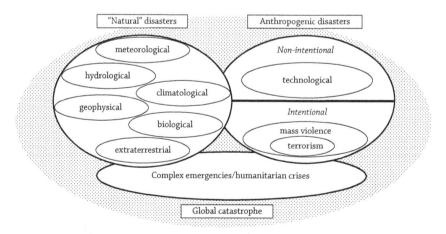

Figure 17.2 **Disaster classification.**

aviation ushered in the era of commercial air crashes. The mass asphyxiation event in Bhopal, India, involved the release of aerosolized pesticide from an abandoned chemical plant. The highest fatality peacetime radiation incident resulted from a reactor meltdown at the Chernobyl nuclear power plant.

Intentional human-caused disasters merit separate classification. These insidious perpetrated acts may involve explosives or weapons of mass destruction. During the September 11, 2001, attack, terrorists "weaponized" commercial aircraft and flew them into the World Trade Center towers, the US Pentagon, and a small community in Pennsylvania.

2 Public Health Consequences of Disasters

Among prominent public health consequences, disasters kill, injure, sicken, and displace human populations and disrupt or destroy health care systems.[3,7]

2.1 Mortality

Disasters kill tens of thousands every year.[3,7] During the first decades of the 2000s, the deadliest disasters were the 2004 Southeast Asia earthquake and tsunami (280,000 deaths), the 2010 Haiti earthquake (220,000), and 2008 Cyclone Nargis in Myanmar (138,000).[3,5] However, the "Great Influenza" of 1918/1919, a natural biological disaster that claimed 50–100 million lives globally, was deadlier than any other historical disaster event.

2.2 Injury

Injury patterns vary according to the nature of the disaster hazards. For example, earthquakes cause widespread structural collapses, resulting in crush injuries and limb trauma among survivors rescued from the rubble. Tsunami waves propel rapidly moving debris flows; survivors who have been submerged in these onrushing waters may develop "tsunami lung" (aspiration pneumonia). The availability of effective tropical cyclone warning systems has decreased death and injury as the storms are passing through; instead, the major burden of storm-related injury takes place during the cleanup phase. For technological disasters, injury patterns match the type of exposure (e.g., collision, collapse, explosion, radiation).

2.3 Infectious Disease

Following a natural disaster, widespread damage to dwellings may leave survivors exposed to insect-borne infectious diseases (e.g., Zika virus, dengue) as exemplified by Hurricane Maria striking Puerto Rico in 2017.[8] Water-borne or food-borne disease outbreaks may erupt due to cross-contamination of water supplies with sewage or hazardous wastes, lack of refrigeration, or inability to properly cook and store foods.

2.4 Chronic Disease Exacerbation

The prognosis for persons with chronic conditions may worsen in the aftermath of disaster if vital, life-sustaining services are disrupted, such as renal dialysis, oxygen for patients with chronic obstructive pulmonary disease (COPD), and critical cancer therapies. Routine medication management of common conditions such as hypertension and diabetes may be jeopardized if patients are unable to refill prescriptions. Damage to the power grid may expose survivors to extreme heat or cold for extended periods, placing the frail elderly and persons with chronic diseases at elevated risk.[8,9]

2.5 Mental Health

Mental health and psychosocial consequences are among the most pervasive health outcomes.[10,11] Survivors who were directly subjected to the forces of harm (e.g., strong winds, ground-shaking, explosion), especially those who believed they were going to die, may experience disturbing memories, sleep disruption, and possible progression to posttraumatic stress disorder (PTSD).[10,11] Survivors who lost a loved one, were displaced from their homes, or experienced other significant life changes are at elevated risk for major depression. Alcohol consumption often increases in the aftermath. Children's mental health and likelihood of exhibiting behavioral problems are significantly influenced by how well their caregivers are able to cope and function after the disasters.

2.6 Impact on Healthcare Systems

Disasters frequently place extraordinary burdens on the local healthcare services. Healthcare systems directly in the path of the hazard may sustain severe damage and be rendered inoperable in the aftermath. Prolonged power outages may severely restrict available services. Healthcare systems that remain functional may experience a mass casualty incident as a surge of disaster-injured patients arrives seeking care or a fear-propelled onrush of citizens converges on the emergency department, believing they have been exposed to a hazardous agent.

3 Urban Settings and Disasters

Disasters require the overlap of hazards and people. Regarding the place dimension, the urban disaster risk landscape is literally defined by where and how human populations settle.

3.1 Place: Where Hazards Prevail

Prominent types of disasters flourish in specific regions of the planet.[12] Tropical cyclones form above warm oceans, and the rotating planet spins them westward and poleward. Therefore, the greatest risk for landfall is borne by urban coastal and island populations living along the western-most portions of the great oceans, in tropical or subtropical latitudes. In contrast, strong earthquakes and tsunamis that can topple or inundate urban centers are generated along the seismically active boundaries between the Earth's tectonic plates.

Only rare, exceptional events have truly global reach. Most notable among hazards that circumnavigate the globe are "slate-wiper" communicable diseases like the 1918/1919 pandemic influenza and epoch-changing planetary impacts.

3.2 Place: Where People Live

Talking about disaster hotspots moves us farther into discussion of urbanization and disasters.[12] The global population has quadrupled in the past 100 years and progressively migrated to urban environments.[4,5] Urbanization interacts in a complex fashion with disaster risk; some aspects of city living amplify disaster risks while others allow cities to prepare and respond better than dispersed rural populations.[4-6]

3.2.1 Population Density

Urbanization concentrates people geographically. This is where the overlap of hazards and people becomes prominent; a focal disaster impact on a densely populated urban center amplifies the likelihood of harm on a mass scale. Consider the destruction of Port-au-Prince during the 2010 Haiti earthquake or the inundation of New Orleans during 2005 Hurricane Katrina.

Teeming urban settings complicate the logistics for staging a mass evacuation or marshalling people into community shelters as a disaster is approaching. In 2017, Hurricane Harvey intensified so rapidly that Houston had to jettison strategies for evacuation, thereby subjecting the metropolitan population to pummeling rains and deadly flooding. In contrast, as Hurricane Irma menaced the peninsula, highly stressed Floridians clogged all north-bound highways as they evacuated the state en masse.

3.2.2 Mass Gatherings

Urban environments are magnets for events that convene large crowds in open air or enclosed venues. Even as fairs, festivals, expos, sporting events, and concerts spark camaraderie—or spirited competition—these mass gatherings are inherently dangerous due to risks for the crushing movement of stampeding crowds and vulnerability to perpetrated attacks.

3.2.3 Urban Poverty

Urban environments worldwide are comprised of smaller sectors, municipalities, or neighborhoods that are distinctive in terms of age, population make-up, and position on the wealth-to-poverty continuum. Poverty is concentrated in ecologically unsuitable urban sectors where the poor are susceptible to the ravaging effects of natural disasters coupled with prolonged disruption of fragile infrastructure.

3.2.4 *Built Environment*

The quality and durability of housing stock and commercial buildings play important roles in exacerbating or mitigating urban risks when disaster strikes. Depending upon structural integrity, occupants may be at risk for collapse, fire or explosion; loss of roof; shattering glass; flooding pipes; or hazardous electrical circuitry. High-rise buildings carry special risks for wind damage and raging fires and pose extraordinary challenges for vertical disaster response. Mass transit systems, including tunnels and subways, are prone to flooding, as was showcased dramatically in New York City during Hurricane Sandy in 2012.

3.3 Hazard-People Interactions

Type of hazard influences the nature of disaster impacts on urban populations, as four examples illustrate. The dense clustering of population in urban slums greatly increases the spread of infectious diseases, as vividly witnessed in 2014, when Ebola surged through the capital cities of West Africa.[13] Seismic events are among the deadliest, particularly when they raze structures throughout a large urban cityscape (e.g., Port-au-Prince, Haiti, 2010). Flood events routinely displace residents of river communities, as happens with periodic floods extending for hundreds of miles along the Mississippi River. Tropical cyclone storm surge may overrun and submerge coastal cities, as dramatically evidenced by 2013 Super Typhoon Haiyan inundating the Philippines.

Anthropogenic disasters threaten urban populations with the possibility of rapidly exposing large numbers of inhabitants to human-generated hazards. For example, the rupture of a chlorine tanker may form a caustic chemical plume moving over densely populated urban areas. The 2010 Deepwater Horizon oil spill brought public health and ecological harm to coastal urban residents in four states bordering the Gulf of Mexico.

4 Disasters and Climate Change

According to CRED, climate-related natural disasters are the composite of hydrological, meteorological, and climatological events.[3] CRED recorded 240 climate-related disasters annually prior to 2000, but more than 340 annually during the early decades of the 2000s, a 44% increase.

Climate change is occurring with an accelerating pace and is approaching critical tipping points that threaten the global population, but more so those who live in urban centers. Globally, among the 10 hottest years on record, nine occurred during the 13-year period, 2005–2017. The primary cause of climate variability is emissions of greenhouse gases and related human activities, where about 80% comes from cities. Simultaneously, while the global sea level has risen a modest 7–8 inches since 1900, a further rise of 1–4 feet is predicted by 2100, with an outside possibility of an 8–foot rise.

Climate change is anticipated to increase disaster frequency and severity with disproportionate impacts on urban areas. Anticipated effects include increased incidence of daily tidal flooding, increased frequency and intensity of heavy rainfall, increased flooding due to extreme precipitation, major increases in potentially deadly heatwaves associated with ongoing rises in global temperatures, increased frequency of wildfires that threaten urban areas and profoundly modify local ecosystems, long-duration hydrological drought, increases in tropical cyclone intensity and precipitation rates, increases in the frequency of high-intensity tropical cyclones, possible increases in tornadoes, and increases in the severity of land-falling atmospheric rivers.[14]

While this discussion of disasters concentrates on discrete, time-bound incidents, climate change also portends longer duration trends, particularly droughts and desertification, that pose major threats for urban food security. Even more challenging in a warming, drying planet is the maintenance of adequate supplies of clean, fresh water. Already, in 2018, Cape Town, South Africa is approaching a "Day Zero" phenomenon of complete water shortage. Water stress may ultimately be the major urban survival threat in upcoming decades, a disaster scenario with existential implications.

Urbanization and climate change interact synergistically to increase disaster threats for urban residents.[15,16] A sophisticated analysis projected weather-related disaster events for Europe throughout the remainder of the twenty-first century. The authors predict that the proportion of the European population annually exposed to a weather-related disaster will increase by a factor of 12, from 5% to 65% by the end of the century, and the corresponding annual mortality from these weather-related events will be 50 times higher.[17]

5 Disaster Risk Reduction and Resilience in Urban Environments

Much attention has been paid to the role of resilience in disasters.[6] From a psychological vantage, resilience is the modal outcome; most individual survivors muster the resources to cope, regain function, and resume activities. Most rebound relatively rapidly, while far fewer progress to debilitating mental health outcomes. Beyond the individual, a focus on resilience is now actively promoted at the community level and can be scaled up to the large city level as well. Multiple characteristics of urban living are amenable for strengthening urban resilience.[6]

5.1 Disaster Forecasting and Warning

When analyzing potential risks, disaster forecasting is a key component of the planning process. Warning systems can be especially effective in urban settings where the geographic proximity of population members ensures that warnings are received, giving citizens the lead time to take self-protective actions.

5.2 Engaging the Urban Emergency Management Environment to Promote Resilience

One key urban advantage is the prospect of putting lessons learned from previous disasters to work in a manner that promotes community disaster resilience while safeguarding the city from future hazard encounters. Optimally, cities operate as learning collaboratives. Having experienced a disaster event, cities undergo a recovery and reconstruction process that, if sufficiently resourced, translates into quantifiable improvements in emergency management expertise, emergency response capability, construction code enforcement, and hardening of healthcare and vital infrastructure to better withstand future disaster threats.

5.3 Engaging the Urban Social Environment to Promote Resilience

It may be possible to harness the social ties of urban community living to facilitate resilience through citizen agency. Homeowners associations, civic groups, citizen response teams, and voluntary organizations active in disasters (e.g., Red Cross) can stimulate community engagement in preparing for known and anticipated hazards.

As an example of community resilience, Fargo, North Dakota, anticipates an annual flood threat along the Red River of the North during the spring snowmelt. In 2009, as Red River waters rose to record flood stage, 85,000 "flood fighters" stepped up, working ceaselessly in blizzard conditions to fill and place 8.5 million sandbags around the city's perimeter. The result? Flooding inside the city limits was prevented completely.

5.4 Urban Population Disaster Protection and Preparedness

Enlightened city planning would prioritize disaster risk reduction and achieve stepwise improvements to the structural integrity of the city's built environment, decrease housing and environmental disparities for the resident population (particularly those that relate directly to disaster hazards), create robust shelter environments, and develop effective evacuation strategies.

5.5 Urban Disaster Mitigation

Emergency management entities can seek funding for urban disaster mitigation projects. For example, in Florida, many coastal communities use local mitigation funds to create massive flood control projects that significantly safeguard their citizens during episodes of hurricane-triggered inland flooding.

5.6 Real-World Experience, Drills, and Simulations

As one component of evolving urban resilience, disaster response continuously improves in effectiveness and capacity through well-executed and frequently rehearsed responses to routine emergencies. These can be scaled up to accommodate a larger event when disaster strikes. Urban centers are ideally suited for conducting training exercises and simulations that recalibrate the repertoire of responder skills to handle mass casualty scenarios. Large-population urban environments provide economies of scale, allowing emergency management to coordinate and redistribute personnel and call on a depth of resources to meet the emergency needs of a specific disaster event.

5.7   Force Protection as a Resilience Strategy

A related element of urban resilience is developing strategies and support resources for emergency response personnel whose duties expose them to physically grueling and psychologically challenging calls (e.g., death of a child, inability to resuscitate a patient) as well as urban disasters. "Force protection" is a recognized priority for achieving urban disaster resilience by keeping responders safer.

5.8   Emergency Response Coalitions and Mutual Aid

Using incident management system protocols, response operations can be structured effectively based on targeting trained personnel and resources to areas with identified needs. This process is strengthened through mutual aid agreements across jurisdictions. Many disasters are "concentric," with a defined area of maximal impact surrounded by areas that are progressively less affected. In a catastrophic event, when response assets are incapacitated at "ground zero," nearby resources can be deployed to the most affected areas. A recent advance has been the regional consolidation of area hospitals into healthcare disaster response coalitions; during a disaster, coalition member hospitals distribute incoming patients, medical personnel, supplies, and assets across the region to balance out the demands of a mass casualty event.

6   Conclusion

Population increase, urbanization, and climate change are progressing simultaneously and inexorably, magnifying the effects of each other. These features shape the disaster risk landscape experienced by urban residents and highlight the urgency to prepare cities and communities for significant public health impacts. Cities must anticipate not only more severe versions of past disaster events, but also a future punctuated by evolving threats. There is equal urgency to create resilient urban communities that can prevent and mitigate disaster threats as well as recover from and build back better after disaster strikes. This will pay dividends in terms of improving life and health in urban settings during most days when no active disaster events are impacting the cityscape, and, when disaster does happen, cities will be better equipped.

References

1. Shultz JM, Galea S, Espinel Z, Reissman DE. Disaster ecology. In Ursano RJ, Fullerton CS, Weisaeth L, Raphael B, eds. *Textbook of disaster psychiatry*. 2nd ed. Cambridge: Cambridge University Press; 2017.
2. Helbing D. Globally networked risks and how to respond. *Nature*. 2013; 497: 51–59.
3. Wahlstrom M, Guha-Sapir D. *The human cost of natural disasters 2015: a global perspective*. Brussels, Belgium: Centre for Research on the Epidemiology of Disasters (CRED); 2015.
4. McLean D, ed. *World disasters report 2010: focus on urban risk*. Geneva, Switzerland: International Federation of Red Cross and Red Crescent Societies (IFRC); 2010.

5. Dickson E, Baker JL, Hoornweg D, Tiwari A. *Urban risk assessments: understanding disaster and climate risk in cities.* Washington, DC: World Bank Group; 2012.

6. Global Facility for Disaster Reduction and Recovery. *Investing in urban resilience: protecting and promoting development in a changing world.* Washington, DC: World Bank Group; 2015.

7. Glasser R, Guha–Sapir D. *Poverty and death: disaster mortality, 1996–2015.* Brussels, Belgium: Centre for Research on the Epidemiology of Disasters (CRED); 2016.

8. Shultz JM, Kossin JP, Shepherd JM, Ransdell JM, Walshe R, Kelman I, Galea S. Risks, health consequences, and response challenges for small-island-based populations: observations from the 2017 Atlantic hurricane season. *Disaster Med Public.* 2018; 6:1–13.

9. Lee JY, Kim H. Projection of future temperature-related mortality due to climate and demographic changes. *Environ Int.* 2016; 94: 489–494.

10. Galea S, Nandi A, Vlahov D. The epidemiology of post-traumatic stress disorder after disasters. *Epidemiol Rev.* 2005; 27(1): 78–91.

11. Goldman E, Galea S. Mental health consequences of disasters. *Annu Rev Public Health.* 2014; 35:169–183.

12. Dilley M, Chen RS, Deichmann U, et al. *Natural disaster hotspots: a global risk analysis.* Washington, DC: World Bank Group; 2005.

13. Shultz JM, Espinel Z, Espinola M, Rechkemmer A. Distinguishing epidemiological features of the 2013–2016 West Africa Ebola virus disease outbreak. *Disaster Health.* 2016; 3(3):1–11.

14. Wuebbles DJ, Fahey DW, Hibbard KA, Dokken DJ, Stewart BC, Maycock TK, eds. *Climate science special report: fourth national climate assessment, volume I.* Washington, DC: US Global Change Research Program, 2017: 257–276.

15. Patz JA, Frumkin H, Holloway T, et al. Climate change challenges and opportunities for global health. *JAMA.* 2014; 312(15):1565–1580.

16. Kelman I. Linking disaster risk reduction, climate change, and the sustainable development goals. *Disaster Prev Manag.* 2017; 26:254–258.

17. Forzieri G, Cescatti A, Batista E, Silva F, Feyen L. Increasing risk over time of weather-related hazards to the European population: a data-driven prognostic study. *Lancet Planet Health.* 2017; 1(5): e200–e208. doi:10.1016/S2542-5196(17)30013-X

SECTION III

METHODS AND APPROACHES TO UNDERSTANDING HEALTH IN CITIES

18

Urban Public Health

A Historical Perspective

RICHARD RODGER

1 Introduction

Historical perspectives on urban public health have concentrated mainly on interventionist strategies deployed by agencies, usually towns and cities, authorised to act within their boundaries for the common good. This is not to deny the contribution of medical advances, particularly military surgical developments, or the scientific study of pathogens and their transmission, or of palliative care undertaken in the community and in religious foundations were unimportant. Public health, however, made the greatest impact on life expectancy for the urban population over time. When dealing with epidemic disease (plagues) and endemic environmental conditions hostile to life expectancy (tuberculosis, cholera, typhus, typhoid), it was public measures coupled with improvements in the standard of living—resulting specifically in better nutritional standards—that have been identified as the major forces explaining the historical decline of mortality rates. The chapter adopts a largely chronological perspective on public health developments from medieval to early modern, and then moves to a consideration of the major shifts in public health that occurred in the eighteenth and nineteenth centuries. Though most attention is devoted to European trends, the colonization of the Americas, Africa, and Asia ensured networks of knowledge were, by contemporary standards, quite quickly disseminated, though locally taken up at very variable rates. The historical study of public health is, therefore, an inherently worldwide one, with the important qualification that the pace of change and uptake of ideas was uneven.

2 Medieval Mindsets

It is important to recognize that public health is a concept that is culturally constructed and mutates over time. Though the discourse of public health emerged in a recognizably modern garb in the eighteenth and nineteenth centuries, in earlier periods, too, urban authorities enacted measures to protect, promote, and restore the health of fellow citizens albeit based on rather different intellectual premises than those of today. To depict medieval cities as unregulated spaces of dirt and pollution where streets were lined with dung heaps and rotting vegetable matter, where piped water was an occasional luxury and rivers ran with effluent, where disease was countered by herbal remedies or irrational superstition, and where any concept of public health was conspicuous by its absence is to decontextualize public health efforts. The ancient, medieval, and early modern city was unquestionably a dirty and dangerous place, but any teleological, progressive interpretation of the development of public health constitutes a caricature of the "Dark Ages" and obscures some fundamental continuities in the urban experience of health and disease.[1]

The management of the physical environment has, therefore, a long pedigree in urban communities. Particularly well documented in the most densely urbanized areas of the medieval world, the cities of northern Italy and the Low Countries, are the codified regulations issued by monarchs and civic rulers intended to manage waste disposal, public lavatories, interments in extramural cemeteries, and infectious diseases such as leprosy. Supplies of clean water, essential to modern notions of public health, were more restricted, but its significance was recognized in authorities' investment in piped water in many medieval cities. "Nuisances," identified as infringements of space, paving, light, and amenity, including structural strength, were recorded in the *Nychtbourheid Buik* (Neighborhood Book) in a number of sixteenth- and seventeenth-century Scottish towns, and reflected local concern for issues of community health and well-being. An entry in Edinburgh on November 14, 1677, stated that "the expense of street cleansing, the removal of middens" was justified in terms of "keeping the town neat and clean in tyme coming." The concern for the physical environment and the importance attached to cleanliness was a long-standing issue for civic government. But there was also a perceived continuum between the physical and spiritual health of the community, and any attempt to manage the environment was closely connected with attempts to manage morality. Humoral imbalance in bodily fluids based on four psychological temperaments—melancholic, choleric, phlegmatic, and sanguine—was considered to be caused by foul air in an early variant of the miasmatic theory of infection. This imbalance, it was thought, contributed to immoral behavior (intemperance, promiscuity, self-indulgence) that further weakened resistance to disease. Morality, religious instruction, and environmental living conditions were, therefore, never far apart.[2]

3 Epidemics

In the Middle Ages and early modern period, urban populations were held in check by a combination of endemic and epidemic diseases, and by harvest failures. Between 1347 and 1351, the bacterium *Yerisina pestis* spread first from China to the Middle East and then throughout Europe. Bubonic plague, or the "Black Death" as the pandemic was later known, was transmitted by fleas in rats and other species and in the blood and sputum of humans; it has been estimated to have killed up to 20% of the world population. In England, estimates vary locally from 25% to 60%. The Black Death is the best-known pandemic, but subsequent outbreaks of epidemic disease were common. These affected Paris (1464–66), Venice (1576–77), Castile (1596–99), London (1603–11, 1664–67), Algiers (1620–21), Naples (1656–67), Prague (1681), Baghdad (1689–90,

1772), Marseille (1720), and Moscow (mid-1770s), as well as many other lesser known urban settlements throughout Europe and the Middle East. Some towns and cities endured multiple visitations. Constantinople, because of its climate, size, and major strategic trading location, recorded more than 30 epidemics in the second half of the eighteenth century alone. Epidemic disease literally decimated urban populations, and, perhaps more seriously, indirectly weakened survivors so that they succumbed more easily to other illnesses, irrespective of their social class. Urban authorities regularly enacted measures to prevent the spread of plague—through quarantine, temporary use of *cordons sanitaires*, and the cleansing of streets of rubbish and animals—though such measures were of limited efficacy and urban population levels were largely static until well into the eighteenth century. Nowhere was this more evident than in the decline in new foundations of Central European towns (Figure 18.1).

Responses to plague—by the crown, the church, and by civic authorities—were limited in their effectiveness, resting as they did on a flawed understanding of its transmission and cause, but nonetheless they constituted proactive measures to halt the spread of the disease in the interest of the wider community. The sense of crisis generated by the threat of plague enabled urban authorities to frame and implement regulations that restricted the movement of people and permitted officials to enter and inspect private property for the existence of plague. In the larger Italian cities, health boards were established to implement regulations. In such crises, however, the preservation of public health was also a matter of the spiritual and moral reformation of the people: if disease was a punishment from God, a moral reformation was seen by many as the best preventative public health measure.

The effect of plagues and harvest failure, mitigated to a limited extent by public health initiatives, can be summarized in the long-run average life expectancy of four countries: England/Great Britain, Sweden, the United States, and Japan (Figure 18.2). Until the late eighteenth century, both Britain and Sweden, the countries with the longest data series, experienced an average age expectancy of 30–40 years. Thereafter, life expectancy began to rise, albeit with more variability in Sweden; and then, from 1850, the long-run upward drift was fairly steady in these and many other European countries. By 2000, only Japan, South Korea, Hong Kong, and Singapore had an average life expectancy at birth of 80, closely followed after 2000 by most western European countries, Canada, Australia, New Zealand, Macao, and Israel. These averages do not take into account the female-to-male advantage of about 4% in the average life span between 1850 and 2010, the different pace of urbanization in various countries (Figure 18.2), and that, although life expectancy was generally higher in the rural sector, it was offset by harvest failures and natural disasters. Despite this, life expectancy provides some indication of the overall progress of the public's health across time and urban space.

4 Population Growth and Urbanization

What had changed in the middle of the eighteenth century was the relationship between food supplies and population levels. Malthus's formulation of a long-run equilibrium was overturned·in England by an unprecedented increase in agricultural productivity associated with new rotations and organizational changes in land and labor.[3] The transition has been described as, "A low-intensity agricultural system . . . replaced by a high

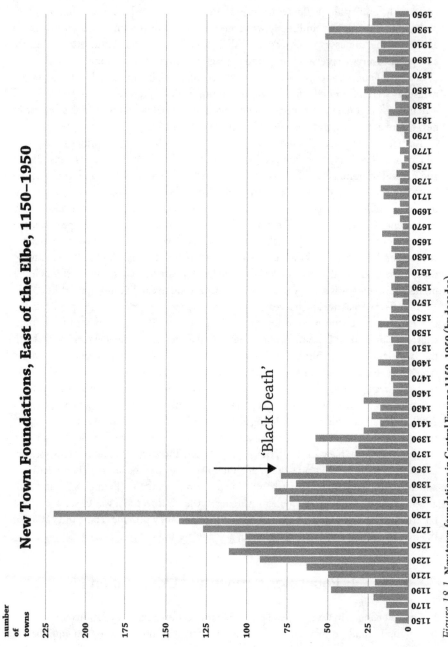

Figure 18.1 New town foundations in Central Europe 1150–1950 (by decades).

Source: Stoob H. *Forschungen zum Städewesen in Europa*, volume 1. Cologne, Germany: Böhlau Verlag; 1970.

Life Expectancy (in years)

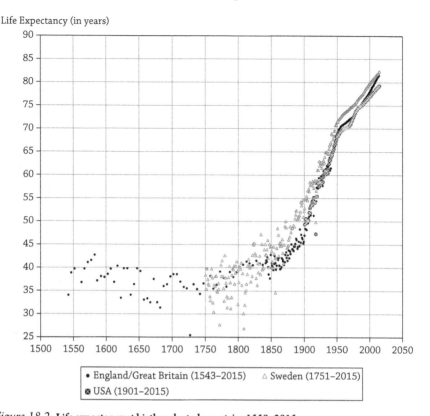

Figure 18.2 **Life expectancy at birth: selected countries 1550–2015.**
Sources: Zijdeman R, Ribeiro da Silva F. Life expectancy since 1820. In: Luiten van Zanden J, Baten J, Mira d'Ercole M, Rijpma A, Smith C, Timmer M, eds. *How was life? Global well-being since 1820.* Paris, France: OECD Publishing; 2014: 101–116. Data from 1950 use the United Nations Population Division data website. Available at https://esa.un.org/unpd/wpp/Download/Standard/Population/. Accessed May 3, 2018.

intensity system based on arable crops." Unrest in France and in the German states in the late eighteenth and early nineteenth centuries over social inequalities resulted in revolution and the abolition of feudalism and serfdom in eastern Europe and also produced agrarian efficiency gains sufficient to supply the expanding urban sector. Greater scientific and technical knowledge contributed to a belief that positive measures could be taken to improve the health of the population. Statistical and spatial data underpinned political arithmetic and led to a realization that the productive capacity of a healthy population contributed to the creation of wealth. Higher death rates in cities compared to rural areas—the urban penalty—convinced many that sanitary reform specifically and public health more generally were worthwhile investments.[4]

In parallel with scientific and technological changes in the late eighteenth and early nineteenth centuries was an intense interest in the health of cities. The political economy of Adam Smith's *Wealth of Nations* (1776) was interdependent with the health of nations, and so it was unsurprising that a surge of specialist publications developed. Foremost among them was Johan Peter Franck's nine-volume *System einer vollständigen medicinischen Polizey* (*A Complete System of Medical Policy*) published between 1779 and 1827. It was a comprehensive treatise on hygiene and public health based on Franck's experience gained as sanitary inspector general for Lombardy and on his prestigious royal appointments in London, Vienna, and St. Petersburg. Using detailed records, Franck fused physiological conditions with "medical policing," an approach also prevalent in Scottish medical education, where medical jurisprudence—recommendations for public health administration and policy based on medical information—was a compulsory course of study for all medical graduates. In France, too, Alexandre Parent-Duchâtelet, Louise-René Villermé, and a wider group of hygienists were active after 1814 in the Paris Health Council and published the journal *Annales d'hygiène publique* to disseminate the latest findings. Perhaps predictably, there was a post-Revolution dialectic between statists, that is, those hygienists who considered that the state should assume the main role in public health reform, and liberals, who argued that change was best achieved by individuals, reserving thereby a residual role in public health for the state.

With their strong emphasis on statistics, hygienists questioned both the prevailing miasmatic theories of disease causation and the role of climate. This rejection of conventional approaches to public health, epidemics, and disease can be seen as a product of Enlightenment thought, exemplified not just by French hygienists, but also by Franck, Andrew Duncan in Edinburgh, and Auguste Tissot in Switzerland. Their approach to public health revolved around rational analysis, education, and administrative arrangements enshrined in law. Empiricism and humanitarianism were combined to focus on preventive measures rather than ones reactive to emergencies. Public health policy was linked, therefore, to the Enlightenment idea of progress and the "civilizing" process associated with it and eventually embraced longer term cultural initiatives—museums, reading rooms, lectures, galleries, and parks in conjunction with sermons and urban missions—with the intention to address the deeply rooted social and sanitary problems of nineteenth-century urban life.[5]

Against this background, European towns and cities were confronted with rapid urbanization (Figure 18.3) associated with industrialization and the equally rapid deterioration of living conditions.[6] Natural increase and immigration overwhelmed the existing infrastructural investment in housing, sewers, and streets, and the process only accelerated with the arrival of the railway companies and the demolition of entire districts in major European cities. Though the timing differed, the process of urban environmental degradation was experienced in towns and cities throughout Europe and North America.[7]

To address the insanitary city, reports by Edwin Chadwick's *Sanitary Condition of the Labouring Population* (1842) and Lemuel Shattuck's *Report of the Sanitary Commission of Massachusetts* (1850) were influential in Britain and North America.[8] Chadwick's proposal for a national agency, the General Board of Health, to coordinate public health reform in England and Wales encountered serious opposition locally, but Shattuck's recommendation for state and local boards of health was more durable precisely because it preserved local control over local public health issues. Shattuck stressed the importance of six elements in effective public health administration: vital statistics, control of infectious diseases, maternal and child health, health education, public health laboratories, and integrated sanitary systems for the community. Generously, Shattuck acknowledged the contributions of French and British sanitary reformers, one of whom, William Henry Duncan, held the first appointment in Britain of a Medical

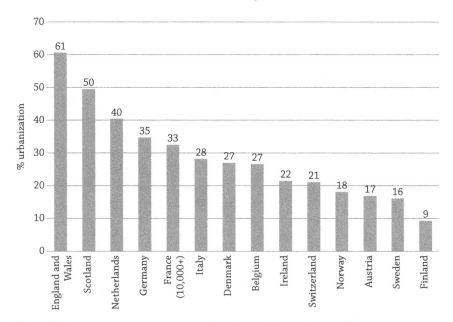

Figure 18.3 **European urbanization, 1911 (population of towns of 20,000+).**
US census data uses a threshold of 2,500 to define "urban." In 1910, on this more modest basis, the
United States was 46% urban. A 10,000-population threshold in 1911 to define urban meant that
England and Wales were 79% urban and France 33%.
Source: de Vries J. *European Urbanisation 1500–1800*. London: Routledge; 1984: 39–48.

Officer of Health (Liverpool, 1847–63) and sent Shattuck parcels of public health
documents on Liverpool in 1849 and forwarded others from health professionals in
Manchester, Edinburgh, and Glasgow. This professional networking was highly significant. Knowledge and best practice were shared, and key texts such as William Gairdner's
Public Health in Relation to Air and Water (1865) remained the standard work of reference for students of public health for many years. The diffusion of expertise extended
to the colonial areas administered by European powers since trained public health staff
imported the precepts and principles of public health and deployed these in an imperial
setting. On the occasion when Henry Littlejohn, Medical Officer of Health and university professor in Edinburgh, obtained public recognition from the state after 36 years
of service, 3,500 of his former medical students scattered all over the world provided
their own appreciation. Public health administration in the Empire owed much to the
durable networks established during training in Britain.[9]

5 Public Health and Community Health

By the 1850s and 1860s, public health professionals had shown that foul-smelling air
(miasma) and individual character flaws were symptoms, not causes, of ill health. Poverty
was at the root of the problem. Low wages—between 1770 and 1830 in England real
wages for those in work were virtually static—and irregular employment diminished
the ability of the breadwinner and family members to withstand disease, particularly

epidemic disease, and so adversely affected quality of life. Public health in the second half of the nineteenth century was focused less on sanitary strategies and increasingly on specialist areas of public health. Initiatives were very varied. They included services associated with occupational health; mental health; vaccination and compulsory notification of infectious diseases; controls on the adulteration of food; public laboratories to analyze samples; tighter regulation of markets, especially slaughter-markets; interments and, in the twentieth century, facilities for cremation.[10] Mother and child increasingly became a major focus of public health policy in Europe in the last quarter of the nineteenth century through the introduction of district nursing, health visitors, and midwifery services and an increase in the number of infant welfare centers, milk dispensaries, and school medical inspections, which, in Germany, contributed (Figure 18.4) to a significant one-third reduction in infant mortality in the 20 years from 1900 to 1920. France was considered to have a world-leading program in this area by 1900.

Most important of all, living standards improved appreciably in the last quarter of the nineteenth century and early twentieth century boosted by cheap food made more accessible through significant advances in international marine transport. The abundant grain produced in the American Midwest and the Ukraine and refrigerated meat from Australasia and South America meant rising real wages did more to improve the health of nations more than any single, or perhaps several, health initiatives. Set against these general national trends, it should be noted that class differentials *within* countries were considerable. For example, infant deaths in families where the father was in unskilled work were almost 40% higher in 1895 in England than for families where the father was in professional work. Furthermore, a genetic urban penalty applied, too. Thus, parents

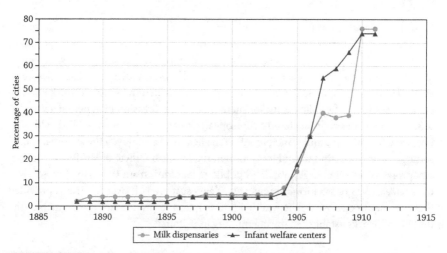

Figure 18.4 **German cities with milk depots and infant centers 1885–1911.**

Note: The vertical axis refers to the percentage of 45 German cities with populations of at least 50,000 in which there was one or more milk dispensary or infant welfare center.

Source: Brown J. Economics and infant mortality decline in German towns, 1889–1912: household behaviour and public intervention. In: Sheard S, Power H, eds. *Body and city: histories of urban public health*. London: Aldershot; 2000: 182.

who could afford a four-room flat in Glasgow produced girls of school age in 1907 who were about 6% heavier and taller than those born to parents of two-room flats and were also less likely to suffer from skeletal, dental, and skin problems because of their diets and living conditions in larger, wealthier households.

The landscape of public health in the last third of the nineteenth century was fundamentally altered in Europe, North America, and a few other locations, and was largely based on nutritional and urban environmental improvements made possible by sustained real wage gains, which in Britain cumulatively amounted to about 70% between 1850 and 1914. This underlying economic condition was complemented by organizational changes within towns and cities, many of which acquired extensive administrative powers legitimating the use of local taxes to finance capital projects such as reservoirs, baths, wash houses, slaughterhouses, refuse disposal, city-wide sewage systems, embryonic town planning projects, and a multitude of controls over nuisances. Medical knowledge advanced in relation to the treatment of infectious diseases, and Robert Koch's pioneering work in microbiology in the 1880s and 1890s firmly established links between microorganisms and specific diseases, notably tuberculosis and cholera, both of which were traced to infectious bacteria. A major breakthrough was achieved in the use of agar to develop and isolate pure cultures, and, with improvements in laboratory microscopes, the germ theory of disease was established as a result of Koch's research, thereby replacing earlier impressionistic ideas regarding foul air and spontaneous generation of disease.

Municipal intervention in public health had a long pedigree, and the tentacles of officialdom have become increasingly extensive. Formal structures have evolved through religious foundations and charities, and, for the comfortably off, through private insurance schemes, to cover illness and infirmity. To motivate workers and to imbue work with a sense of entitlement to health, social insurance schemes of various types and generosity developed. The German Chancellor Otto von Bismarck introduced a social insurance scheme for those older than 70 in 1883. This sickness insurance scheme was based on mandatory contributions from workers, employers, and the government. Together with a workmen's compensation scheme (1884), it gave Germans long-term security of income based on social insurance principles. Other countries developed variants of this arrangement: Sweden (1891), Denmark (1891), Britain (1908), France (1928), and the United States (1935). For large areas of the world, such arrangements are unimaginable, confronted as they are with ongoing concerns regarding water quality and malnutrition and susceptibility to major epidemics: Ebola, cholera, viral meningitis, dengue fever, yellow fever, avian flu, poliomyelitis; Lassa fever; *Escherichia coli*, AIDS, and many others. Such outbreaks occur in parts of the world where public health provisions and funding are fragile and where life expectancy is, at best, half that of European, North American, and East Asian countries. Political stability, educational instruction, the availability of inexpensive basic medicines, and robust public health administration are essential to an improvement in the healthfulness of such countries.

6 Conclusion

From a reactive mode of public health interventions designed essentially as emergency measures to contain epidemic disease, there emerged in the mid-nineteenth century an increasingly sophisticated and ultimately comprehensive system of public health administration. The transition was driven by overcrowding in insanitary cities arising from population growth which, in turn, was generated by a combination of agricultural innovation, New World wealth, and the appeal of factory employment in cities. The pace of such change was beyond the resources of towns and cities to adapt their existing infrastructural investment in sanitation and sewers, with devastating effects in the event of any outbreak that threatened the health of the public. In the course of many decades, and certainly extending well into the twentieth century in Europe and North America, initiatives to develop hydraulic engineering to improve water supply and disposal, suburbanization to reduce overcrowding, public analysis to monitor food quality, and a barrage of community and educational strategies relating mainly to maternal and child health, each contributed to sustained improvements in mortality and morbidity rates. Perhaps the impact of public health programs was best captured in a pamphlet published during World War I which linked the economic and military condition of servicemen: "you cannot expect to get an A1 population out of C3." homes.

References

1. Geltner G. Public health and the pre-modern city: a research agenda. *History Compass.* 2012; 10(3):219–230.
2. Rawcliffe C. *Urban bodies: communal health in late-medieval English towns and cities.* Woodbridge, UK: Boydell Press; 2013.
3. Clark G, Alter G. The demographic transition and human capital, 1700–1870. In Broadberry S, O'Rourke K, eds. *The Cambridge economic history of modern Europe vol. 1: 1700–1870.* Cambridge: Cambridge University Press; 2010: 43–69.
4. Lepetit B. *The pre-industrial urban system: France, 1740–1840 (Themes in international urban history).* Cambridge: Cambridge University Press; 1994. Originally published as *Les villes dans la France moderne (1740–1840).* Paris; 1988.
5. Laxton P, Rodger R. *Insanitary city: Henry Littlejohn and the condition of Edinburgh.* Lancaster, UK: Carnegie Publishing; 2014.
6. de Vries J. *European urbanisation, 1500–1800.* London: Routledge; 1984.
7. Melosi MV. *The sanitary city: urban infrastructure in America from colonial times to the present.* Baltimore, MD: Johns Hopkins University Press; 1999.
8. Hamlin C. *Public health and social justice in the age of Chadwick: Britain, 1800–1854.* Cambridge: Cambridge University Press; 1998.
9. Kidambi P. *The making of an Indian metropolis: colonial governance and public culture in Bombay, 1890–1920.* Burlington, VT: Ashgate Publishing Company; 2007.
10. Sheard S, Power H (eds.). *Body and city: histories of urban public health.* London: Aldershot; 2000.

19

A Systems Science Approach to Urban Health

DANIELLE C. OMPAD AND YESIM TOZAN

1 Definition of Systems and Complex Systems

Scholars from a variety of scientific disciplines increasingly make use of the concept of a "system." However, there is no single definition of the concept. Some scholars define systems very generally as "a set of objects together with relationships between the objects and between their attributes," while others see systems as evolving and complex, with "many components that adapt and learn as they interact."[1] The latter definition highlights the growing interest across multiple disciplines in the notion of complexity that may address some of the shortfalls of the reductionist approach to scientific inquiry.[2]

Although these diverse perspectives make it difficult to define what exactly constitutes a complex system, there are a set of properties that are widely associated with them.[3] Complex systems are made up of a multitude of elements that are in flux and interact over time.[4] These interactions are often nonlinear and may involve significant time delays.[4] Furthermore, they may be best described as circular chains of causal relationships (e.g., feedback loops) rather than unidirectional relationships. Feedback loops can be self-reinforcing (i.e., producing hard-to-predict, path-dependent, unstable dynamics such as sequelae of natural disasters) or self-correcting (i.e., producing strong resistance to change and intervention, such as the development of black markets in response to increases in taxes or tariffs). Individual elements and feedback loops within systems are not established and maintained in isolation, and they often interact with each other.[4] Interactions among these feedback loops produce an emergent system behavior that cannot be explained by an understanding of the individual elements alone.[3] This dynamic behavior persists over time and adapts to changing conditions.[4] In systems science, we are mainly concerned with building an understanding of these phenomena so that we can manage complex systems effectively.

1.1 Urban Settings as Complex Systems

In the urban health literature, cities have historically been thought of as complex systems with many interrelated features on multiple dimensions such as the physical environment including the built environment, climate, and geography; the social environment including social networks and civil society structures; politics and governance; and the economy.[5,6] In the mid-1960s, Berry described "cities as systems within systems of cities," while Forrester, a computer scientist who founded the field of system dynamics, defined urban settings as "a system of interacting industries, housing, and people."[7,8]

The complex nature of urban settings is characterized as both an asset and a deficit for urban health, with researchers making reference to both urban health advantages and penalties, ordered complexity, and disorder and chaos.[9-16] The University College London *Lancet* Commission on Healthy Cities recognized that, because cities are complex systems, health outcomes in cities are challenging to predict due to the many interactions and feedback loops that shape their occurrence, and unintended (and often adverse) consequences can arise.[17] For example, Crush and Frayne frame the complexity of urban food systems as a challenge to be overcome to ensure food security in urban settings.[18] In contrast, Fournier and Touzard posit that the complexity of food systems is actually an asset that can promote food security through the use of different production and exchange models.[19]

Cities are also recognized as dynamic settings that change in time under the effect of a variety of internal (i.e., city level) and external forces (i.e., international, regional, country, and local levels).[20] For example, while population changes such as births, deaths, and migration in and out of cities may shape cities internally and can result in concentrations of poor individuals in some areas and gentrification in others, external forces such as social movements, climate change, proximal inequities, and decentralization of governance may impact cities by interacting with various parts of the system.[5,21] Under the influence of such forces, different parts of the system receive feedback and can take prominence at different time periods depending on how they have interacted with other interrelated parts in a previous time period.

Complexity and dynamism are implicit in prominent urban health conceptual frameworks, and this perspective is strongly featured in the Healthy Cities Movement. Duhl and Hancock described urban settings as "partly organism, partly ecosystem" and hailed them as the example par excellence of complex systems: "emergent, far from equilibrium, requiring enormous energies to maintain themselves, displaying patterns of inequality and saturated flow systems that use capacity in what appear to be barely sustainable but paradoxically resilient networks."[14] Urban health scholars are increasingly examining urban health problems through the lens of complex adaptive systems, but this is a nascent area of inquiry. Moreover, systems science is relatively new to public health science. The utility of systems thinking for improved understanding and action in public health was first explored in response to the threat of emerging infectious diseases.[22] Over the past decade, the application of system science methodologies to public health problems has grown, focusing on areas such as pandemic flu, HIV/AIDS, diabetes, and substance abuse.[22-25] During the same time frame, several leading public health agencies have endorsed the principles and methodologies of systems thinking and have issued funding opportunities to stimulate research and application.[26-33] Yet systems science approaches are still underutilized in the public health field, and the scope, depth, and potential value of systems science for advancing solutions to complex problems related to public health remain to be seen.[34,35]

1.2 Systems Science

Systems science grew out of general systems theory approaches that emerged in the 1930s.[36] Systems science is characterized by a set of methodologies to study complex systems in society and nature.[37] These methodologies are particularly well-suited to developing a holistic view of a system or a problem by synthesizing a large amount of knowledge across a multitude of domains in a model in order to investigate its underlying dynamics. System science models rely on a conceptual or mental model and use both qualitative and quantitative data sources. These models produce generative explanation and emphasize emergent behaviors of systems. Therefore, system science methodologies are often employed for policy analysis and design where the tradeoffs and unintended consequences of different policy options are examined in a virtual experimentation environment, thus saving resources and time.[20,38] They can also be used for generating and testing dynamic hypotheses related to system behavior and forecasting plausible future scenarios under specified conditions or explicit assumptions.

2 Systems Science Methodologies

There are three commonly used systems science methodologies in urban health studies: systems dynamics (SD), agent-based modeling (ABM), and network analysis (NA).[38] SD and ABM use formal models to simulate change in a system and test the impact of different interventions on elements of the system. NA is focused on describing and analyzing the relationships between entities in a network; in public health studies these entities are typically people (as in studies of social networks) but could also be genes, animals, or organizations.[38] Here, we will provide an overview of each method and provide an example of the method applied to an urban health research question.

2.1 Systems Dynamics

The SD approach uses computer simulation models to study complex systems and is focused on understanding how the elements of a system interact with each other to produce the complex behavior of a system.[39,40] SD is somewhat unique among the methods used in public health because it allows for the analysis of feedback loops (i.e., circular chains of causal relationships), nonlinear relationships, and time delays between different variables.[20,38] Data in the model can be qualitative and quantitative and from primary and secondary sources. SD also lends itself to community participation as group model building is very much the norm.[41,42] In urban health studies, SD has been used to examine a variety of issues including bicycling, oral health, and waste disposal.[43–46]

Macmillan et al. modeled commuter bicycling policies using SD in Auckland, New Zealand.[43] At the time of the study, Auckland had experienced substantial increases in car ownership with decreases in bicycling and the use of public transportation.[47] To develop the SD models, the team used data from semi-structured interviews and a multidisciplinary literature review to create preliminary feedback loops. Feedback loops describing commuting trends over time, and with a causal loop specific to commuter bicycling, were refined in two workshops and meetings with more than 30 stakeholders. The simulation model was then populated with epidemiological and administrative data; expert opinion was used when data were not available.

Simulations modeled three types of policy scenarios: a regional cycle network (i.e., marked bicycle lanes, shared bus and bicycle lanes, and off-road shared footpaths), arterial (i.e., roads that carry high through-traffic volumes) segregated bicycle lanes, and self-explaining roads (i.e., roads that elicit safe behaviors by design).[43,48,49] A combination of arterial segregated bicycle lanes and self-explaining roads was also modeled. The benefits outweigh the harms for all scenarios, but a combination of segregated bicycle lanes for main roads and speed reductions on local roads was deemed the most beneficial.

2.2 Agent-Based Modeling

ABM also uses computer simulation models to understand systems by studying the behavior of individual elements (i.e., agents) in the system and how they interact with other agents and with structures of the environment.[38] Agents may be people, animals, or any other individual element in a system that is capable of autonomous action to meet its objectives.[50] For the simulations, agents are programmed to behave in particular ways and to interact with other agents as well as with the environment. In public health, ABM has been most often used to study epidemics and infectious disease dynamics.[51-53] More recently, ABM has been applied to the study of posttraumatic stress disorder, food insecurity, dietary behaviors, and alcohol-related harms.[54-59]

Li et al. used ABM to model fruit and vegetable consumption in New York City (NYC).[57] The agents for their simulation were adults in NYC, and data for the agents were extracted from the 2010 US Census, the 2010 NYC Community Survey, and the Food Attitudes and Behavior Survey, as well as other published studies.[60-62]

Agents were defined by demographics (i.e., age, gender, and educational attainment), taste preferences, health beliefs related to healthy eating, and food-related price sensitivity. Agents were placed in NYC boroughs or neighborhoods that were characterized by the location of food outlets (i.e., limited-service restaurants, supermarkets, and fruit and vegetable markets) as well as by the ratio of healthy to unhealthy food outlets.

The ABM assessed the impact of increasing the number of fruit and vegetable vendors (i.e., mobile carts and markets) by 10% or 20% and decreasing the price of fruits and vegetables by 10% or 20% (alone and in combination) on fruit and vegetable consumption.[57] The model demonstrated increases in the consumption of two or more servings of fruits and vegetables from the baseline model that ranged from 0.93% to 6.16% depending on intervention scenario and borough. Further analyses revealed that the most comprehensive intervention (i.e., 20% increase in food vendors coupled with a 20% decrease in fruit and vegetable costs) would have the largest impact in neighborhoods with the lowest levels of educational attainment and smaller ratios of healthy to unhealthy food outlets.

2.3 Network Analysis

NA aims to understand relationships among different types of entities. Three main approaches are used to study networks: visualization, description, and statistical modeling.[38] Descriptions focus on specific features of networks, such as their size, composition, density, strength of the relationships, and dynamics.[63] Unlike SD and ABM, which are methods unto themselves, NA uses a variety of statistical approaches to analyze network composition, characteristics of relationships, and changes in features of networks and relationship over time.[64]

Merrill et al. used organizational NA to examine communication and information flows in an urban/suburban health department.[65] There were 156 employees in the health department, and most (93%) completed a survey that measured relationships and communication in the workplace, with questions about work-related information flows (i.e., from whom they received information and to whom they gave information), who was important in helping them think about complex issues in the workplace, and perception of the knowledge and skills possessed by their specific co-workers. They also assessed public health tasks, knowledge, and resources within the network.

In their analysis of the department, Merrill et al. found subgroups of employees working in three general areas: public health nursing and related programs, environmental health, and administration/programs.[65] The department had a centralized network structure—that is, communication and decision-making was controlled by a central group—and there was less communication between different programs in the department than within them. The research team brought the results back to the health department, and this resulted in some changes in the organization's processes as well as cross-training of staff and development of workgroups that cut across different programs to increase communication and effectiveness.

Social NA (SNA) focuses on relationships among people and the materials and support transmitted across network ties (i.e., relationships). SNA can focus on egocentric, dyadic, triadic, or complete networks. Egocentric networks are centered on one person (i.e., the *ego*), and all the other people with whom he or she has relevant relationships (i.e., the *alters*).[64] For example, studies of HIV risk may focus on sexual partners or people with whom the ego injects drugs. Dyadic and triadic NAs are focused on pairs and trios of individuals, respectively, while complete NAs are concerned with an entire network of individuals and the ties within the network.[64]

3 Conclusion

Interest in systems science and its applications to public health has been growing in the past few decades. A number of high-profile health agencies, including the National Institutes of Health, the Institute of Medicine, and the Centers for Disease Control and Prevention, have formally recognized the utility and value of systems science in studying complex public health problems and have committed resources to support both research and training programs in this area. Yet the application is limited, and systems science theories, methods, and tools are not part of academic curricula and training in most schools of public health.

In public health, we are equally concerned with research and practice. Systems science methodologies have clear advantages over traditional study design and data analysis approaches used in public health as these methodologies account for complexity and explain how complex systems work. For example, a common frustration is the slow scale-up of interventions that have been shown to be effective and cost-effective, particularly in resource-constrained settings. Paina and Peters recently argued that the pathways involved in the process of scaling up are as different as the local contexts in which they emerge and that a lack of understanding of the adaptive properties of these dynamic pathways involved in scale-up often leads to a rapid, short-term change at the expense of building a sustainable health system in the long term.[66] This example summarizes the level of complexity that characterizes the problems we face in population health. System science methodologies provide an opportunity to foster collaboration among researchers, practitioners, and policymakers from different disciplines and to investigate the systemic nature of complex urban health issues, and we expect a growing demand for their use in urban health research and practice.

References

1. Holland JH. Studying complex adaptive systems. *J Syst Sci Complex.* 2006; 19(1):1–8.
2. Gallagher R, Appenzeller T, Normile D. Beyond reductionism. *Science.* 1999; 284(5411):79.
3. Ladyman J, Lambert J, Wiesner K. What is a complex system? *Eur. J. Philos.* 2013; 3(1): 33–67.
4. Meadows DH, Wright D. *Thinking in systems: a primer.* White River Junction, VT: Chelsea Green Publishing; 2008.
5. Galea S, Freudenberg N, Vlahov D. Cities and population health. *Soc Sci Med.* 2005; 60(5):1017–1033.
6. Lawrence RJ. Urban health: an ecological perspective. *Rev Environ Health.* 1999; 14(1):1–10.
7. Berry BJ. Cities as systems within systems of cities. *Pap Reg Sci.* 1964; 13(1):147–163.
8. Forrester JW. *Urban dynamics.* Cambridge, MA: MIT Press; 1969.
9. Bocquier P, Madise NJ, Zulu EM. Is there an urban advantage in child survival in sub-Saharan Africa? Evidence from 18 countries in the 1990s. *Demography.* 2011; 48(2):531–558.
10. Matthews Z, Channon A, Neal S, Osrin D, Madise N, Stones W. Examining the "urban advantage" in maternal health care in developing countries. *PLoSMed.* 2010;7(9):e1000327. doi:10.1371/journal.pmed.1000327
11. Goebel A, Dodson B, Hill T. Urban advantage or urban penalty? A case study of female-headed households in a South African city. *Health Place.* 2010;16(3):573–580.
12. Rice J, Rice JS. The concentration of disadvantage and the rise of an urban penalty: urban slum prevalence and the social production of health inequalities in the developing countries. *Int J Health Serv.* 2009; 39(4):749–770.
13. Kearns G. The urban penalty and the decline in mortality in England and Wales, 1851-1900. *Ann Demogr Hist (Paris).* 1993:75–105.
14. Duhl LJ, Hancock T. *Promoting health in the urban context.* Copenhagen, Denmark: World Health Organization; 1988.
15. Wilson AG. Ecological and urban systems models: some explorations of similarities in the context of complexity theory. *Environ Plan A.* 2006; 38:633–646.
16. Batty M. The size, scale, and shape of cities. *Science.* 2008; 319(5864):769–771.

17. Rydin Y, Bleahu A, Davies M, et al. Shaping cities for health: complexity and the planning of urban environments in the 21st century. *Lancet.* 2012; 379(9831):2079–2108.

18. Crush JS, Frayne GB. Urban food insecurity and the new international food security agenda. *Dev So Afr.* 2011; 28(4):527–544.

19. Fournier S, Touzard J-M. The complexity of food systems: an asset for food security? *Vertigo La Revue Electronique en Sciences de l'environnement.* 2014; 14(1). Available at http://vertigo. revues.org/14840.

20. Tozan Y, Ompad DC. Complexity and dynamism from an urban health perspective: a rationale for a system dynamics approach. *J Urban Health.* 2015; 92(3):490–501.

21. Vlahov D, Agarwal SR, Buckley RM, et al. Roundtable on urban living environment research (RULER). *J Urban Health.* 2011; 88(5):793–857.

22. Glasser JW, Hupert N, McCauley MM, Hatchett R. Modeling and public health emergency responses: lessons from SARS. *Epidemics.* 2011; 3(1):32–37.

23. Morris M, Kretzschmar M. Concurrent partnerships and transmission dynamics in networks. *Soc Networks.* 1995; 17(3-4):299–318.

24. Jones AP, Homer JB, Murphy DL, Essien JD, Milstein B, Seville DA. Understanding diabetes population dynamics through simulation modeling and experimentation. *Am J Pubic Health.* 2006; 96(3):488–494.

25. Hoffer LD, Bobashev G, Morris RJ. Researching a local heroin market as a complex adaptive system. *Am J Community Psychol.* 2009; 44(3-4):273–286.

26. Mabry PL, Olster DH, Morgan GD, Abrams DB. Interdisciplinarity and systems science to improve population health: a view from the NIH Office of Behavioral and Social Sciences Research. *Am J Prev Med.* 2008; 35(2S): S211–S224.

27. Best A, Clark PI, Leischow SJ, Trochim WMK, eds. *Greater than the sum: systems thinking in tobacco control.* Bethesda, MD: National Cancer Institute; 2007.

28. Scutchfield FD, Perez DJ, Monroe JA, Howard AF. New public health services and systems research agenda: directions for the next decade. *Am J Prev Med.* 2012; 42(5 S1):S1–S5.

29. Thomas CW, Corso L, Monroe JA. The value of the "system" in public health services and systems research. *Am J Public Health.* 2015; 105 S2:S147–S149.

30. de Savigny D, Taghreed A, eds. *Systems thinking for health systems strengthening.* Geneva, Switzerland: World Health Organization; 2009.

31. Gerberding JL. Protecting health: the new research imperative. *JAMA.* 2005; 294(11):1403–1406.

32. Hussey P, Bankowitz R, Dinneen M, et al. From pilots to practice: speeding the movement of successful pilots to effective practice. *Discussion paper.* 2013. Available at http://nam.edu/wp-content/uploads/2015/06/Pilots.pdf. Accessed 27 June 2018.

33. Institute of Medicine (US) Committee on Valuing Community-Based Non-Clinical Prevention Policies and Wellness Strategies. *An integrated framework for assessing the value of community-based prevention.* Washington, DC: National Academies Press; 2012.

34. Mabry PL, Milstein B, Abraido-Lanza AF, Livingood WC, Allegrante JP. Opening a window on systems science research in health promotion and public health. *Health Educ Behav.* 2013; 40(1S):5S–8S.

35. Ip EH, Rahmandad H, Shoham DA, et al. Reconciling statistical and systems science approaches to public health. *Health Educ Behav.* 2013; 40(1S):123S–131S.

36. Von Bertalanffy L. The history and status of general systems theory. *Acad Manag J.* 1972; 15(4):407–426.

37. Sterman JD. Learning from evidence in a complex world. *Am J Public Health.* 2006; 96(3):505–514.

38. Luke DA, Stamatakis KA. Systems science methods in public health: dynamics, networks, and agents. *Annu Rev Public Health.* 2012; 33:357–376.

39. Richardson GP. The feedback concept in American social science with implications for system dynamics. 1983 System Dynamics Conference; 1983; Chestnut Hill, MA.

40. Richardson GP. Reflections on the foundations of system dynamics. *System Dynamics Review.* 2011; 27(3):219–243.

41. Apostolopoulos Y, Lemke MK, Barry AE, Lich KH. Moving alcohol prevention research forward-Part II: new directions grounded in community-based system dynamics modeling. *Addiction.* 2018; 113(2):363–371.

42. Proust K, Newell B, Brown H, et al. Human health and climate change: leverage points for adaptation in urban environments. *Int J Environ Res Public Health.* 2012; 9(6): 2134–2158.

43. Macmillan A, Connor J, Witten K, Kearns R, Rees D, Woodward A. The societal costs and benefits of commuter bicycling: simulating the effects of specific policies using system dynamics modeling. *Environ Health Perspect.* 2014; 122(4):335–344.

44. Macmillan A, Woodcock J. Understanding bicycling in cities using system dynamics modelling. *J Transp Health.* 2017; 7(Pt B):269–279.

45. Metcalf SS, Northridge ME, Widener MJ, Chakraborty B, Marshall SE, Lamster IB. Modeling social dimensions of oral health among older adults in urban environments. *Health Educ Behav.* 2013; 40(1 Suppl):63s–73s.

46. Guo H, Hobbs BF, Lasater ME, Parker CL, Winch PJ. System dynamics-based evaluation of interventions to promote appropriate waste disposal behaviors in low-income urban areas: a Baltimore case study. *Waste Manag.* 2016; 56:547–560.

47. Mees P. *Transport for suburbia: beyond the automobile age.* New York: Earthscan; 2010.

48. Carroll MA, Yamamoto EC. Level of service concepts in multimodal environments. In Pande A, Wolshon B, eds. *Traffic engineering handbook.* Hoboken, NJ: John Wiley & Sons; 2016.

49. Theeuwes J, Godthelp H. Self-explaining roads. *Safety Sci.* 1995; 19(2–3):217–225.

50. Siegfried R. *Modeling and simulation of complex systems: a framework for efficient agent-based modeling and simulation.* Berlin: Springer Vieweg; 2014.

51. Burke DS, Epstein JM, Cummings DA, et al. Individual-based computational modeling of smallpox epidemic control strategies. *Acad Emerg Med.* 2006; 13(11):1142–1149.

52. Lee BY, Bedford VL, Roberts MS, Carley KM. Virtual epidemic in a virtual city: simulating the spread of influenza in a US metropolitan area. *Transl Res.* 2008; 151(6):275–287.

53. Reiner RC, Jr., Stoddard ST, Scott TW. Socially structured human movement shapes dengue transmission despite the diffusive effect of mosquito dispersal. *Epidemics.* 2014; 6:30–36.

54. Cerda M, Tracy M, Keyes KM, Galea S. To treat or to prevent? Reducing the population burden of violence-related post-traumatic stress disorder. *Epidemiology.* 2015; 26(5):681–689.

55. Koh K, Reno R, Hyder A. Designing an agent-based model using group model building: application to food insecurity patterns in a U.S. Midwestern Metropolitan City. *J Urban Health.* 2018; 95(2):278–289.

56. Li Y, Zhang D, Pagan JA. Social Norms and the consumption of fruits and vegetables across New York City neighborhoods. *J Urban Health.* 2016; 93(2):244–255.

57. Li Y, Zhang D, Thapa JR, et al. Assessing the role of access and price on the consumption of fruits and vegetables across New York City using agent-based modeling. *Prev Med.* 2018; 106:73–78.

58. Zhang D, Giabbanelli PJ, Arah OA, Zimmerman FJ. Impact of different policies on unhealthy dietary behaviors in an urban adult population: an agent-based simulation model. *Am J Public Health.* 2014; 104(7):1217–1222.

59. Scott N, Hart A, Wilson J, Livingston M, Moore D, Dietze P. The effects of extended public transport operating hours and venue lockout policies on drinking-related harms in Melbourne, Australia: results from SimDrink, an agent-based simulation model. *Int J Drug Policy.* 2016; 32:44–49.

60. *2010 US Census.* Washington, DC: US Census Bureau; 2010.

61. *New York City Community Health Survey (CHS).* New York: New York City Department of Health and Mental Hygiene; 2010.

62. *Food attitudes and behaviors survey.* Rockville, MD: National Cancer Institute; 2015.

63. Mobus GE, Kalton MC. Networks: connections within and without. In Mobus GE, Kalton MC, eds. *Principles of systems science.* New York: Springer; 2015.
64. Knoke D, Yang S. *Social network analysis.* 2 ed. Thousand Oaks, CA: Sage; 2008.
65. Merrill J, Caldwell M, Rockoff ML, Gebbie K, Carley KM, Bakken S. Findings from an organizational network analysis to support local public health management. *J Urban Health.* 2008; 85(4):572–584.
66. Paina L, Peters DH. Understanding pathways for scaling up health services through the lens of complex adaptive systems. *Health Policy Plan.* 2012; 27(5):365–373.

20

Sociology

LEI JIN, CHENYU YE, AND ERIC FONG

1 Introduction

Sociologists have long been interested in urbanization and the ways in which urban living influenced people's life outcomes, including their health and well-being. These interests intersect with other core sociological concerns, such as socioeconomic inequality, racial and ethnic relations, migration, social cohesion, and social control to inform unique sociological perspectives urban health. In this chapter, we first review sociological perspectives that have helped us understand how urban communities affect people's health and well-being. We then discuss the current methods used and methodological challenges and innovations. Last, we briefly outline the directions of future research.

2 Sociological Perspectives on Urban Communities and Health

The field of urban sociology was developed from the efforts to understand the causes and consequences of the drastic changes that have been taking place in cities all over the world since the early twentieth century. Much of the empirical work in this area has had a distinct American focus, but the theoretical insights have been applied and adapted in many other social contexts. A substantial body of the research in urban sociology focused on health and well-being as outcomes. In the first half of the twentieth century, the Chicago School of sociology pioneered the ecological model and examined social pathologies arising from the urban landscape.[1,2] Drawing inspiration from earlier studies, sociological research on the effects of neighborhood per se and their social mechanisms has flourished since the mid-1990s. This body of research has revealed the unique opportunities and risks afforded by urban living; in particular, motivated by both the social reality in contemporary cities and other important empirical and theoretical concerns in sociology, it delineated three sets of social characteristics of the urban community that may be consequential to people's health and well-being: concentrated disadvantage, racial residential segregation, and collective efficacy. In the remainder of this section, we will review the theories and empirical research that connect these characteristics of community social context to individual health and well-being.

2.1 Concentrated Disadvantage

The concentrated disadvantage thesis argues that the aggregate socioeconomic conditions of a community affect the health and well-being of its residents above and beyond individual socioeconomic status. This argument became particularly salient when, starting from the 1970s, large cities in the United States, especially Chicago and Detroit, experienced rapid shifts in the structure of their economies and an exodus of middle-class and working-class families. Consequently, neighborhoods in traditional city centers became characterized by high levels of poverty, racial segregation, disrupted families, and residential instability. Residents who were trapped in these inner-city neighborhoods became the new "underclass."[3,4] In his seminal work, Wilson documented the plight of the urban underclass and explored its causes and consequences.[4] Subsequent research has focused on the detrimental effects of concentrated disadvantage in inner-city communities.

The concentration of poverty is consequential to individuals' health and well-being through a multitude of environmental, institutional, and social factors. In poverty-stricken neighborhoods, the dilapidated physical environment and lack of attractive green spaces discourage residents from engaging in physical activity, which has been shown to be crucial to both physical and mental well-being. Moreover, the dilapidated environment may affect individual health and well-being through psychological pathways, such as causing stress and anxiety, lowering self-esteem and efficacy, and heightening hostility.[5]

High-poverty communities are also less capable of providing resources to crucial institutions such as schools. Moreover, the peers of children in high-poverty neighborhoods are likely from poor families and at high risk of failure in schools. Therefore, individuals from high-poverty communities tend to have lower levels of educational attainment than those from more affluent communities, and a large body of research has shown that education is connected to healthier lifestyles and better health outcomes.[6] Poor communities are also less attractive to businesses and investors, which implies that there is a shortage of local jobs; unemployment in turn has negative material and psychological consequences for individual well-being.[4] In addition, the lack of business competition may lead to higher prices and lower quality goods and services compared to more affluent neighborhoods.[7] For example, studies have shown that it is more difficult to maintain a healthful diet in high-poverty neighborhoods partly because healthy foods are more expensive and less accessible in these places.[8]

The concentration of poverty also has consequences for individuals' social networks and the prevailing social norms they experience.[9] Residents in high-poverty neighborhoods are geographically isolated from middle-class and working-class individuals, and, consequently, their social networks are more restricted and tend to contain a high percentage of ties to others who are equally disadvantaged. These resource-poor social networks may not be able to provide social support to buffer shocks and stresses or transmit social influences that are conducive to behavioral patterns that promote health. The absence of middle-class individuals in high-poverty neighborhoods may lead to a lack of role models that embody mainstream attitudes, behaviors, and aspirations.[4] In sum, individuals in these neighborhoods experience a collective socialization that may not inculcate healthful practices.

2.2 Racial and Ethnic Segregation

Residential segregation by racial and ethnic groups has been a long-standing feature of the social landscape of modern cities. The sociologists of the early Chicago School described how new European immigrants would disperse from enclaves in the center of the city to the periphery as they and their offspring experienced upward mobility and assimilation.[1] Later studies of residential segregation in the United States mostly focused on African Americans. With the influx of Hispanic and Asian immigrants during the past three decades, the composition of minority groups in the United States has changed. More recent studies started to assess the residential segregation of other ethnic or racial minority groups and found different patterns and consequences of segregation. It has been argued that because the historical processes that led to segregation differed among racial and ethnic groups, the effects may also vary.

For African Americans, residential segregation grew and persisted throughout most of the twentieth century. In the era of legal discrimination (1910–1960), African Americans faced many barriers and restrictions in finding housing in US cities. Institutionalized and sanctioned racism led to patterns of residential segregation that persist to this day. Since the 1970s, with the advent of the Civil Rights Movement and a changing political environment, African American residential segregation decreased moderately, but the level of segregation remained high in inner-city neighborhoods in many metropolitan areas. This period also witnessed the loss of manufacturing jobs and an exodus of middle- and working-class black families from city centers to suburbs. As a result, inner-city neighborhoods were plagued by high levels of poverty.[10]

In this context, high degrees of African American residential segregation have been hypothesized to be detrimental to individual health, and the primary mechanism pertains to the indirect effects of concentrated poverty.[11] Most empirical studies have provided evidence that linked higher levels of black–white segregation to worse health outcomes, but these studies tended to conflate the effects of residential segregation and concentrated poverty since the two processes are highly correlated with each other for African Americans.[11-13] Few studies have explicitly and rigorously conceptualized and investigated the effects of residential segregation independent of concentrated poverty. Interestingly, a number of studies of black–white segregation found that such segregation produced protective effects; particularly, black individuals living in segregated neighborhoods were less likely to experience discrimination and reported better mental health.[14-16] This evidence on the resilience of segregated black communities points to the need to clearly theorize and test mechanisms of African American residential segregation apart from concentrated poverty.

The segregation processes for racial and ethnic groups such as Hispanics and Asians are different from that of African Americans. Because of cultural barriers and limited resources, Hispanic and Asian immigrants often chose to live in neighborhoods with a high concentration of co-ethnics.[17,18] In these ethnic enclaves/communities, immigrants may receive more social support, engage in more social activities, obtain more useful information regarding jobs and access to services, and experience less discrimination than in racially integrated neighborhoods.[12] Although discrimination against non-black minorities may have contributed to the segregation process, the formation of ethnic enclaves/communities was also due to the preferences of new immigrants. Empirical research has found that Hispanics living in areas where Hispanics were segregated from whites exhibited more health-promoting behavior and better health outcomes than those living in more integrated places.[19–21] Only a few studies examined the health effects of Asian residential segregation, and they found that, similar to Hispanics, living among co-ethnics seems to foster both healthful behavior and better health outcomes.[21,22]

2.3 Collective Efficacy

The theory of concentrated disadvantage emphasizes community-level socioeconomic characteristics and the resources individuals can derive from the communities in which they live. Although the study of concentrated disadvantage has been fruitful, researchers have sought to go beyond neighborhood socioeconomic conditions and the focus on individual resources. Motivated by the research on neighborhood social disorganization and social capital, the theory of collective efficacy was developed to signify how communities can act as a collective to benefit their residents.

In their classic work on crime and delinquency in Chicago neighborhoods, Shaw and McKay (1943) formulated the concept of neighborhood social disorganization; it refers to "the inability of a community structure to realize the common values of its residents and maintain effective social control."[2] Shaw and McKay and other scholars found that, in addition to delinquency, communities characterized by social disorganization suffered disproportionately ill outcomes, many of which were health-related.[23,24] These studies highlighted the importance of collective social processes at the level of the neighborhood in shaping individuals' life chances.

Although the theory of social capital was not developed in the study of urban communities, it is highly relevant to understanding community-level collective processes. Coleman defines social capital as resources arising from the structure of social relationships that can be used to achieve specific goals.[25] Sampson suggested that, in this formulation, at the level of the community, social capital may facilitate collaboration and enforce informal social control in the forms of reciprocal obligations, intergenerational closure, and voluntary associations. Sampson argues that social capital is closely related to durable social networks, often strong social ties. In contemporary urban communities, close-knit and locally situated ties are no longer typical features of people's social networks; however, these communities may still be capable of mounting collective action and maintaining social control that benefit their residents. On the contrary, communities that feature strong local ties may discourage collective responses to local problems.[26]

Based on these critiques of the social capital theory, Sampson sought to redefine and clarify the role of social capital in the context of urban communities. Drawing inspiration from Putnam's efforts to expand the concept of social capital to include shared norms and mutual trust that may facilitate cooperation and collaboration, Sampson proposed the theory of *collective efficacy*.[27] Collective efficacy is "a task-specific construct that refers to shared expectations and mutual engagement by residents in local social control"; it emphasizes "shared beliefs in a neighborhood's conjoint capability for action to achieve an intended effect, and hence an active sense of engagement on the part of residents."[28] Sampson argued that collective efficacy does not have to be linked to communities with strong and dense local ties. It has been posited that communities with greater collective efficacy are better able to mobilize collective action, for example to improve local schools or prevent the opening of fast food restaurants, enforce social norms and social control, and provide assistance to residents in need.[23,29]

In a 1995 survey of 8,782 residents from 343 Chicago neighborhoods, collective efficacy was operationalized as shared expectations about informal social control and social cohesion and generalized trust. Residents were asked to rate the likelihood that their neighbors would intervene in situations such as children skipping school and hanging out on a street corner or children spray-painting a local building and to report their agreement with statements such as "people in this neighborhood can be trusted." Studies based on these data found that collective efficacy was associated with less violence and better physical and mental health after other community and individual characteristics were accounted for. In particular, collective efficacy mediated some of the negative effects of concentrated disadvantage; that is, high-poverty neighborhoods also tended to have lower collective efficacy, which in turn is connected to worse health of residents. However, collective efficacy also had an independent effect after measures of concentrated disadvantages were controlled for; that is, equally disadvantaged neighborhoods may have different levels of collective efficacy and therefore different levels of resident well-being.[28,30,31]

Notably, collective efficacy is considered to have a proxy measure: income inequality. The relationship between income inequality and health was initially examined in a cross-national comparison, but researchers soon started to assess income inequality at different levels of geographical units, including the neighborhood.[32] It has been hypothesized that, in addition to inducing negative social comparison and stress, income inequality may also damage social capital and collective efficacy. High levels of income inequality may increase the social distances among residents who are then less likely to form enduring social ties. Moreover, groups with different levels of income are less likely to share common interests and therefore less likely to collaborate in collective action.[33] Empirical research assessing neighborhood income inequality and individual health, however, has produced mixed findings.[32] The hypothesis about the detrimental health effects of neighborhood income inequality is not entirely compatible with the prediction of concentrated disadvantage.[34] This inconsistency points to the need to consider more detailed measurements of the distribution of economic resources in a community, their associated material and psychological pathways, and the heterogeneity in the effects.

3 Methods Used in the Sociological Study of Urban Health

Early sociological studies of urban communities typically employed qualitative methods such as ethnography and interviews to provide in-depth descriptions of how people lived their lives in their communities and how they interacted with their neighbors and neighborhood institutions.[35] Since the mid-1990s, quantitative studies using multilevel models have dominated the research of neighborhood effects.[36] These studies combine data on the characteristics of individuals, such as their socioeconomic status and health status, with data on neighborhood characteristics, typically derived from administrative records or aggregated from information on individuals in a neighborhood. Then these data are analyzed using random-effects models (alternatively termed *hierarchical linear models*). Multilevel modeling has the advantage of being able to account for the interdependence of individuals in the same neighborhood arising from mutual influence and shared environment. It can also assess the relationship between individual outcomes and community characteristics controlling for other individual- and community-level factors, thereby avoiding the so-called *ecological fallacy* that plagued studies linking aggregate neighborhood outcomes (e.g., infant mortality rate in a neighborhood) and community characteristics. Multilevel models can also be used to examine the interactions between individual- and community-level factors.[37]

3.1 Methodological Issues and Innovations

At the time, the proliferation of multilevel modeling represented a major methodological innovation. However, neither multilevel models applied to cross-sectional data nor studies using ethnography and interviews can address a long-standing challenge; that is, identifying the causal effects of neighborhoods on individual outcomes. People sort themselves into different neighborhoods, and, as a result, high-poverty and affluent neighborhoods contain individuals who differ in many observed and unobserved ways. Because of the selection bias, when multilevel models use cross-sectional data, the neighborhood effects they identify may be attributed to unobserved differences in individuals living in high-poverty and more affluent neighborhoods.[38] The statistical method cannot adequately separate neighborhood effects from the individual differences. Two methods have been used to address the causation problem.

The first pertains to assigning individuals to neighborhoods in a random or semi-random fashion to minimize the role of individual choice in neighborhood selection. The most extensive effort is the Moving to Opportunity (MTO) Study. The MTO study randomized 4,604 households living in high-poverty neighborhoods in five large US cities to three groups: one group received vouchers to subsidize rents in lower poverty neighborhoods and housing-mobility counseling (experimental group); the second group received rent-subsidizing vouchers without any relocation restrictions (voucher-only group); and the third is the control group. Ten to fifteen years after the MTO assignment, follow-up studies examined physical and mental health and labor-market outcomes among adults, and physical and mental health, educational attainment, and risky behavior among youth. The findings showed that, on average, adults in the experimental group enjoyed better mental and physical health than those in the control group (namely, less psychological stress and lowest rates of extreme obesity and diabetes), whereas the voucher-only group in general did not fare better in terms of health outcomes compared with the control group. Among youth, however, the health-promoting effects of moving to a lower poverty neighborhood are observed only in girls but not in boys; in fact, overall, boys in the experimental group had slightly worse outcomes compared to those in the control group. The precise cause for the gender difference is unclear, but it is possible that the drop in relative status associated with moving to more affluent neighborhoods is more detrimental to boys than to girls. Ultimately, the MTO experiment showed that neighborhood socioeconomic conditions had moderate but significant effects on people's health, but these effects vary with gender and age.[39] The MTO study was a milestone in the study of neighborhood effects, but it was criticized for not being generalizable and not inducing enough changes in the neighborhood socioeconomic environment to truly estimate neighborhood effects.[40] Moreover, the MTO was only designed to assess the average treatment effects, but the mechanisms of neighborhood socioeconomic status were left unexplored.[40] The resources and time that are required to carry out such large-scale social experiments are also prohibitive.

The second approach to addressing the issue of causal inference involves the use of fixed-effects models. These studies took advantage of longitudinal data and focused on individuals who moved during the study period, and, as a result, their neighborhood environment changed. In these models, individuals are used as their own controls and individual-level time-invariant characteristics are accounted for.[35] Studies using fixed-effects models have so far produced mixed findings with regard to the neighborhood effects on health.[41] The fixed-effects approach has been criticized because mobile individuals may differ significantly from those who did not move, and therefore inferences based on mobile individuals may not be generalizable. Researchers have only recently started to use longitudinal data to assess neighborhood effects, and, although it offers a promising approach to tackle the challenge of causal inference, the underlying assumptions of the approach and the potential violation of those assumptions need to be taken seriously.

The second long-standing methodological challenge in the study of neighborhood effects relates to the definition of the neighborhood and community, and this challenge is especially acute in quantitative studies. In these studies, *neighborhoods* are typically defined according to administrative boundaries such as zip codes or census tracts. However, these administrative spatial units may not correspond to the neighborhood as it is experienced. Moreover, it has been argued that, in addition to their residential neighborhoods, individuals may be exposed to multiple contexts that can influence their well-being. To tackle these issues, recent methodological innovations involve gauging individuals' perception of the boundaries of their neighborhoods and gathering detailed information on the contexts in which individuals conducted their routine activities; measurements of perceived neighborhoods and neighborhood exposure can then be constructed.[42,43] Empirical studies comparing the conventional administrative spatial units with an alternative delineation of neighborhood experience suggest that the amount of resources available to individuals implied in different types of neighborhood measures can be substantially different.[44] This approach offers a promising direction to avoid arbitrarily setting the boundaries of communities of the study subjects. However, introducing more individual discretion into the definition of neighborhoods may further complicate the efforts to clearly identify the causal influence of neighborhoods, which needs to be reconciled in future research.

4   Directions for Future Research

Sociology has a long tradition of assessing how urban communities influence people's health and well-being. The research on identifying the unique effects of urban neighborhoods has flourished since the 1990s. Sociologists have contributed to this area of research by focusing on the social context of people's residential neighborhoods and, in particular, have extensively theorized on and empirically examined three aspects of the social context and their associated pathways, including concentrated disadvantage, racial and ethnic residential segregation, and collective efficacy. The empirical studies have been faced with the challenges of ascertaining the causal influence and identifying meaningful boundaries of urban communities. Methodological advancements have been made to address these issues, but more still needs to be done. Additionally, the mechanisms through which neighborhood social characteristics affect individual health and well-being need to be investigated systematically and rigorously.

Finally, researchers have started to recognize that the effects of neighborhood social context may vary for different social groups and across different social contexts; however, more studies are needed to systematically address this heterogeneity.[35] In particular, most theories and evidence concerning the health effects of urban communities were initially developed in the social context in US cities, especially Chicago.[35] A substantial body of research has also been done in Western Europe and uncovered patterns of the health effects of neighborhood social characteristics that are different from those in the United States.[34] Studies of community social contexts in low-income countries are relatively rare, although cities and neighborhoods in low-income countries can be vastly different from their European and North American counterparts. For example, compared with US cities that inspired much of urban sociology, Asia's mega cities typically do not have economically deprived urban centers or racial and ethnic residential segregation. Instead, these cities are characterized by high population density, expanding income inequality, and large populations of rural-to-urban migrants who are often segregated from urban natives. These urban environments would present a different set of benefits and risks for their inhabitants. Although researchers have started to examine the health consequences of living in these urban environments, much more future research needs to focus on urban communities in more diverse social contexts.[45]

References

1. Park RE, Burgess EW, McKenzie RD. *The city*. Chicago, IL: University of Chicago Press; 1925.
2. Shaw CR, McKay HD. *Juvenile delinquency and urban areas: a study of rates of delinquents in relation to differential characteristics of local communities in American cities*. Chicago, IL: University of Chicago Press; 1943.
3. Massey DS. The age of extremes: concentrated affluence and poverty in the twenty-first century. *Demography*. 1996; 33(4):395–412.
4. Wilson WJ. *The truly disadvantaged: the inner city, the underclass, and public policy*. 2nd ed. Chicago, IL: University of Chicago Press; 1989.
5. Cohen DA, Mason K, Bedimo A, Scribner R, Basolo V, Farley TA. Neighborhood physical conditions and health. *Am J Public Health*. 2003; 93(3):467–471.
6. Wodtke GT, Harding DJ, Elwert F. Neighborhood effects in temporal perspective: the impact of long-term exposure to concentrated disadvantage on high school graduation. *Am Sociol Rev*. 2011; 76(5):713–736.
7. Fellowes M. From poverty, opportunity: putting the market to work for lower income families. *Brookings*. July 1, 2016. Available at: https://www.brookings.edu/research/

from-poverty-opportunity-putting-the-market-to-work-for-lower-income-families/. Accessed September 9, 2018.

8. Larson NI, Story MT, Nelson MC. Neighborhood environments: disparities in access to healthy foods in the US. *Am J Prev Med.* 2009; 36(1):74–81.

9. Cattell V. Poor people, poor places, and poor health: the mediating role of social networks and social capital. *Soc Sci Med.* 2001; 52(10):1501–1516.

10. Kramer MR, Hogue CR. Is segregation bad for your health? *Epidemiol Rev.* 2009; 31(1):178–194.

11. White K, Borrell LN. Racial/ethnic residential segregation: framing the context of health risk and health disparities. *Health Place.* 2011; 17(2):438–448.

12. Yang T-C, Zhao Y, Song Q. Residential segregation and racial disparities in self-rated health: how do dimensions of residential segregation matter? *Soc Sci Res.* 2017; 61:29–42.

13. Acevedo-Garcia D, Lochner KA. Residential segregation and health. In Kawachi I, Berkman LF, eds. *Neighborhoods and health.* New York: Oxford University Press; 2003.

14. Bell JF, Zimmerman FJ, Almgren GR, Mayer JD, Huebner CE. Birth outcomes among urban African-American women: a multilevel analysis of the role of racial residential segregation. *Soc Sci Med.* 2006; 63(12):3030–3045.

15. Hutchinson RN, Putt MA, Dean LT, Long JA, Montagnet CA, Armstrong K. Neighborhood racial composition, social capital and black all-cause mortality in Philadelphia. *Soc Sci Med.* 2009; 68(10):1859–1865.

16. Yuan ASV. Racial composition of neighborhood and emotional well-being. *Sociol Spectr.* 2007; 28(1):105–129.

17. Iceland J. *Where we live now: immigration and race in the United States.* Berkeley: University of California Press; 2009.

18. Logan JR, Zhang W, Alba RD. Immigrant enclaves and ethnic communities in New York and Los Angeles. *Am Sociol Rev.* 2002; 67(2):299–322.

19. Lee M-A, Ferraro KF. Neighborhood residential segregation and physical health among Hispanic Americans: good, bad, or benign? *J Health Soc Behav.* 2007; 48(2):131–148.

20. Mobley LR, Root ED, Finkelstein EA, Khavjou O, Farris RP, Will JC. Environment, obesity, and cardiovascular disease risk in low-income women. *Am J Prev Med.* 2006; 30(4):327–332.

21. Yang T-C, Shoff C, Noah AJ, Black N, Sparks CS. Racial segregation and maternal smoking during pregnancy: a multilevel analysis using the racial segregation interaction index. *Soc Sci Med.* 2014; 107:26–36.

22. Walton E. Residential segregation and birth weight among racial and ethnic minorities in the United States. *J Health Soc Behav.* 2009; 50(4):427–442.

23. Morenoff JD, Sampson RJ, Raudenbush SW. Neighborhood inequality, collective efficacy, and the spatial dynamics of urban violence. *Criminology.* 2001; 39(3):517–558.

24. Faris R, Dunham H. *Mental disorders in urban areas: an ecological study of Schizophrenia and other psychoses.* Oxford: University of Chicago Press; 1939.

25. Coleman JS. Social capital in the creation of human capital. *Am J Sociol.* 1988; 94:S95–S120.

26. Sampson RJ. The neighborhood context of well-being. *Perspect Biol Med.* 2003; 46(3):S53–S64.

27. Putnam RD. *Bowling alone: the collapse and revival of American community.* New York: Simon & Schuster; 2001.

28. Sampson RJ. Neighborhood-level context and health: lessons from sociology. In Kawachi I, Berkman LF, eds. *Neighborhoods and health.* New York: Oxford University Press; 2003.

29. Sampson RJ, Morenoff JD, Gannon-Rowley T. Assessing "neighborhood effects": social processes and new directions in research. *Annu Rev Sociol.* 2002; 28(1):443–478.

30. Browning CR, Cagney KA. Moving beyond poverty: neighborhood structure, social processes, and health. *J Health Soc Behav.* 2003; 44(4):552–571.

31. Wen M, Cagney KA, Christakis NA. Effect of specific aspects of community social environment on the mortality of individuals diagnosed with serious illness. *Soc Sci Med.* 2005; 61(6):1119–1134.

32. Pickett KE, Wilkinson RG. Income inequality and health: a causal review. *Soc Sci Med.* 2015; 128(0):316–326.

33. Wilkinson R, Pickett K. *The spirit level: why greater equality makes societies stronger.* New York: Bloomsbury Press; 2009.
34. Galster GC. The mechanism(s) of neighbourhood effects: theory, evidence, and policy implications. In van Ham M, Manley D, Bailey N, Simpson L, Maclennan D, eds. *Neighbourhood effects research: new perspectives.* Dordrecht, Netherlands: Springer; 2012:23–56.
35. Small ML, Feldman J. Ethnographic evidence, heterogeneity, and neighbourhood effects after moving to opportunity. In van Ham M, Manley D, Bailey N, Simpson L, Maclennan D, eds. *Neighbourhood effects research: new perspectives.* Springer, Dordrecht; 2012:57–77.
36. Arcaya MC, Tucker-Seeley RD, Kim R, Schnake-Mahl A, So M, Subramanian SV. Research on neighborhood effects on health in the United States: a systematic review of study characteristics. *Soc Sci Med.* 2016; 168:16–29.
37. Fitzmaurice GM, Laird NM, Ware JH. *Applied longitudinal analysis.* 2 ed. Hoboken, NJ: Wiley; 2011.
38. Hedman L, van Ham M. Understanding neighbourhood effects: selection bias and residential mobility. In van Ham M, Manley D, Bailey N, Simpson L, Maclennan D, eds. *Neighbourhood effects research: new perspectives.* Dordrecht, Netherlands: Springer; 2012:79–99.
39. Ludwig J, Duncan GJ, Gennetian LA, et al. Long-term neighborhood effects on low-income families: evidence from Moving to Opportunity. *Am Econ Rev.* 2013; 103(3):226–231.
40. Sampson RJ. Moving to inequality: neighborhood effects and experiments meet social structure. *Am J Sociol.* 2008; 114(1):189–231.
41. Jokela M. Are neighborhood health associations causal? A 10-year prospective cohort study with repeated measurements. *Am J Epidemiol.* 2014; 180(8):776–784.
42. Sharp G, Denney JT, Kimbro RT. Multiple contexts of exposure: activity spaces, residential neighborhoods, and self-rated health. *Soc Sci Med.* 2015; 146:204–213.
43. Vallée J, Le Roux G, Chaix B, Kestens Y, Chauvin P. The 'constant size neighbourhood trap' in accessibility and health studies. *Urban Stud.* 2015; 52(2):338–357.
44. Perchoux C, Chaix B, Brondeel R, Kestens Y. Residential buffer, perceived neighborhood, and individual activity space: new refinements in the definition of exposure areas: the RECORD Cohort Study. *Health Place.* 2016; 40:116–122.
45. Wen M, Fan J, Jin L, Wang G. Neighborhood effects on health among migrants and natives in Shanghai, China. *Health Place.* 2010; 16(3):452–460.

21

Urban Planning

Leveraging the Urban Planning System to Shape Healthy Cities

HELEN PINEO, NICI ZIMMERMANN, AND MIKE DAVIES

1 Introduction

Given the strong influence of the urban environment on population health and well-being, urban planning offers a strategic and impactful opportunity to improve urban health. The purpose of planning is to manage urban change in a way that is sustainable, equitable, and efficient. The practice of planning involves creating and delivering land-use management and other place-based policies and programs (such as those for housing, transportation, and employment) in collaboration with the community and private- and public-sector stakeholders. Planning activities have a larger leverage on health than the physical and natural environment alone, for example, through integrated policies which seek to ensure that schools, jobs, and recreational activities are created alongside quality affordable housing and transportation services. Furthermore, planning activities which prioritize sustainable development (through reducing environmental footprints and increasing resilience to environmental change) play a significant role in planetary health and associated health impacts. Scholars and practitioners of population health can contribute to the planning process at multiple stages to shape places that will positively influence health and well-being for decades.

Although planning can support health objectives, there are a number of characteristics of the planning system that create challenges. Urban planning may appear to be a highly technical and scientific field, easily adaptable to the evidence-based approach of the health professions, but, in reality, planning policy and decision-making is highly complex and contingent on economic forces and the democratic system in which it operates. Understanding and addressing these complexities is essential to work effectively with the planning system to promote health.

This chapter will equip readers with the knowledge required to engage with urban planning services to improve population health and well-being. Public health and urban planning fields have shared beginnings and values.[1,2] Herein, we review historic urban planning/design solutions to health challenges and highlight a way forward for future planning and development. We give an overview of the planning process and suggest stages at which health interventions could be most effectively deployed. We also explore some of the complex challenges for healthy urban planning, providing a selection of frameworks as potential solutions. We describe urban planning theories, practice, and terminology based on our experience of the planning systems in the United Kingdom, North America, and Australia. The chapter is of relevance to a global audience; however, it is most relevant in high-income countries where planning is part of a democratic system of government.

2 Learning from Past Attempts to Improve Health Through Urban Form

The foundations of public health and urban planning linked health with the social and physical environment in overcrowded and polluted nineteenth-century cities. A number of planning and design solutions have been trialed and adopted over the past century with the aim of improving urban health. The early town planner Ebenezer Howard proposed removing people from squalid living conditions to health-promoting "utopian" Garden City settlements in the countryside.[3] The Swiss-born architect Le Corbusier proposed vertical cities in the form of tall buildings with multiple healthy design measures.[4] Many architects of British and American 1950s and 1960s high-rise housing estates were purportedly inspired by his ideas but failed to implement features that he deemed essential, such as the provision of management services, and infamous examples like the Pruitt-Igoe projects in St. Louis, Missouri, have since been demolished.[4] Contemporary developments still struggle with adequate provision and management of amenities and facilities, resulting in avoidable health impacts. For example, residents living in communities with poor access to recreation facilities and parks are more likely to be overweight and are less physically active than residents with greater access.[5]

Urban sprawl is a widely acknowledged failure of twentieth-century development, often blamed on urban planning, but driven by many factors.[6] Compact city development with mixed land uses and public transportation is now globally recognized and advocated as a healthy form of urban development.[7] However, a complex range of factors continue to result in the development of communities that are physically and socially disconnected from urban centers and associated opportunities, including jobs and education. Socioeconomically disadvantaged communities tend to live in the least accessible neighborhoods and those most afflicted with environmental nuisances (noise, pollution, etc.), thus creating numerous physical and mental health impacts.[8]

In the 1980s and 1990s, global initiatives such as the World Health Organization's Healthy Cities Movement and the community-driven Local Agenda 21 created momentum to integrate health and sustainable development objectives into the activities of municipal built environment departments, including planning, housing, regeneration, and transportation.[9,10] The 2015 global commitment to the United Nation's Sustainable Development Goals (SDGs) marks a push to renew links between sustainable development, health, and city planning.[11,12] The Copenhagen Consensus of Mayors, an initiative of the WHO Healthy Cities Network in Europe, demonstrates clear leadership to improve urban health through policies that prioritize people and the planet (in alignment with the SDGs), including through urban planning.[13] Today's planners are aware of the successes and failures of the past and are interested in working alongside health professionals to create health-promoting cities. Yet many would argue that more advocacy, training, and leadership is required to ensure that health is a core objective in urban planning and related fields.[14]

3 Integrating Health in Urban Planning Activities

Planning policies and decisions will guide investment, design, and construction for 15–20 years, with subsequent health impacts lasting for decades. Figure 21.1 shows a simplified version of the urban planning system. The planning process stages (central circles) in this diagram should not be viewed as discrete tasks. Planning is an iterative process that should be informed by its successes and failures and adapt accordingly. Community and stakeholder engagement are integral to planning and will occur throughout the development and delivery of local plans. Planning activities are informed and constrained by social, economic, and environmental factors and overseen by elected politicians. The form and function of local planning systems are set out by national (and/or state) regulations and policies. Each stage in this diagram represents an opportunity to influence the built environment to improve health and well-being.

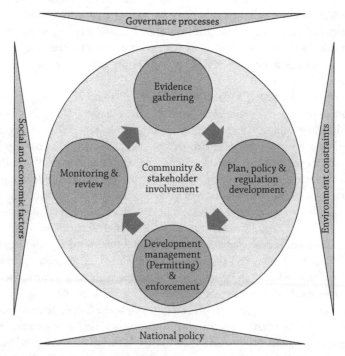

Figure 21.1 **Simplified process of urban planning system.**

3.1 Community and Stakeholder Involvement

Community participation and political decision-making are built into planning legislation ensuring that land-use and investment decisions have been reached through a democratic process. This aligns with contemporary health practice (and policy-making generally), which promotes public participation to engage local communities in the decision-making process and ultimately to improve decisions and outcomes by taking into account a wide range of views.[15] Planners collaborate with local organizations and developers during plan development, and they also elicit the direct involvement of the community through collaborative planning exercises.

Observations about place are complex, and there may be conflicting views among community members and experts about what is required. There are a range of methods to gather community perceptions about health and place, including asset mapping, workshops, photo-surveys, participatory mapping, street audits, and digital engagement.[16] Beyond their roles as stakeholders in the planning process, health professionals may also be able to assist with these engagement activities.

The democratic nature of planning can create challenges when stakeholders within the community represent competing interests. These tensions can be directly related to health. For example, a group of residents living in derelict housing may resist urban renewal with concerns of raising property prices. Politicians may also prioritize the short-term objectives of economic growth over the costs of creating high-quality sustainable environments. These complex problems require diverse stakeholders (the community, the local authority, developers, and other partners) to debate priorities and collaboratively create solutions; in practice, this is difficult to achieve.

3.2 Evidence Gathering

Evidence for planning purposes consists of data about the current and projected circumstances of a place and its residents. Data may come from government statistics agencies, surveys, and topic-based studies (such as a housing needs assessment). Health professionals can provide valuable data about the current and projected health needs of the local population and how this relates to the built environment. For example, a high prevalence of noncommunicable diseases can be used to advocate for features which support physical activity, including active transport infrastructure, playgrounds, greenspaces, and sports facilities. A health impact assessment can also be used as evidence for a proposed plan or new development.

3.3 Plan, Policy, and Regulation Development

The contents of a local plan and the extent to which it addresses health and well-being topics will depend on legislation and local requirements. The plan will usually include sections on employment, economy, transportation, housing, education, healthcare, green/blue spaces, environmental issues (e.g., flooding), and other topics of local importance. From a social determinants of health lens, it is clear that planning policies cover many factors that can influence health and well-being. Health professionals and planners should work together to ensure health considerations are integrated throughout the local plan.

3.4 Development Management

The process of development management (as it is termed in the United Kingdom) involves reviewing applications for proposed changes to the built environment and working with developers to achieve growth requirements in line with policy objectives. In low- and middle-income countries, much development happens without planning consent, and enforcement activities rarely occur, thus creating a number of health risks.[9]

Healthy design measures can be incorporated into multiple stages of the development management process (Figure 21.2 outlines a UK example). It is important to influence the design and application process at the earliest stages to achieve healthy planning aims. Planners may negotiate with developers about the interpretation of local policies on a specific project, including the way in which health-related objectives (such as adequate daylighting) are translated into detailed designs. There are a number of tools to assist this process: healthy planning checklists, health impact assessment, and certification systems (e.g., WELL, Leadership in Energy and Environmental Design [LEED], and Building Research Establishment Environmental Assessment Method [BREEAM]).

Planning authorities may require developers to pay a fee toward the cost of new infrastructure, such as sidewalks and parks. Charging arrangements will be set out in policy documents, although contributions are often negotiated on a site-by-site basis. It is not usually possible to achieve all policy aspirations on a single site for many reasons, often related to cost (known as *economic viability*). A significant challenge for development management planners, and a core task of urban planning, is thus to balance multiple competing interests and objectives.

3.5 Monitoring and Review

The final stage in the cycle of urban planning involves reviewing the success of local policies against the plan's objectives. Many policies will be associated with monitoring indicators which should be reported publicly to increase transparency in local government. Unfortunately, this stage is not usually well-resourced and may be done poorly or not at all. A recent review of indicator tools about the physical environment impact on health found that a growing number report data at the neighborhood scale, allowing communities and policymakers to explore spatial and health equity issues within cities.[17] Public health teams can offer significant support to planners in analyzing and interpreting municipal data related to health and the built environment, which then becomes evidence for future plan preparation.

4 Frameworks for Addressing the Complexity of Healthy Urban Planning

The relations between the urban environment, health, and policy solutions are complex, creating challenges for understanding and managing healthy cities. Complex

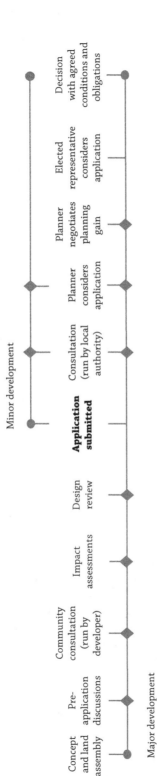

Figure 21.2 **Development management process for developer-led minor and major development in England and Wales.** Diamonds indicate points at which health and well-being considerations could be integrated.

systems are characterized as being uncertain, resistant to policy interventions, and likely to produce unintended consequences.[18] There are a number of challenges associated with urban planning that contribute to the complexity of creating and delivering health-promoting policy and design interventions, including competing objectives and demands (e.g., sustainability and economic growth), tensions with market-led versus public sector-led development, political decisions and priorities, short-term versus long-term considerations, and representation of community interests in land use. In addition, the complexity of the urban health system makes it difficult to investigate specific cause-and-effect relations and interconnections across features in the built environment.[9] A number of frameworks have been proposed to address the complexity of urban health and associated planning policy responses.

Cummins et al. argue that a "relational" view of place and population health is needed for both policy and research purposes, specifically to address health inequalities. This approach would involve a more detailed investigation of people and place by rethinking spatial boundaries, the impact of social networks, and the dynamic nature of places.[19] Corburn proposes this approach for healthy urban planning due to the many social, political, and governance processes involved.[20]

Corburn also proposes an adaptive management framework to address the complexity of healthy urban planning and particularly health equity. Adaptive management acknowledges and works with complexity and uncertainty by closely monitoring policy interventions (through indicators and an evaluation framework) and making adjustments where necessary. A range of stakeholders should be involved in developing a model for change, considering and prioritizing policy interventions, monitoring impacts over time, and adjusting policy responses as necessary.[21]

In line with the adaptive management approach, Rydin et al. also recommend experimenting with local policy solutions and closely monitoring policy impacts. They also propose that cities undertake complexity analyses to understand the connections between features of the urban environment and health and related policy interventions.[9]

A final healthy urban planning framework is the Health Map, proposed by Barton and Grant as a tool to promote dialogue and local investigation into health and place.[22] This tool is informed by the Dahlgren and Whitehead social determinants of health model with reference to sustainable development principles.[23] The Health Map seeks to address the complexity of this policy area by improving understanding and collaboration across health and planning professionals. Beginning with people, the Health Map moves through social, economic, and environmental components of a settlement and encourages consideration of how each of these spheres impacts health and well-being. A combination of the tools and frameworks discussed here can be applied by urban planners and public health professionals in the process of healthy city planning.

5 Conclusion

Barton argues in a *City of Well-Being* that planning needs to get back to its century-old roots when "promoting a healthy environment was not viewed in opposition to economic development. Rather, it was seen as a prerequisite for it, increasing productivity and creativity."[24]

Today's planners are charged with many tasks. Improving health and well-being is among these, but this may not be considered the most important by politicians, communities, or planners themselves. The task of planners and health professionals who seek to promote healthy urban planning is to raise the status of healthy design on the agenda of local leaders and the community. Advocating for active transport, greenspace, and high-quality buildings requires a clear estimation of the co-benefits that these features create for local economies (jobs and productivity), social justice, and the environment, as well as the health benefits. In addition, planners in low- and middle-income countries play a key role in coordinating essential infrastructure requirements to meet the demands of rapidly growing cities such as water, waste, and sanitation services. Just as in high-income countries, planners need to consider infrastructure resilience to the effects of climate change and natural disasters, such as structural safety, overheating, drought, and adaptability to flooding. Our chapter has provided a summary of the planning system and a selection of frameworks to help health professionals harness the power of the planning system to shape healthy cities for the future.

References

1. Dannenberg AL, Frumkin H, Jackson R, eds. *Making healthy places: designing and building for health, well-being, and sustainability.* Washington, DC: Island Press; 2011.
2. Barton H, Thompson S, Burgess S, Grant M, eds. *The Routledge handbook of planning for health and well-being: shaping a sustainable and healthy future.* New York: Routledge; 2015.
3. Howard E. *Garden cities of to-morrow.* Revised ed. Eastbourne, UK: Attic; 1985.
4. Marmot AF. The legacy of Le Corbusier and high-rise housing. *Built Environment.* 1981; 7(2):82–95.
5. Gordon-Larsen P, Nelson MC, Page P, Popkin BM. Inequality in the built environment underlies key health disparities in physical activity and obesity. *Pediatrics.* 2006; 117(2):417–424.
6. Howard, F. *Urban sprawl and public health: designing, planning, and building for healthy communities.* Washington, DC: Island Press; 2004.
7. *Global report on urban health: equitable, healthier cities for sustainable development.* Geneva, Switzerland: World Health Organization; 2016: 242.
8. *Addressing the social determinants of health: the urban dimension and the role of local government.* Copenhagen, Denmark: World Health Organization; 2012.
9. Rydin Y, Bleahu A, Davies M, et al. Shaping cities for health: complexity and the planning of urban environments in the 21st century. *Lancet.* 2012; 379(9831):2079–2108.
10. Kickbusch I, Gleicher D. *Governance for health in the 21st century.* Copenhagen, Denmark: World Health Organization; 2013.
11. Giles-Corti B, Vernez-Moudon A, Reis R, et al. City planning and population health: a global challenge. *Lancet.* 2016; 388(10062):2912–2924.
12. *Resolution adopted by the General Assembly on 25 September 2015: transforming our world: the 2030 agenda for sustainable development.* New York: United Nations General Assembly; 2015.
13. *Copenhagen consensus of mayors: healthier and happier cities for all.* Copenhagen, Denmark: World Health Organization; 2018.
14. Grant M, Brown C, Caiaffa WT, et al. Cities and health: an evolving global conversation. *Cities & Health.* April 2017:1–9. doi:10.1080/23748834.2017.1316025
15. Martin GP. Public and user participation in public service delivery: tensions in policy and practice. *Sociol Compass.* 2009; 3(2):310–326.
16. Pineo H. *Healthy planning and regeneration: innovations in community engagement, policy and monitoring.* Watford, UK: Building Research Establishment; 2017. doi:10.13140/RG.2.2.22459.11048

17. Pineo H, Glonti K, Rutter H, Zimmermann N, Wilkinson P, Davies M. Urban health indicator tools of the physical environment: a systematic review. *J Urban Health;* 2018; 95(5):613–646.
18. Sterman JD. Learning from evidence in a complex world. *Am J Public Health.* 2006; 96(3):505–514.
19. Cummins S, Curtis S, Diez-Roux AV, Macintyre S. Understanding and representing "place" in health research: a relational approach. *Soc Sci Med.* 2007; 65(9):1825–1838.
20. Corburn J. Urban inequities, population health and spatial planning. In Barton H, Thompson S, Grant M, Burgess S, eds. *The Routledge handbook of planning for health and well-being: shaping a sustainable and healthy future.* New York: Routledge; 2015: 37–47.
21. Corburn J. *Healthy city planning: from neighborhood to national health equity.* New York: Routledge; 2013.
22. Barton H, Grant M. A health map for the local human habitat. *J R Soc Promot Health.* 2006; 126(6):252–253.
23. Whitehead M, Dahlgren G. Concepts and principles for tackling social inequities in health: levelling up Part 1. Copenhagen, Denmark: World Health Organization; 2007.
24. Barton H. *City of well-being: a radical guide to planning.* New York: Routledge; 2017.

Health Services Research

Studying Healthcare Services in the City

MICHAEL K. GUSMANO

1 Defining Health Services Research

Health services research draws on multiple disciplines to better understand how the organization and financing of health services can improve the delivery of healthcare services. In 2000, the Association of Health Services Research convened a panel of experts in the field who developed a broad definition of health services research as "a multidisciplinary field of scientific investigation that studies how social factors, financing systems, organizational structures and processes, health technologies, and personal behaviors affect access to health care, the quality and cost of health care, and ultimately our health and well-being. Its research domains are individuals, families, organizations, institutions, communities, and populations."[1] As this definition suggests, health services research has a clear focus on healthcare systems, but includes studies that examine how broader economic, political, and social determinants influence the use of healthcare and population health. The growth of a distinctive *urban* health services research reflects the recognition that most of the world's population lives in cities, that the process of urbanization can have an effect on global public health, and that city public health and healthcare systems can help to address health system challenges.[2–4] The field of health services research is driven by a desire to base healthcare services on good evidence.[5] During the past several decades, it has become an enormous field of research with a professional association (AcademyHealth, formerly known as the Association for Health Services Research) and a flagship journal (*Health Services Research*), along with a host of other academic and professional journals that publish health services research and government agencies that are focused primarily on generating and supporting health services research. These include country-specific agencies like the Agency for Healthcare Research and Quality in the United States or INSERM, the French National Institute of Health and Health Research. There are also multicountry efforts, including European Commission–funded health services research.[6] While some health services research is focused on cities, a large portion of it ignores the issue of place entirely.

In this chapter, I will highlight the development of health services research with a particular focus on the United States, but there is an enormous body of research that examines health systems around the world and growing attention to the relationship between urban health services and global health. In addition to the fact that health services research explores health systems across the world, the range of topics in this field is remarkably broad. These topics include studies that compare healthcare financing, including the implications of health insurance coverage for the use of healthcare and the economic well–being of families.[7-9] Other studies try to understand the influence of economics and politics on government support for healthcare services.[10] There are studies that examine the size and nature of the healthcare workforce, including those that examine the globalization of the healthcare workforce.[11] Along with research that describes healthcare systems, the field includes studies that compare the relationship between social and economic determinants of health and the use of healthcare services in different countries and regions, those that seek to understand the contributions of health services to health outcomes, the evaluation of public health and healthcare interventions on outcomes, and comparisons of the performance of entire health systems using a variety of indicators.[12-17]

2 A Brief History of Health Services Research in the United States

Studies that examine the organization, delivery, financing, and performance of health services are widespread, but the field of health services research is relatively young. In the US, there was relatively little attention paid to these issues until the federal government expanded its role in paying for health services. With the adoption of Medicare and Medicaid in 1965, the US federal government dramatically expanded its role in financing healthcare services in the United States. This quickly led to concerns about the impact of these programs on the federal budget and the discovery of a healthcare spending "crisis."[18] While economists typically argue that there is no level of healthcare spending that is "too much," questions remain about whether we are spending available resources efficiently and generating "value for money."[19,20]

In the late 1960s, researchers in medicine, economics, and other fields started raising questions about the value of healthcare spending in the United States. Since the late 1960s, there has been growing political skepticism about the value and effectiveness of healthcare services.[21] These concerns came from both ends of the political spectrum and helped fuel a burgeoning new field of inquiry that came to be known as health services research.[22]

Some of the early work in health services research focused on the organization and delivery of healthcare. Kerr White, a physician and economist, was a pioneer in the new field of health services research. His research established support for the idea that better access to primary care could reduce rates of hospitalizations.[23] Barbara Starfield, who studied under White, continued work on the role of primary care and the organization of health systems.[24] Another physician influenced by White was John Wennberg, whose work further developed the field of health services research.[24] In 1973, Wennberg and Alan Gittelsohn, a statistics professor, documented wide, unexplained variations in medical resources, medical expenditures, and the use of medical care by 13 different "hospital services area" in Vermont.[25] They argued that the magnitude of the differences they observed were unlikely to be explained by differences in patient need or outcome. Instead, physician uncertainty about the efficacy of different treatments was a more likely explanation of geographic variation in the use of healthcare services. Similarly, research by Robert Brook and his colleagues at RAND in the late 1970s and early 1980s suggested that physician recommendations were not always based on good scientific evidence.[26–29] During the past 40 years, researchers have continued to document small area variation in the use of healthcare services, and there is still an active debate about the factors that explain it.[30] The interest in small area variation in the use of healthcare is only one dimension of health services research, but its focus on place helped to reinforce the importance of local context for better understanding how health systems work. The appreciation for the role of place helps to justify the development of a research in health services that focuses on cities.

3 Urbanization and Urban Health Services Research

The increased focus on cities by those who conduct health services research reflects the urbanization of the world. More than half of the world's population lives in cities, and, by 2050, the United Nations projects that two-thirds of the world's population will live in cities.[31] Along with studies that examine city health systems in the wealthy countries of the world, there is a growing literature on health services in cities in low- and middle-income countries.[32–35] An important theme of this work is concern about the quality of healthcare available to residents of these cities.[36,37]

3.1 The Focus of Urban Health Services Research: Safety-Net Hospitals and Clinics

The urban health services research literature concentrates on the use of health services among vulnerable populations and the organizations that care for them.[38] This literature has made important contributions to our understanding of the nature of the healthcare safety net in cities, the barriers to access faced by these vulnerable populations, the use of health services among vulnerable populations, and the value of innovations in health policy and health services delivery for these populations.

Along with research on access to and the use of healthcare services for poor and vulnerable populations, urban health services research also examines the performance and well-being of healthcare safety-net institutions in cities.[39,40] The US healthcare safety net includes institutions and programs that are funded, in part, by city and other local governments, including city and county public hospitals, community health centers, local health departments, and a variety of local programs for the uninsured and individuals in the community who do not qualify for Medicare, Medicaid, or other forms of public health insurance. These include a host of city and county programs for undocumented patients, many of whom are concentrated in large cities like Chicago, Houston, Los Angeles, Miami, New York, and San Francisco.[41] Not surprisingly, most of these cities (or their surrounding counties) have developed programs that finance healthcare services for undocumented patients.

A third category of studies investigates the implications of national policies for poor and underserved people and communities. For example, in recent years, there have been a large number of studies that examine the implementation of the Patient Protection and Affordable Care Act, including the expansion of Medicaid, and other federal, state, and local programs. These studies demonstrate how local policies and the nature of the healthcare delivery systems influence the implementation and impact of these federal and state programs.

3.2   Features of the City: Geography, Physical Barriers, and Social Factors

Some of these studies use city-level data because they represent purposive sampling frames for studying populations and treatments of interest, but they do not necessarily investigate the features of cities or neighborhoods that may influence the use of healthcare.[42,43] Others, however, investigate how neighborhood characteristics influence the need for healthcare and its use.[44,45] For example, a growing body of studies examine how public transportation and housing influence the use of healthcare services.[46-49] There are also studies that evaluate programs for subpopulations in cities (e.g., for people with tuberculosis and HIV/AIDS, needle exchange and other programs for IV drug-using populations, and interventions to address the use of drugs, including methamphetamine and opioids).[50-51] Some notable efforts to investigate how the organization and financing of health services relate to characteristics of cities, as discussed later, often rely on insufficient data about urban and health system characteristics.[52,53]

4   Disentangling the Impact of Healthcare from the Social and Economic Determinants of Health

One of the biggest challenges facing those who conduct health services research is how to identify the contributions of healthcare to health. Critics of the high costs of healthcare frequently point out that behavioral, economic, environmental, and social factors have a greater impact on individual health than does healthcare. Yet while the role of healthcare in improving population health is small compared to interventions aimed at social and environmental determinants, healthcare still matters to patients who are suffering from disease.

4.1   Using Indicators to Identify the Value of Healthcare Services

But if we accept the premise that healthcare can alleviate suffering and, for some patients, extend life, how can we measure access to appropriate care? Many studies rely either on comparisons of "inputs" (e.g., physicians, hospital beds) or on survey data to measure the use of healthcare. Understanding these inputs and the volume of care that is available and used is important, but it is difficult to answer questions about the appropriateness or efficiency of care with such data.

Another approach focuses on barriers in accessing healthcare that is known to prevent disease, reduce avoidable hospitalizations, and decrease premature mortality. One measure that has been used in several studies to assess urban health systems is *mortality amenable to medical care*.[54] This is a broad measure, one that relies on mortality data that captures the consequences of poor access to disease prevention and primary care, as well as to specialty services. For example, public health interventions like tobacco regulations may reduce premature death by reducing the prevalence of cancer and heart disease. Expanding access to primary care may lead to an increase in routine screening for breast and colon cancers, which may also reduce premature death. Finally, improving access to and/or the quality of specialty care services may increase the use of life-extending technologies (e.g., chemotherapy for patients with cancer or revascularization for patients with heart disease). While this measure is useful, it does not allow one to disentangle the consequences of poor access to disease prevention versus primary or specialty healthcare services.

A second frequently used measure is *hospitalization for ambulatory care sensitive conditions* (ACSC).[55,56] Access to ambulatory care reduces the probability of hospitalization for medical conditions that can be treated effectively outside the hospital. These include hospitalizations for conditions like bacterial pneumonia, congestive heart failure, diabetes, and asthma. Although some studies question whether ACSC can reliably distinguish health system characteristics from the socioeconomic status of their populations, there is agreement that differences in rates of ACSC among neighborhoods reflect disparities in access to ambulatory care, not population health status.[57]

In addition to offering insights into the extent to which urban health systems are providing timely and appropriate access to healthcare services, both mortality amenable to care and ASCS measures are convenient because they rely on administrative data that are routinely collected for other purposes, and it is possible to use these measures to compare access across and within cities. At the same time, mortality and hospital administrative data have limits. Mortality data provide very limited information about individuals beyond age, primary cause of death, gender, and neighborhood of residence. Mortality amenable to medical care may be more plausibly linked to the use of healthcare than total mortality, but it is impossible to examine the use of healthcare over a life course among people who die from an amenable cause. Similarly, the hospital administrative data used to calculate ACSC do not include clinical information and only include limited information about the socioeconomic status of the patients, so it is difficult to identify with any precision the contributions of healthcare to this outcome.

5 Placing a Greater Priority on Additional Data

One of the ongoing challenges to advancing health services research is the lack of available and comparable data on urban and health system characteristics of cities, particularly data that provide information about both individual and neighborhood characteristics. In the United States, Medicare and Veterans Administration claims data can be used to compare the use of healthcare services across and within cities. Restricted versions of datasets allow researchers to access geocoded data and use multilevel models to identify the potential contributions of neighborhoods on health, but, like the hospital administrative data just described, they are not as rich as clinical datasets and include limited information about the socioeconomic status of individuals.[58] Furthermore, neither dataset offers information about the entire population of a city. Neither can be used to explore access to, the use of, or consequences of health services among younger city residents.

Other large national datasets, like the Behavioral Risk Factor Surveillance System, allow for comparisons between people living in urban versus non-urban settings but do not provide information about the specific urban area or details about its attributes or local policies. Smaller studies that rely on original surveys, mixed methods, and qualitative interviews provide rich information that allows researchers to develop hypotheses about potential barriers to care but often do not have large enough samples to allow for geographic comparisons within or across cities.[59-61]

To advance health services research on cities, it will be crucial to develop better data to improve our capacity to compare urban health and health systems. Across the world, most of the routine health and healthcare surveys that are used to assess access, self-reported health status, and the use of healthcare services are conducted at the national level, with samples that do not allow for city-level comparisons. Even when these surveys do produce estimates at the city level, they do not allow for neighborhood-level estimates that would allow researchers to examine disparities within cities or investigate the degree to which neighborhood characteristics may contribute to these outcomes. There are a few notable examples, including the New York City Community Health Survey and the Los Angeles County Health Survey, which both provide detailed information about self-reported health status, social and demographic factors that may influence health and the use of healthcare services, and geographic identifiers that allow researchers to compare the contexts in which people live. But even in other world cities in wealthy nations, there is a limit to how far it is possible to find data of this sort. Mortality and hospital administrative data often provide geographic identifiers that allow for neighborhood-level analysis, but these sources provide almost no information about individual factors that may influence health or the use of healthcare services like education, income, marital status, or work history. In low- and middle-income countries, there is often a lack of basic information, including accurate mortality statistics with information about the cause of death. As a result, it is difficult for researchers and officials to engage in routine monitoring of health system performance or to identify factors that are contributing to health system problems.[62] With few exceptions, urban health services research relies on data that are insufficient to evaluate the performance of health systems, particularly if we hope to identify the unique contributions of health services and neighborhood characteristics to health.[63] The cost of collecting data of this sort is not trivial, and it is often difficult to make the case for spending on public health infrastructure. Without it, however, policymakers are operating in the dark, making it difficult to know how to direct limited resources in ways that improve public health.

6 Conclusion

Spending on healthcare services has been increasing rapidly. The world's highest income countries have experienced high healthcare spending for decades, but the recent push for universal health coverage (UHC) has led to increased spending on health services in low- and middle-income countries as well. Because governments are committing a growing share of society's resources to health services, there has been, understandably, a subsequent growth in research designed to better understand the organization, financing, and delivery of these services. The urbanization of the world's population means that much of this new spending on health services takes place in cities.

The field of health services research has a long history of studying health systems in cities and in comparing health services in urban and rural settings. Although some of this research examines cities simply because they are convenient places to sample vulnerable populations or to better understand the institutions and programs that serve them, a growing body of research recognizes that features of the city—and the physical and social environments of neighborhoods—are likely to influence health, health behaviors, access to healthcare, and the use of health services. Unfortunately, the information that would allow researchers to test hypotheses about the contributions of the physical and social environments of cities is limited. Investments in public health surveillance, which includes better information about the environments in which people live and make use of health services, would help to improve urban health services research and, most importantly, the healthcare systems that serve city residents.

References

1. Lohr K, Steinwachs DM. Health services research: an evolving definition of the field. *Health Serv Res.* 2002; 37(1):15–17.
2. Marinacci C, Demaria M, Melis G, et al. The role of contextual socioeconomic circumstances and neighborhood poverty segregation on mortality in 4 European cities. *Int J Health Serv.* 2017; 47(4):636–654.
3. Krawczyk N, Kerrigan D, Bastos FI. The quest to extend health services to vulnerable substance users in Rio de Janeiro, Brazil in the context of an unfolding economic crisis. *Int J Health Serv.* 2017; 47(3):477–488.
4. Stuber J, Galea S, Ahern J, Blaney S, Fuller C. The association between multiple domains of discrimination and self-assessed health: a multilevel analysis of Latinos and blacks in four low-income New York City neighborhoods. *Health Serv Res.* 2003; 38:1735–1760.
5. Gray BH. The legislative battle over health services research. *Health Aff (Millwood).* 1992; 11(4): 38–66.
6. Hansen J, ed. *Health services research into European policy and practice: final report of the HSREPP project.* Utrecht, Netherlands: Netherlands Institute for Health Services Research; 2011.
7. Rivera-Hernandez M, Rahman M, Mor V, Galarraga O. The impact of social health insurance on diabetes and hypertension process indicators among older adults in Mexico. *Health Serv Res.* 2016; 51(4):1323–1346.
8. Baird K. High out-of-pocket medical spending among the poor and elderly in nine developed countries. *Health Serv Res.* 2016; 51(4):1467–1488.
9. Parmar D, Reinhold S, Souares A, Savadogo G, Sauerborn R. Does community-based health insurance protect household assets? Evidence from rural Africa. *Health Serv Res.* 2012; 47(2):819–839.
10. Cylus J, Mladovsky P, McKee M. Is there a statistical relationship between economic crises and changes in government health expenditure growth? An analysis of twenty-four European countries. *Health Serv Res.* 2012; 47(6):2204–2224.
11. Devlo D. Migration of nurses from Sub-Saharan Africa: a review of issues and challenges. *Health Serv Res.* 2007; 42(3):1373–1388.

12. Roos LL, Walld R, Uhanova J, Bond R. Physician visits, hospitalizations, and socioeconomic status: ambulatory care sensitive conditions in a Canadian setting. *Health Serv Res.* 2005; 40(4):1167–1185.

13. McClure EM, Garces A, Saleem S, et al. Global network for women's and children's health research: probable causes of stillbirth in low- and middle-income countries using a prospectively defined classification system. *BJOG.* 2018;125(2): 131–138.

14. Haider SJ, Chang LV, Bolton TA, Gold JG, Olson BH. An evaluation of the effects of a breastfeeding support program on health outcomes. *Health Serv Res.* 2014; 49(6):2017–2024.

15. Poznyak D, Peikes DN, Wakar BA, Brown RS, Reid RJ. Development and validation of the modified patient-centered medical home assessment for the comprehensive primary care initiative. *Health Serv Res.* 2018; 53(2):944–973.

16. Rieckmann T, Renfro S, McCarty D, Baker R, McConnell KJ. Quality metrics and systems transformation: are we advancing alcohol and drug screening in primary care? *Health Serv Res.* 2018; 53(3):1703–1726.

17. Schoen C, Osborn R, Squires D, Doty MM. Access, affordability, and insurance complexity are often worse in the United States compared to ten other countries. *Health Aff (Millwood).* 2013; 32(12):2205–2215.

18. Marmor TR. Rethinking national health insurance. In Marmor TR, ed. *Political analysis and American medical care: essays.* Cambridge: Cambridge University Press; 1983:187–206.

19. Fogel RW. The extension of life in developed countries and its implications for social policy in the twenty-first century. *Popul Dev Rev.* 2000; 26:310.

20. Gusmano MK, Callahan D. Value for money: use with care. *Ann Intern Med.* 2011; 154(3):207–208.

21. Starr P. *The social transformation of American medicine: the rise of a sovereign profession and the making of a vast industry.* New York: Basic Books; 1982.

22. Callahan D. *Taming the beloved beast: how medical technology is ruining our health system.* Oxford: Oxford University Press; 2009.

23. White KL, Williams TF, Greenberg BG. The ecology of medical care. 1961. *Bull N Y Acad Med.*1996; 73(1):187.

24. Berkowitz E. History of health services research project interview with Barbara Starfield. U.S. National Library of Medicine website. Available at https://www.nlm.nih.gov/hmd/nichsr/starfield.html. 2003. Accessed June 1, 2018.

25. Wennberg J, Gittelsohn A. Small area variations in health care delivery: a population-based health information system can guide planning and regulatory decision-making. *Science.* 1973; 182(4117):1102–1108.

26. Brook RH. Practice guidelines and practicing medicine: are they compatible? *JAMA.* 1989; 262:3027–3030.

27. Brook RH, Williams KN, Rolph JE. Controlling the use and cost of medical services: the New Mexico experimental medical care review organization: a four year case study. *Med Care.* 1978; 16(9S):1–76.

28. Brook RH, Lohr K, Chassin M, Kosecoff J, Fink A, Solomon D. Geographic variations in the use of services: do they have any clinical significance? *Health Aff (Millwood).* 1984; 3(2):63–73

29. Brook RH, Chassin MR, Fink A. A method for detailed assessment of the appropriateness of medical technologies. *Int J Technol Assess Health Care.* 1986; 2:53–63.

30. Wennberg J. Forty years of unwarranted variation—and still counting. *Health Policy.* 2014; 114:1–2.

31. Department of Economic and Social Affairs. *World urbanization prospects: the 2014 revision.* New York: United Nations; 2014.

32. Puthenparambil MJ, Kröger T, Van Aerschot L. Users of home-care services in a Nordic welfare state under marketisation: the rich, the poor and the sick. *Health Soc Care Community.* 2017; 25:54–64.

33. Perelman J, Rosado R, Amri O, et al. Economic evaluation of HIV testing for men who have sex with men in community-based organizations: results from six European cities. *AIDS Care.* 2016; 29:8,985–989.

34. Bradley EH, Canavan M, Rogan E, et al. Variation in health outcomes: the role of spending on social services, public health, and health care, 2000–09. *Health Aff (Millwood)*. 2016. 35:5,760–768.

35. Montgomery M, Stren R, Cohen B, Reid HE. *Cities transformed: demographic change and its implications in the developing world*. New York: Routledge; 2013.

36. Puri L, Das J, Pai M, et al. Enhancing quality of medical care in low income and middle income countries through simulation-based initiatives: recommendations of the Simnovate Global Health Domain Group. *BMJ Simul Technol Enhanc Learn*. 2017; 3:S15–S22.

37. Sobel HL, Huntington D, Temmerman M. Quality at the centre of universal health coverage. *Health Policy Plan*. 2016; 31(4):547–549.

38. Kuang X, Johnson, KR, Schetzina K, Kozinetz C, Wood DL. An ecological model of health care access disparities for children. *Int J Public Health Res*. 2017; 9(2):169–180.

39. Dubay L, Kenney GM. Health care access and use among low-income children: who fares best? *Health Aff (Millwood)*. 2001; 20:1,112–121.

40. Makaroun LK, Bowman C, Duan, K, et al. Specialty care access in the safety net-the role of public hospitals and health systems. *J Health Care Poor Underserved*. 2017; 28(1): 566–581.

41. Berlinger N, Calhoon C, Gusmano MK, Vimo J. *Undocumented immigrants and access to health care in New York City: identifying fair, effective, and sustainable local policy solutions: report and recommendations to the Office of the Mayor of New York City*. New York: The Hastings Center and the New York Immigration Coalition; 2015.

42. Benjamins MR, Hunt BR, Raleigh SM, Hirschtick JL, Hughes MM. Racial disparities in prostate cancer mortality in the 50 largest US cities. *Cancer Epidemiol*. 2016; 44:125–131.

43. Reilly KH, Neaigus A, Wendel T, Marshall DM 4th, Hagan H. Bisexual behavior among male injection drug users in New York City. *AIDS Behav*. 2016; 20(2):405–416.

44. DeGuzman PB, Cohn WF, Camacho F, Edwards BL, Sturz VN, Schroen AT. Impact of urban neighborhood disadvantage on late stage breast cancer diagnosis in Virginia. *J Urban Health*. 2017; 94:199–210.

45. Haley DF, Linton S, Luo R, et al. Public housing relocations and relationships of changes in neighborhood disadvantage and transportation access to unmet need for medical care. *J Health Care Poor Underserved*. 2017; 28(1):329–349.

46. Hindhede A, Bonde A, Schipperijn J, Scheuer S, Sørensen S, Aagaard-Hansen J. How do socio-economic factors and distance predict access to prevention and rehabilitation services in a Danish municipality? *Prim Health Care Res Dev*. 2016; 17(6):578–585.

47. Zhang X, Dupre ME, Qiu L, Zhou W, Zhao Y, Gu D. Urban-rural differences in the association between access to healthcare and health outcomes among older adults in China. *BMC Geriatr*. 2017;17(1):151.

48. Culhane DP, Metraux S, Hadley T. Public service reductions associated with placement of homeless persons with severe mental illness in supportive housing. *Housing Policy Debate*. 2002; 13(1):107–163.

49. Kersten EE, LeWinn KZ, Gottlieb L, Jutte DP, Adler NE. San Francisco children living in redeveloped public housing used acute services less than children in older public housing. *Health Aff (Millwood)*. 2014; 33(12):2230–2237.

50. Bowser B, Fullilove R, Word C. Is the new heroin epidemic really new? Racializing heroin. *J Natl Med Assoc*. 2017; 109(1):28–32.

51. White C, Ready J, Katz CM. Examining how prescription drugs are illegally obtained: social and ecological predictors. *J Drug Issues*. 2016; 46(1):4–23.

52. Andrulis DP. The public sector in health care: evolution or dissolution? Three scenarios for a changing public-sector health care system. *Health Aff (Millwood)*. 1997; 16(4):131–140.

53. Dunham JD. *The data management system. Project on Human Development in Chicago neighborhoods: Technical Report I*. Washington, DC: United States Department of Justice, National Institute of Justice; 1997.

54. Gusmano MK, Rodwin VG, Weisz D, Ayoub R. Health improvements in BRIC Cities: Moscow, São Paulo and Shanghai, 2000–2010. *World Med Health Policy*. 2016; 8(2):127–138.

55. Gusmano MK, Rodwin VG, Weisz D. A new way to compare health systems: avoidable hospital conditions in Manhattan and Paris. *Health Aff (Millwood)*. 2006; 25(2):510–520.

56. Gusmano MK, Rodwin VG, Weisz D. Persistent inequalities in health and access to health services: evidence from NYC. *World Med Health Policy*. 2017; 9(2):186–205.

57. Wennberg J. Population illness rates do not explain population hospitalization rates. *Med Care*. 1987; 25(4):354–359.

58. Byrne T, Nelson RE, Montgomery AE, Brignone E, Gundlapalli AV, Fargo JD. Comparing the utilization and cost of health services between veterans experiencing brief and ongoing episodes of housing instability. *J Urban Health*. 2017; 94(1):54–63.

59. DeVoe JE, Graham AS, Angier H, Baez A, Krois L. Obtaining health care services for low-income children: a hierarchy of needs. *J Health Care Poor Underserved*. 2008; 19(4):1192–1211.

60. Maeva J, Grassineau D, Balique H, et al. Improving access and continuity of care for homeless people: how could general practitioners effectively contribute? Results from a mixed study. *BMJ Open*. 2016; 6(11). doi:10.1136/bmjopen-2016-013610

61. Shaw S. The pharmaceutical regulation of chronic disease among the U.S. urban poor: an ethnographic study of accountability. *J Critical Public Health*. 2018; 28(2):165–176.

62. Gusmano MK, Rodwin VG, Weisz D. Delhi's health system exceptionalism: inadequate progress for a global capital city public health. *Public Health*. 2017; 145:23–29.

63. Gusmano MK, Rodwin RG. Needed: global cooperation for comparative research on cities and health. *Int J Health Policy Manag*. 2016; doi:10.15171/ijhpm.2016.39

23

Environmental Health Impact Assessment

CARLOS DORA

1 Introduction

Urban development interventions in a variety of sectors, including in transport, housing, land-use planning, waste management, and energy, can generate substantial health benefits to affected communities. These opportunities for health can be overlooked and unnecessary health risks and costs caused and potential benefits foregone if health issues are not explicitly considered as part of urban projects, plans, and strategies. The health sector has acquired an appreciation of the social and environmental determinants of health and has advocated for the need to include health in the development of other sector policies, a concept known as *Health in All Policies* (HiAPs).[1-3] How HiAP is implemented remains a work in progress. One tool, the *health impact assessment* (HIA), is key for assessing the health benefits and risks of a proposed programmatic or policy intervention. The HIA considers in advance the possible unintended consequences, thus leading to recommendations on how to avoid health risks and increase health gains from the intervention.[4]

This chapter briefly describes a rationale for how HIA can influence other sector policies to protect and promote public health and goes on to explain HIA, including the key steps in its implementation procedure, the origins of HIA, and its links to other assessments of policies, plans, and projects (PPPs). It outlines some of the methodological debates and recent advances; provides examples of its use over time, including in cities; and provides insights from urban HIA evaluations. The chapter makes the point that although HIA is a robust methodology that is increasingly used in some countries, it is essential that it becomes part of the core health systems functions and be implemented everywhere in order to deliver the opportunities offered by HiAPs. Cities and urban populations in particular can benefit from the HIA's use of scientific evidence to guide local policy while engaging with stakeholders and incorporating their views and perspectives. The chapter concludes by identifying challenges and opportunities for making full use of HIA as a core urban public health tool.

2 Rationale for and Definition of HIA

Early identifications of health risks and benefits that can result from city PPPs can help ensure that related health gains are obtained, that risks are avoided, that diseases are prevented, that related health costs are not transferred to society or to health systems, and that health inequalities are reduced. Foresight through early investment in an HIA of public policies and decisions is an effective way to do this.[4,5]

HIAs provide a systematic procedure and methodologies to identify how a PPP in any sector is expected to impact health and to identify those likely to be affected[6] (see Box 23.1 and Figure 23.1) as a convener brings together experts and stakeholders to deliberate on the issues. HIA also offers an opportunity to listen to the communities and stakeholders potentially affected by the policy or project and to include their questions and concerns in the context of the assessment. HIA considers stakeholder perspectives, expectations, and hopes, engaging them throughout the stages of implementation as well as facilitating their ownership of results.[7] Through active civic engagement, HIA is a framework and a mechanism to provide information, accountability, and transparency on the health consequences of public and private policy and investment decisions.

The HIA team draws on scientific evidence about how the proposed PPP may affect health determinants among different population groups, provides knowledge of baseline exposure to those determinants, and estimates changes expected to take place because of the PPPs, including opportunities to improve health (e.g., access to healthy food or cleaner air) or increases in health risks (e.g., from injuries or social isolation). HIA results can inform all stakeholders about the anticipated impacts of a proposed PPP on health for different population groups likely to be affected and summarize implications for health equity.[8] HIA methods can assure that health is considered in municipal or national deliberations of PPP proposals through a thorough analysis and the inclusion of health considerations among tradeoffs (e.g., impacts on jobs, environment, costs, and savings). HIA methods enable the use of scientific and local data to provide information such as health impact scenarios for the PPPs being analyzed and compared.[9] Those analyses and deliberations can inform urban development debates and decisions in land use, transportation, or building codes.

3 Uses of HIA

The decision to support HIA is usually developed in cooperation with the organization responsible for the PPP being assessed. There are also other uses for and types of HIA, including mandated (to fulfill a regulatory requirement), advocacy (led by individuals who are neither the proponents nor the decision-makers, but with the goal of influencing those decisions), and community-led (to help define and understand issues affecting them).[10]

A large proportion of implemented HIAs have focused on urban policies. For example, 60% of HIAs in Australia and New Zealand during the period 2005–2009 were performed in urban development policies and projects.[11] In France, most HIAs are performed in urban projects.[12] The US Centers for Disease Control and Prevention

---

Box 23.1 **Implementing Health Impact Assessments**

Health impact assessments (HIAs) aim to inform policy or project alternatives, and HIA results need to feed into policy debates. Considerations of context and stakeholder interests are therefore essential for the HIA to be fit for purpose. These are normally described under stakeholder participation and engagement, and its importance cannot be overemphasized.

Listed here are the five steps usually described for HIA. I would add an additional early step—policy and stakeholder analysis—which helps identify questions and frame the analyses so they respond to the crucial policy debates and create plans for engagement and the communication of findings throughout the HIA process.

1. *Screening to identify if a project, policy, or plan* (PPP) is likely to affect health determinants and requires a brief or more extensive HIA. This is done by expert assessment, using checklists or by defining types of interventions which will always require an HIA.
2. *Scoping* identifies the PPP alternatives to be assessed, the range of health determinants and outcomes, the populations affected, time and place considerations, and other issues as well as methods and tools to be used in the HIA. This step defines the Terms of Reference for the impact assessments or studies needed and defines the stakeholder engagement plan.
3. *Impact analysis or appraisal* involves a rapid or more in-depth estimation of the expected health impacts in different population groups using qualitative and quantitative methods and tools. Results will include baseline conditions, analyze direction, gauge the likelihood and importance of impacts, and consider alternatives to change the PPP to improve its health performance. Results are issued in an HIA report.
4. The *HIA report* is considered in the PPP impact mitigation or enhancement action plans along with other considerations.
5. *Monitoring and reporting* the process and outcomes establish if the recommendations were accepted by decision-makers, if proposed changes were implemented, and if stakeholders understood the health issues at stake, and this stage also tracks changes in relevant health determinants and health outcomes.

Source: WHO.

(CDC) had a program that provided tools and training for healthy urban planning and healthy community design, and it supported the development of HIA at the local level, including through direct funding of and technical assistance with a number of HIAs for local-level planning.[13] The majority of case studies on its website dealt with transport and land use. In Europe, the World Health Organization (WHO) EURO Health Cities program's Networks of Healthy cities adopted HIA as a key tool for implementing

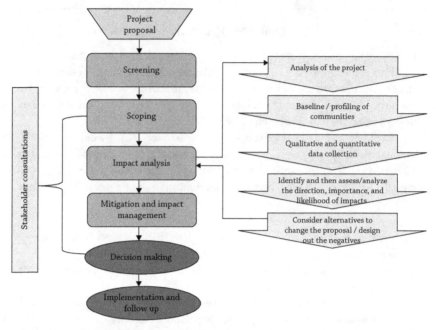

Figure 23.1 **Health impact assessment (HIA) process.**

HiAP.[14] Considerable experience exists with HIAs in urban development, and there are a large number of tools and guidelines for that purpose.[15]

Although the HIA can be a valuable process, the implementation of HIAs remains voluntary, and it is seen mostly in places where there is clear leadership, adequate access to expertise, and dedicated resources. HIAs are not yet a core part of health systems' roles and responsibilities, nor are they implemented on a wide scale or mainstreamed into regular public functions. A broader embrace of HIA could provide opportunities through the systematic use of a tool that practitioners could use for tackling the social and environmental determinants of health to promote health equity.

4 Origins of HIA

The first assessments aimed at anticipating and preventing the negative impacts of development projects on the environment were launched in the US National Environmental Policy Act in 1969. These *environment impact assessments* (EIAs) reference health as a key justification and expected outcome from implementing the procedure.[16] EIAs, however, did not consider social determinants or the positive health outcomes that can result from proposed projects, nor did they include health expertise in the assessment procedure. *Social impact assessment* and *integrated assessments* were developed later, enlarging the range of impacts considered but still making limited reference to health.

Strategic environment assessments (SEAs), developed by the late 1990s, proposed to address some of the EIA's limitations, such as accounting for the cumulative effect of separate projects. The SEA protocol of the United Nations Economic Commission for Europe (UNECE) Environment Impact Assessment Convention received substantial inputs from the health sector (health ministries, experts, and the WHO) and specified when and how to consider health at different stages of the assessment and the need to consider health goals and consult with health authorities.[17,18]

Early HIAs were used in low- and middle-income countries around large infrastructure projects (such as for water and sanitation—see World Commission on Dams), covering mostly vector-borne diseases and other physical and biological risks to health.[19]

5 Development of HIA

Academia, WHO, and pioneer experts in a few countries, along with annual meetings of professional associations of HIA practitioners, played an important role in clarifying the methods and good practice used in procedure implementation. The International Association of HIA Practitioners has transformed into the health chapter of the International Association of Impact Assessment (IAIA). IAIA also convenes practitioners in an environment and a social chapter and holds yearly conferences. Short courses on HIA (e.g., in the United Kingdom, Canada) contributed to early capacity building, and these courses are still offered today. These debates led to greater clarity on what is unique about HIA and how it can be linked to other assessments (EIAs in particular). These debates included, for example, the use of qualitative and/or quantitative methods, the depth of analysis (when to use rapid or in-depth analysis), the need to include social determinants of health in addition to environmental determinants, the inclusion of a focus on health equity, and the benefits of having HIAs that are independent from EIAs. Often those were seen as either-or questions, but, by and large, they have evolved on when to consider each method and how to include equity, for example, thus leading to a higher standard of practice. Still there are practitioners who tend to cover more thoroughly the environmental determinants of health or those that can be easily quantified, and good practice standards point to the need to consider all impacts and use appropriate methods for estimating each one.

Adoption of HIA as national policy followed a landmark WHO workshop in Europe which clarified the definitions of social, economic, and environmental determinants of health (Goteborg Consensus paper).[6] Legislation requiring stand-alone HIAs as part of a drive for HiAPs were adopted in Quebec and in Thailand.[20,21] Wales screened parliamentary decisions for potential health impacts and now has an HIA requirement inscribed into its Public Health Law, and several countries put greater emphasis on health equity (e.g., *health equity impact assessments*).[22–24]

HIA has been used to influence urban environments for health in many parts of the developed world, including Australia, Europe, London, and cities in the United States.[25–27] Learning by doing has embedded HIA in health and non-health agencies in NSW Australia.[28] This movement toward HIA comes in response to evidence that urban design and sprawl affect determinants of noncommunicable diseases, the realization that retrofitting a built environment to make it healthier is difficult and costly, and that there is a need to reconquer the city.[29,30]

In low- and middle-income countries, HIAs are still largely missing from the program and policy arena unless required by an external project driver such as a development bank, and usually only for large infrastructure projects in transport, the extractive industry (e.g., oil and mining), or water projects.[31] Some of these banks, like the International Finance Corporation (IFC), the private-sector lending arm of the World Bank, have added health assessments to their investment safeguards as a positive step to anticipate and avoid health risks linked to their lending.[32]

The HIA model has been used to frame analyses of health benefits from climate change mitigation, as in the Health in a Green Economy WHO analyses, and HIA was proposed as a core tool for implementing HiAP in urban areas at the Habitat III World Summit.[33,34] Recent progress on methods include quantitative modeling of the expected health impacts of policy decisions.[35] HIA practice and scholarship have advanced our understanding of the context and the mechanisms by which HIA can contribute to HiAP.

6 Institutionalization of HIA

To generate health benefits, HIAs need to be implemented regularly in a multitude of policy decisions and not only occasionally. How to ensure that when, in most countries, there are no legal requirement for HIAs, is a core challenge. There are a number of examples of how HIA has been institutionalized.[36]

Importantly, EIAs are required by law in most countries worldwide. One strategy to extend the use of HIAs is to strengthen health assessments within environmental assessments.[37] The European Commission directive on EIAs, for example, now requires human health assessment to be included, possibly in response to earlier concerns that health promotion was being limited by not including health in EIAs.[16,38] The health assessments adopted by the IFC safeguards have also been adopted by other banks following the Equator Principles for financing large projects by private-sector lenders, as well as by the International Council on Mining and Metals.[32,39,40]

EIA regulations already reference human health, but, in practice, coverage of health within EIA is often limited to considerations of the physical environment (e.g., air, water soil, and pollution/emissions-related issues) usually measured against a national or international (e.g., WHO) threshold value or limit. The concern is that by integrating HIA into EIAs one could limit the extent of the health assessment, hide tradeoffs, or give the false impression that health is being adequately considered.

Good practice examples, guidance, and advocacy for integrating health within the EIA propose that EIAs must ensure that health implications are being assessed with an adequate degree of depth, consider positive health outcomes as well as negative ones, be based on health expertise, relate to accepted public health goals, and consult with health stakeholders. Additionally, good practice suggests that the results from the health assessment must be communicated and remain open to public scrutiny, as is the case with EIA results.

Stand-alone HIAs (i.e., those not linked to other assessments) have been introduced in several high-income countries, mostly by health departments, as a tool for HiAPs. Healthy Cities in Europe also had a specific focus on HIAs during their 2003–2008 implementation period, and cities like London have examined mayoral strategies through a HIA lens.[41,42] HIA adoption in the United States increased following a National Academy of Sciences report and support from philanthropic organizations and the CDC.[43-45] These HIAs consider social and environmental determinants of health and focus on the distribution of those impacts (health equity). Some of these countries and cities have applied HIAs to policies and plans, many develop guidance for the conduct of HIAs and carry out training and pilot implementation, and a few have created repositories of the evidence base needed for HIAs and examples of HIA practice (e.g., the HIA Gateway in the United Kingdom).

The implementation of HIA in those countries and cities has fluctuated over time, responding to contextual and historical circumstances.

7 Evaluations of HIA Implementation

An analysis of HIAs in Australia and New Zealand, countries which led important developments in this area, recognizes that there is still "limited legislative support for its use" and that "HIAs remain poorly integrated into policy development and decision making."[46] This is attributed to lack of structures and procedures to include HIA recommendations into policies and programs in other sectors, reluctance to add another impact assessment to an already crowded space, and lack of clarity about who funds and implements HIAs. Some technical issues, shared with other impact assessments, remain. Examples include the predictive nature of HIA, difficulty in documenting events, and lack of follow-up to examine if anticipated impacts took place.

A few countries like Thailand and regions like Quebec and British Columbia in Canada have embedded HIA into laws and regulations and mainstreamed the procedure as part of their commitment to HiAPs. An analysis of a Thai case points to the need for the "provision of policy and a regulatory framework for HIA implementation, capacity building and knowledge production at all levels and providing human resources for HIA practice and development."[47] A reflection on the Canadian experience identifies that, at both the federal and provincial levels, significant gains have been made but have not necessarily been sustained.[48] The Canadian government has produced an internationally recognized guide, two provinces have legislated HIA within the context of renewed Public Health Acts, and various public health units are exploring the implementation of HIA in their regions. Some public health organizations use what is called the *expert-driven model of HIA*, while the Quebec provincial government has structured HIA practice built on the "decision-support" model.

Following the introduction of HIA by Healthy Cities Europe in phase IV (2003–2008) as one of four core themes, HIA implementation continued during phase V (when it was not formally continued as a core theme), indicating that there was continued interest in and use of HIA among healthy cities, even though most cities did not feel they had the resources or experience to embark in HIA. The experience among those that did engage in HIA was examined regarding whether the process has opened opportunities for local people to be involved in decision-making.[49]

These were a mix of independent HIAs, HIAs integrated with EIAs or other impact assessments, or those joined to planning or regeneration efforts or other HiAP processes. These HIAs were introduced to respond to health inequities that resulted from the lack of awareness of decision-makers about the health impacts of policy decisions and the lack of a formal opportunity to consider health and health equity during those decisions.

Results identified barriers to implementation: these included lack of data, knowledge, skill, and experience for HIA implementation; lack of a legal basis/requirement; and lack of political support. Being a voluntary and not a statutory requirement may reduce the chances of HIA results being integrated into decisions.

Other evaluations also found that buy-in from other sectors and roles in agenda-setting depended on the inclusion of benefits or cost-saving aspects into the HIA framework and of solid evidence, as well as the adaptation of the tool to users' needs, the engagement of stakeholders, and the use of simple and clear language.[50] It was important that policy authors retained ownership of the policy while understanding its links with health and across other policies.

Feasibility is influenced by support from senior politicians, by allocated time and resources, and by the HIA being a systematic process that is seen as part of a long-term agenda, as well as by effective and regular communication with and engagement of stakeholders.[49] Enabling factors were access to training, access to WHO materials or expertise, and cooperation with academic departments or health authorities, as well as a preexisting culture of working across sectors, a supportive national policy context, and membership in the Healthy Cities network. Sustainability depends on developing an inclusive process and nurturing trust among partners throughout the process to integrate health into the long-term vision. The development of an HIA tool that can be used across a range of policies and the establishment of an HIA review service with local academia encourage generalizability.

8   HIA Today

While there is growing knowledge of and experience with HIA implementation, and there has been progress made in including HIA into EIAs and in carrying out stand-alone HIAs, there is still a big gap in the capacity of health systems to embrace it as a key tool for health protection and disease prevention. The need for "health in all policies" and "intersectoral action" for health are well accepted in the health sector, but the capacity for implementation mechanisms such as HIA is often missing.

HIAs are not yet considered a core function of health systems. The capacity for implementing HIAs still lies largely with academia and consultancy groups responding to demands for EIAs on mostly large infrastructure projects; this is a positive trend, but not enough to respond to some of the largest of today's global health challenges, including urbanization, pollution, and climate change.

There are major opportunities for urban public health through the systematic implementation of HIAs and the integration of health assessments as part of urban planning decisions.

HIA provides a mechanism with which to clarify connections and articulate healthy options in the implementation of the UN's Sustainable Development Goals (SDGs), including not only objectives in goals 3 (Health) and 11 (Cities), but also the goals of other SDGs focused on food and agriculture, energy, climate action, and sustainable consumption, for example.

Health systems are trusted to take a long-term view of the population's health, and they have the knowledge and the indicators to inform and influence other sectors while enhancing accountability over health drivers and outcomes.

The health sector must grasp the opportunities opened up by the expanding number of cities and the growing size of cities worldwide because two-thirds of the world's population is expected to be living in urban areas by 2050.[51] Urban policies, infrastructure, and investments have substantial health implications, but, so far, these are rarely taken into account. The wider use of HIAs to inform urban policies can be one of the key ingredients to promoting public health globally.

The vision is that the health sector will help create an urban development model that enhances cognition and reduces early life risks for children, improves the functional capacity of older persons, prevents injuries and noncommunicable diseases (through cleaner air, opportunities for physical activity, etc.), protects city dwellers from the health impacts of climate change (sea level rise, extreme weather, changes in vector-borne diseases), and promotes mental health (access to green and public spaces), all through an understanding and articulation of the links between urban planning and health and through engagement with other sectors in decision-making (Box 23.2).

9 How to Get There?

To implement HIAs more universally, we need (1) to harness our understanding of the determinants of health in urban areas (knowledge), (2) to provide wide access to the methods and tools for HIA implementation, (3) to create capacity for HIA in health systems (e.g., jobs dedicated to performing HIA and engaging in HiAP), (4) to include HIA as part of the core training provided by schools of public health, (5) to pilot HIA and document how specific policy decisions in a particular city can improve public health, (6) to use health information systems to track the health impacts of other sector policies (using an HIA framework), (7) to understand the regulatory framework that governs urban planning and engage with stakeholders in other sectors to help integrate relevant health knowledge in urban decisions, and (8) to establish robust communication strategies to raise awareness of and commitment to a vision of cities that incorporate health into decisions made across sectors.

There is a need for local and national governments to establish HIA and HiAP mechanisms in city rules and regulations to ensure their systematic and widespread implementation. This would not create health imperialism, as argued by some, in the same way that EIAs have not made environmental criteria overrule other criteria. The effective and systematic implementation of HIAs would, on the contrary, ensure that the health implications of urban decisions are visible and adequately represented in the process of decision-making. Decision-makers may still decide to privilege other competing

---

Box 23.2 **An Agenda for National Healthy Urban Policies**

1. Include Health Impact Assessment (HIA) as part of national urban policies and health policy, making it a requirement for the approval of decisions in urban planning, land use, transport, and housing, among others, parallel to the requirement for environment impact assessments.
2. Facilitate the use of HIA by municipalities and provide cities with a common pool of evidence on the health impacts of public policies relevant to the country/region, as well as methods, tools, case studies, and expertise/training. This will avoid having every city develop its own, thus enabling efficiencies and making best use of resources.
3. Develop a mechanism to track adoption, implementation, and results of HIAs and to estimate how they are affecting public policies. This will provide accountability over how public policies contribute (or not) to public health and enable stakeholders to understand and engage in decision-making that affects health.
4. Include HIA in core health systems functions, along with Health in All Policies (HiAP). The skill mix and experience for that function to be implemented include qualitative methods, such as policy and stakeholder analysis and stakeholder engagement; quantitative methods to estimate whose health will be affected and by how much; communication; advocacy; and health diplomacy.
5. Train HIA and HiAP skills and competencies as part of core public health training.
6. Develop a communication strategy to inform the public about the health impacts of urban policies and decisions and to report on progress and successes.

---

priorities, but, through HIA, health systems would ensure that health issues are given a fair hearing and consideration.

In conclusion, this chapter argues that HIA writ large provides a model for institutionalizing and developing capacity for HiAPs in the health sector, as well as a mechanism for engaging with other sectors in their policy-making by using a type of tool that is familiar to them. HIAs are put forward as a key tool for HiAPs, one that should be incorporated as a core part of health systems. Cities in particular, small and big, stand to benefit most from using sectoral policy decisions and investments as a golden opportunity to promote the health of their populations and create healthy urban futures through a wider use of HIAs.

References

1. *Closing the gaps in a generation: health equity through action on the social determinants of health.* Geneva, Switzerland: World Health Organization; 2008.

2. Milio N. *Promoting health through public policy.* Ottawa, Canada: Canadian Public Health Association; 1986.

3. Leppo K, Ollila E, Pena S, Wismar M, Cook S, eds. *Health in All Policies: seizing opportunities, implementing policies.* Helsinki, Finland: Ministry of Social Affairs and Health of Finland; 2013.

4. Butland B, Jebb S, Kopelman P, et al. *Foresight. Tackling obesities: future choices—project report.* 2nd ed. London: UK Government Office for Science; 2007.

5. Jebb S. Dusting off Foresights' obesity report. UK Government website. 2017. Available at https://foresightprojects.blog.gov.uk/2017/10/04/dusting-off-foresights-obesity-report/. Accessed September 11, 2018.

6. *Health Impact Assessment: main concepts and suggested approach. The Gothenburg Consensus Paper.* Copenhagen, Denmark: World Health Organization; 1999.

7. den Broeder L, Uiters E, ten Have W, Wagemakers A, Schuit AJ. Community participation in health impact assessment. A scoping review of the literature. *Environ Impact Assess Rev;* 2017; 66:33–42.

8. Quigley R, den Broeder L, Furu P, Bond A, Cave B, Bos R. *2006 Health Impact Assessment international best practice principles. Special publication series no. 5.* Fargo, ND: International Association of Impact Assessment; 2006.

9. Kemm J. *Health Impact Assessment. Past achievement, current understanding and future progress.* Oxford: Oxford University Press; 2013.

10. Harris-Roxas B, Harris E. Differing forms, differing purposes: a typology of health impact assessment. *Environ Impact Assess Rev.* 2011; 31(4):396–403.

11. Haigh F, Harris E, NG Chok H, et al. Characteristics of health impact assessments reported in Australia and New Zealand 2005-2009. *Aust N Z J Public Health.* 2013; 37(6):534–546.

12. Roué-Le Gall A, Jabot F, Health impact assessment on urban development projects in France: finding pathways to fit practice to context. *Glob Health Promot.* 2017; 24(2):25–34.

13. Health Impact Assessment. US Centers for Disease Control and Prevention (CDC) website. Available at https://www.cdc.gov/healthyplaces/hia.htm. Accessed September 11, 2018.

14. Ison E. Health impact assessment in the Network of European Cities. *J Urban Health.* 2013; 90(S):105–115.

15. Pennington A, Dreaves H, Scott-Samuel A, et al. Development of an urban health impact assessment methodology: indicating the health equity impacts of urban policies. *Eur J Public Health.* 2017; S2:56–61.

16. Fischer T, Cave B. Health in impact assessments: introduction to a special issue. *Impact Assessments and Project Appraisals.* 2018; 36(1):1–4.

17. *Protocol on strategic environmental assessment.* Geneva, Switzerland: United Nations Economic Commission for Europe; 2003.

18. Dora C. HIA in SEA and its application to policy in Europe. In Kemm J, Parry J, Palmer S, eds. *Health Impact Assessment.* Oxford: Oxford University Press; 2004: 403–410.

19. Birley M. *PEEM guidelines 2: guidelines for forecasting the vector-borne disease implications of water resource developments.* Geneva, Switzerland: World Health Organization; 1991.

20. Benoit F, Druet C, Hamel G, St-Pierre L. *Implementation of Section 54 of Québec's Public Health Act.* Québec, Canada: National Collaborating Centre for Healthy Public Policy; 2012.

21. Phoolcharoen W, Sukkumnoed D, Kessomboon P. Development of health impact assessment in Thailand: recent experiences and challenges. *Bull World Health Organ.* 2003; 81(6):465–467.

22. Public Health (Wales) Act 2017. Available at http://www.legislation.gov.uk/anaw/2017/2/contents/enacted. Accessed September 11, 2018.

23. Health equity impact assessment tool. Canadian Public Health Association website. Available at https://www.cpha.ca/health-equity-impact-assessment-tool. Accessed September 11, 2018.

24. Povall S, Haigh F, Abrahams D, Scott-Samuel A. Health equity impact assessment. *Health Promot Int.* 2014; 29(4):621–633.

25. Thackway S, Milat A, Develin E. Influencing urban environments for health: NSW Health's response. *NSW Public Health Bulletin;* 2017; 18:9–10.

26. NHS London Healthy Urban Development Unit (HUDU) website. Available at http://www.healthyurbandevelopment.nhs.uk. Accessed September 11, 2018.

27. *Eastern neighborhoods community health impact assessment.* San Francisco, CA: San Francisco Department of Public Health; 2007.

28. Harris-Roxas B, Simpson S. The NSW Health Impact Assessment Project. *NSW Public Health Bulletin.* 2005; 16(7-8):120–123.

29. Frumkin H, Frank L, Jackson R. *Urban sprawl and public health: designing, planning and building for healthy communities.* Washington, DC: Island Press; 2004.

30. Ghel J, Gemzoe L. *New city spaces.* Copenhagen, Denmark: Danish Architectural Press; 2003.

31. Winkler MS, Krieger GR, Divall MJ, Cissé G, Wielga M, Singer BH, Tanner M, Utzinger J. Untapped potential of health impact assessment. *Bull World Health Organ;* 2013; 91:237–312.

32. International Finance Corporation Framework—2006 edition. International Finance Corporation World Bank Group website. Available at https://www.ifc.org/wps/wcm/connect/topics_ext_content/ifc_external_corporate_site/sustainability-at-ifc/policies-standards/ifcsustainabilityframework_2006. Accessed on September 11, 2018.

33. Health in the green economy. World Health Organization website. Available at http://www.who.int/hia/green_economy/en/. Accessed September 11, 2018.

34. *Health as the pulse of the new urban agenda. United Nations Conference on Housing and Sustainable Urban Development, Quito 2016.* Geneva, Switzerland: World Health Organization; 2016.

35. Urban health and sustainable development. World Health Organization website. Available at http://www.who.int/sustainable-development/cities/en/. Accessed September 11, 2018.

36. Lee JH, Röbbel N, Dora C. *Cross-country analysis of the institutionalization of Health Impact Assessment.* Geneva, Switzerland: World Health Organization; 2013.

37. Harris P, Viliani F, Spickett J. Assessing health impacts within environmental impact assessments: an opportunity for public health globally which must not remain missed. *Int J Environ Res Public Health.* 2015; 12(1):1044–1049.

38. Tarkowski S, Ricciardi W. Health impact assessment in Europe: current dilemmas and challenges. *Eur J Public Health.* 2012; 22(5):612.

39. Equator Principles website. Available at http://equator-principles.com. Accessed September 11, 2018.

40. Good practice guidance on health impact assessment. International Council on Mining and Metals website. Available at https://www.icmm.com/en-gb/publications/health-and-safety/good-practice-guidance-on-health-impact-assessment. Accessed September 11, 2018.

41. Health impact assessment. World Health Organization website. Available at http://www.euro.who.int/en/health-topics/environment-and-health/urban-health/activities/health-impact-assessment. Accessed September 11, 2018.

42. Mindell J1, Bowen C, Herriot N, Findlay G, Atkinson S. Institutionalizing health impact assessment in London as a public health tool for increasing synergy between policies in other areas. *Public Health.* 2010; 124(2):107–114.

43. National Research Council. *Improving health in the United States: the role of health impact assessment.* Washington, DC: National Academies Press; 2011.

44. The health impact project. The Pew Charitable Trust website. Available at http://www.pewtrusts.org/en/projects/health-impact-project. Accessed September 11, 2018.

45. Healthy places. US Centers for Disease Control and Prevention (CDC) website. Available at https://www.cdc.gov/healthyplaces/fundedhias/default.htm. Accessed September 11, 2018.

46. Haigh F, Harris E, NG Chok H, et al. Characteristics of health impact assessments reported in Australia and New Zealand 2005–2009. *Aust N Z J Public Health.* 2013; 37(6):534–546.

47. Chanchitpricha C. *Effectiveness of health impact assessment (HIA) in Thailand: a case study of a Potash mine HIA in Udon Thani, Thailand.* [Dissertation]. Norwich, UK: University of East Anglia; 2012.

48. St. Pierre L. Health impact assessment in Canada. In Kemm J, ed. *Health impact assessment: past achievement, current understanding, and future progress.* New York: Oxford University Press; 2012.

49. Simos J, Spanswick L, Palmer N, Christie D. The role of health impact assessment in Phase V of the Healthy Cities European Network. *Health Promot Int.* 2015; 30 S1:i71–i85.

50. Harris P, Harris-Roxas B, Wise M, Harris L. Health impact assessment for urban and land-use planning and policy development: lessons from practice. *Planning Practice & Research.* 2010; 25(5):531–541.

51. Department of Economic and Social Affairs. *World urbanization prospects: the 2018 revision.* New York: United Nations; 2018.

24

Multilevel Perspectives
on Urban Health

DUSTIN T. DUNCAN, YAZAN A. AL-AJLOUNI, ILGAZ HISIRCI,
AND BASILE CHAIX

1 Introduction

Urban environments across the globe are unique and highly complex. Traditional public health approaches to studying urban environments are usually far too simple, focusing on only one "level" of influence in addition to standard, individual sociodemographic characteristics, which is one category of determinants in the social ecological model (see Figure 24.1), or examining the urban environments through a single methodological lens. To advance the next generation of urban health research and practice, researchers and practitioners are increasingly following a "multilevel" perspective that recognizes complexity in urban environments.

In examining people who reside or work in cities, the multilevel conceptual model is an organizational framework that takes us beyond questions of whether one factor in the environment is associated with or is a significant predictor of an outcome. It helps us to think about growing our understanding of the factors that influence disease and health. We get to ask questions like, "Does neighborhood matter?" But we also get to look at how the multiple of levels of an environment might be positive for some outcomes while troublesome for others across a range of geographic locations and populations. A multilevel perspective leads us to a more complex understanding of influences on health, but it also lays the foundation for testing the impact of interventions in the environment (such as urban planning initiatives) on multiple health outcomes and health behaviors.

In this chapter, we first describe a useful framework for promoting multilevel thinking (not just the classical multilevel regression analyses) in urban health research and practice. Following that, we provide examples of research and interventions that use multilevel approaches in urban health. We consider two specific health outcomes—HIV risk and sleep—which have received less attention than other urban health issues such as physical activity, food consumption, and obesity, issues that are now more commonly examined through multilevel approaches and analyses.

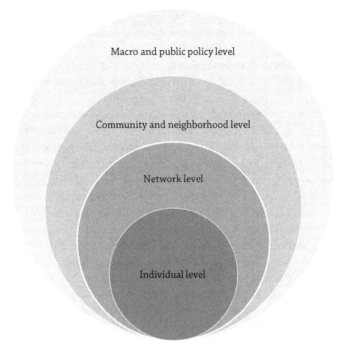

Figure 24.1 **A social ecological model for health.**

2 Framework of Multilevel Public Health and Urban Health

Typically, public health research and practice is poised to address one of the different levels of risks that may influence an individual's health-related behavior or health status in addition to classical sociodemographic factors such as gender, age, and race/ethnicity. A model for multilevel thinking is the *social-ecological model* (see Figure 24.1), which demonstrates that research and intervention designs can address a health behavior/status at one of the different levels of risks: individual level (sometimes referred to as intrapersonal factors), network level (sometimes referred to as interpersonal factors), community/neighborhood level, and macro and public policy level. The early social ecological model of human development was developed by Urie Bronfenbrenner, and there are several variations of this model, including modified models as applied to HIV epidemics.[1]

Research can be designed to investigate an exposure at one of these levels in relation to the health outcome of interest (after controlling for individual sociodemographics if relevant) in order to be able to distinguish the "roots" of specific behaviors (e.g., the health outcome is influenced by community factors vs. social networks) and target intervention strategies to address the behavior at that level. However, these different levels of risk are interconnected and can influence each other. Therefore, researchers need to develop protocols accounting for more than one level, which has direct implications for intervention planning. This is a major issue due to confounding variables that can potentially overestimate the effect of interest.

The individual level, which is the first level of risk, depends primarily on the biological, cognitive, and perceptual or behavioral factors associated with acquisition or transmission of risks. This can include being more vulnerable to a given disease due to genetic factors or self-motivated risk behaviors. The next level of risk is the network level, which can include social networks, family networks, sexual networks, and/or drug-using networks. Networks can influence an individual's behavior in different ways; for example, certain networks, such as parents or partners, can expose individuals to higher risk behaviors while others can be protective against high-risk behaviors through support and access to resources (via social capital). Furthermore, community-level risk, the third level, can play a role in influencing behaviors because it can affect individual-level behavior as well as one's social network and determine one's access to prevention resources, treatment, care services, and other types of resources that are useful to maintain health (e.g., healthy foods, parks, and sport facilities). Moreover, in addition to a range of physical exposures (e.g., air pollutants and noise), the community where residents live can either promote wellness or reinforce stigma and discrimination, which can negatively influence health behaviors and health outcomes.[2] The fourth level of risk that can be addressed in research and intervention is the macro and public policy level. Relevant macro-level factors include overall indicators of economic performance or economic crises and the policies implemented to intervene on population health that can either promote healthy behaviors or decrease risk behaviors. Combined together, these four levels of risk constitute the social-ecological model that seeks to organize the determinants of health behaviors, allowing research to investigate health outcomes at various exposure levels. The stream of research that emerged around the development of multilevel regression analysis in the mid-1990s and 2000s for isolating so-called neighborhood effects from compositional effects represented an initial empirical attempt to move in this direction, but it often neglected social networks and policies at macro levels when relevant.

A methodological approach related to multilevel public health research, included in neighborhood and health studies, is *agent–based modeling*.[3-5] Agent-based models are representations of these complex systems using a computational model that contains the algorithms and equations used to encode the behaviors of agents. A complex system can be defined as one in which the collective behaviors of the system are a result of dynamic interactions between the individual agents operating within that system. From these interactions emerge system-level properties that individual behaviors cannot explain on their own. While agent-based modeling is not meant to replace the empirical collection and analysis of data, it is a complementary approach that promotes a multilevel perspective in public health research.

In the next section, we discuss multilevel approaches to studying HIV risk and sleep, two different, significant public health outcomes. HIV is a global health issue.[6] Approximately 36.7 million people worldwide are estimated to be living with HIV/AIDS. The incident rate for HIV in 2016 was estimated to be 1.8 million, resulting in 5,000 new cases every day. Although perhaps seemingly less severe, poor sleep health is common and carries a multitude of health risks, including mental illness, substance use, diabetes, obesity, and hypertension.[7-10]

We focus on research examining one level of risk for each of the outcomes. We first start with HIV risk research, including studies that focus on gay, bisexual, and men who have sex with men (MSM) as these continue to be groups at greatest risk of HIV infection across the globe, including in the Caribbean, sub-Saharan Africa, Western Europe, and the United States.[11] We discuss one method for assessing risk levels in MSM (i.e., surveys delivered on popular geosocial networking applications for MSM populations).[12]

3 Examples of Different Levels Perspectives in HIV Risk Research

Duncan et al. conducted an individual-level study examining associations between financial hardship, condomless anal intercourse, and HIV risk among a sample of MSM in Paris.[13] The sample, recruited via an ad on a popular geosocial networking smartphone application for MSM, consisted of 580 Parisian users who provided informed consent and completed the survey. Financial hardship was defined as a difficulty in gaining resources to meet the needs to sustain a household. In this study, high financial hardship was associated with engagement in condomless anal intercourse, engagement in condomless receptive anal intercourse, engagement in condomless insertive anal intercourse, engagement in transactional sex, and infection with non-HIV sexually transmitted infections (STIs). This study suggests that individual-level interventions to reduce financial hardships could decrease sexual risk behaviors in MSM.

In another study, Duncan et al. investigated the effect of sexual networks on sexual risk behaviors.[14] This study examined the relationships between experiences of intimate partner violence (IPV) victimization and sexual risk behaviors in a sample of MSM in New York City. In this study, participants were recruited through ads on the geosocial-networking application and asked to complete a survey ($n = 175$). IPV was assessed through six yes–no statements on experiences with IPV in their lifetime, including physical IPV, sexual IPV, and psychological IPV (a combination of emotional, financial, isolation, and intimidation forms of IPV). Results revealed that lifetime experiences of IPV were common: overall, more than one-third of respondents reported having been the victim of at least one form of IPV in their lifetimes. In addition, this study found that 24% reported having been a victim of emotional IPV in their lifetimes, followed by 11.4% reporting having been a victim of sexual IPV. The least commonly reported form of IPV was financial IPV, with a prevalence of 4.6%. Moreover, having experienced any form of IPV victimization was associated with a higher total number of partners for both condomless receptive and insertive anal intercourse. As such, this study demonstrates that prevention methods may influence individual-level health behaviors by intervening on the network level, which is the second risk level in the social-ecological model.

At the community level, this group investigated the association between the types of venues for meeting sexual partners, condomless anal intercourse, engagement in group sex, and HIV/STI risk among a sample of MSM.[15] This study considered venues frequented by individuals to be a community-level risk that can influence an individual's behavior choice. The sample population (n = 580) consisted of geosocial-networking application users based in Paris who were recruited using a text advertisement encouraging them to complete an anonymous web-based survey. After adjustment for sociodemographics, multivariable models were used to assess the association between public venues (e.g., gay clubs, bars, and discos), cruising venues (e.g., gay saunas, beaches, and parks), and Internet-based venues (e.g., Internet chat sites and geosocial-networking apps), condomless anal intercourse, and engagement in group sex, as well as HIV infection and infection with other STIs. Results indicated that seeking sex through cruising venues was associated with risky sexual behavior: condomless receptive anal intercourse, any kind of condomless anal intercourse, multiple partners for both condomless insertive and receptive anal intercourse, engagement in group sex, an STI, and HIV infection. In addition, all venue types were associated with engagement in group sex. These findings revealed that environmental context within the community can foster risk behaviors that are directly linked to negative health outcomes and provides data that can be utilized for prevention at the community risk level.

While most studies assess just one level of health influences (as the examples provided earlier), some are beginning to embrace complexity by examining more than one level. For example, Eritsyan et al. examined the individual-, network-, and city-level factors associated with HIV prevalence among injection drug users (IDU) in eight Russian cities who were recruited via respondent driven sampling (RDS) (n = 2,596).[16] In particular, the multilevel factors included individual-level factors such as duration of injection (years) for a participant and whether or not the participant has been injected with HIV+ IDUs in the past, network-level factors such as mean size of the participant's RDS network in the past 6 months, and city-level factors such as the percentage of the dominant form of commercial heroin in the city and the average length of RDS chains in the city. In bivariate and multivariate models, several individual-, network-, and city-level factors were associated with HIV prevalence.

4 Examples of Different Levels Perspectives in Sleep Research

Research has investigated individual-level factors in poor sleep health, including individual-level race/ethnicity and individual-level private insurance status. For instance, Grandner et al. investigated the effect of race/ethnicity as well as having private insurance status in relation to sleep health.[17] Utilizing data from the 2007–2008 National Health and Nutrition Examination Survey (NHANES), the authors analyzed data from 4,081 individuals. Specifically, the study measured several sleep symptoms, including nonrestorative sleep, daytime sleepiness, snorting/gasping during sleep, and snoring. This study found that black/African American respondents were at increased risk for nonrestorative sleep and sleep latency when compared to non-Hispanic whites. Hispanic/Latino respondents were more likely to report snorting/gasping and snoring when compared to non-Hispanic whites. Additionally, the study found that not having private insurance was associated with poor sleep health. Overall, therefore, this study suggests that individual-level sociodemographic factors can influence sleep health.

In addition to individual-level factors, poor sleep health may be due to network-level factors. As an example, Alcantara et al. conducted a study that examined the association between different stressors (including ethnic discrimination) and sleep health.[18] Participants ($n = 5,313$) were recruited from several urban areas in the United States, including Chicago, Illinois; Miami, Florida; Bronx, New York; and San Diego, California. Participants were Hispanic/Latino adults aged 18–74. Data on ethnic discrimination and sleep health were collected using self-reported data from a survey. Insomnia, daytime sleepiness, and sleep duration were measured as three indicators of sleep health. Ethnic discrimination was found to be associated with several sleep measures, including daytime sleepiness and short sleep duration. The authors concluded that ethnic discrimination, as an example of a network-level factor, was associated with poor sleep in Hispanics/Latinos. Prevention methods that target network-level exposures, therefore, may help improve poor sleep health.

As for the third level of exposures in multilevel research, neighborhood-level exposures, we focus on an example study that investigates neighborhood safety as the main exposure associated with poor sleep health. Hill et al. studied the association between neighborhood safety and sleep health among participants ($n = 39,590$; age range 18–49 years) recruited from different countries, including Mexico, Ghana, South Africa, India, China, and Russia.[19] Sleep health measures included self-reported sleep duration, insomnia symptoms, sleepiness, lethargy, and overall sleep quality. The study found that respondents who feel safe from crime and violence in their neighborhoods tend to exhibit more favorable sleep outcomes than respondents who feel less safe. Perceptions of neighborhood safety were strongly associated with insomnia symptoms and poor sleep quality (past 30 days); moderately associated with sleepiness, lethargy, and poor sleep quality (past 2 days); and inconsistently associated with sleep duration (past 2 days). Interventions to address neighborhood-level exposures (i.e., increase neighborhood safety) therefore may improve sleep health among different populations.

As another example, a study by Oksanen et al. utilized a multilevel perspective, including individual and work-level variables, to examine the co-occurrence of sleep problems and obesity among employees and workplaces in Finland ($n = 39,873$).[20] Individual-level variables were identified as gender, age, and socioeconomic status (SES) through employer records. Work-level variables were identified as occupation type (permanent or temporary) and through survey responses that measured workplace social capital, job strain, and shift work. Results from multilevel logistic regression models for sleep problems and obesity indicated that both individual- and work-level factors influence sleep problems and obesity. For example, job strain was associated with both outcomes.

5 Example of Interventions at Different Multilevels

Multilevel interventions can be implemented to more adequately address public health concerns. For instance, interventions may be applied to target two (or more) levels simultaneously (e.g., intervention targeting both individual-level behaviors and community-level risk factors). These intervention studies are increasingly using the available evidence from observational research to design interventions that simultaneously address more than one level of influence on behavior or health status.

Lippman et al. conducted a multilevel STI/HIV intervention with sex workers in Corumbá, on Brazil's Western border with Bolivia, in order to improve condom use in an attempt to reduce the incidence of STIs.[21] In total, 420 sex workers were enrolled in the study, including 91.7% women, 4.5% men, and 3.8% transvestites. The intervention approach was designed using the social-ecological model described earlier. Intervention strategies targeted the individual level by facilitating participation in STI/HIV testing experiences, targeted the network-level through peer education and counseling, and targeted the community-level through outreach, workshops, and social activities. Concurrently, researchers worked with the city council and health officials to improve the quality of and access to sexual health facilities. Health outcomes of concern included incident chlamydia and/or gonorrhea diagnosis and reported condom use in the 3-month interval following reported intervention exposure. Overall, results indicate that exposure to the intervention was protective against incident STIs and resulted in increased reporting of consistent condom use. Participants exposed to the intervention had significantly higher odds of reporting consistent condom use with regular clients. Additionally, intervention exposure was associated with a significant increase in participation in networks and an increase in perceived social cohesion.

Similarly, Bonuck et al. designed a multilevel intervention approach to improve sleep health outcomes among families with young children, which has currently commenced.[22] This study targets the distal levels of the social-ecological model. For example, at the network level, media campaigns and agency-wide training will be put into place for agency staff and families. Additionally, intervention targeting the community will include forming a Health Services Advisory Council with support from local pediatricians and local sleep medicine specialists who will be available within the participants' community. Knowledge-translation strategies will be implemented on the policy/macro level. Sleep health outcomes will be mainly measured on the individual behavior level using a 7-day sleep log collected at different stages of the study to evaluate the parents' knowledge, attitudes, self-efficacy, and beliefs (a KASB measure), among other factors.

6 Conclusion

We note that a multilevel perspective is best represented by studies using external sources of data on networks, communities, and policies, rather than just self-reported data, in order to eliminate or minimize the risk of same-source bias and reverse causality. It is difficult—although not impossible—to obtain data on social contacts. One well-known example is the Framingham Heart Study, where direct information was collected from people connected with each other. Later researchers conducted social network analyses, including for obesity.[23] We are currently collecting Facebook data and downloading participants' contacts from their smartphones to create an approximated sociometric network in our ongoing longitudinal studies. We also note that some multilevel studies utilize objective measures of neighborhoods, such as police records of neighborhood crime in reported associations with sleep health outcomes in various populations.[24-26]

In summary, multilevel approaches are increasingly used in population health research and practice, including in urban health. While the initial attempts around multilevel regression analysis led to the increasing consideration of both individual and neighborhood factors, future studies need to further integrate the different components of the social ecological model simultaneously, including social networks and policy and other macro-level factors in analysis by using a wider range of methodological approaches (e.g., ABM). This research will ultimately result in more efficient intervention approaches targeting the various spheres of influences, but more research is needed across a range of health outcomes and health behaviors.

Acknowledgments

We thank Byoungjun Kim and Jessica Levitan for providing comments on an earlier version of this chapter.

References

1. Baral S, Logie CH, Grosso A, Wirtz AL, Beyrer C. Modified social ecological model: a tool to guide the assessment of the risks and risk contexts of HIV epidemics. *BMC Public Health.* 2013; 13(1):482.
2. Duncan DT, Kawachi I, eds. *Neighborhoods and health.* 2nd ed. New York: Oxford University Press; 2018.
3. Auchincloss AH, Diez Roux AV. A new tool for epidemiology: the usefulness of dynamic-agent models in understanding place effects on health. *Am J Epidemiol.* 2008; 168(1):1–8.
4. Yang Y, Diez Roux AV, Auchincloss AH, Rodriguez DA, Brown DG. A spatial agent-based model for the simulation of adults' daily walking within a city. *Am J Prev Med.* 2011; 40(3): 353–361.
5. Heaton B, El-Sayed A, Galea S. Agent-based models. In Duncan DT, Kawachi I, eds. *Neighborhoods and health.* 2nd ed. New York: Oxford University Press; 2018.
6. World Health Organization HIV/AIDS fact sheet. World Health Organization website. Available at http://www.who.int/news-room/fact-sheets/detail/hiv-aids. Accessed May 1, 2018.
7. Duncan DT, Goedel WC, Mayer KH, Safren SA, Palamar JJ, Hagen D, Jean-Louis G. Poor sleep health and its association with mental health, substance use, and condomless anal intercourse among gay, bisexual, and other men who have sex with men. *Sleep Health.* 2016; 2(4):316–321.
8. Zizi F, Jean-Louis G, Brown CD, Ogedegbe G, Boutin-Foster C, McFarlane SI. Sleep duration and the risk of diabetes mellitus: epidemiologic evidence and pathophysiologic insights. *Curr Diab Rep.* 2010;10(1): 43–47.
9. Jean-Louis G, Williams NJ, Sarpong D, et al. Associations between inadequate sleep and obesity in the US adult population: analysis of the national health interview survey (1977–2009). *BMC Public Health.* 2014; 14(1):290.
10. Gangwisch JE, Feskanich D, Malaspina D, Shen S, Forman JP. Sleep duration and risk for hypertension in women: results from the nurses' health study. *Am J Hypertens.* 2013; 26(7): 903–911.

11. Beyrer C, Baral SD, Van Griensven F, et al. Global epidemiology of HIV infection in men who have sex with men. *Lancet.* 2012; 380(9839): 367–377.

12. Goedel WC, Duncan DT. Geosocial-networking app usage patterns of gay, bisexual, and other men who have sex with men: survey among users of Grindr, a mobile dating app. *JMIR Public Health Surveill.* 2015; 1(1). doi: 10.2196/publichealth.4353.

13. Duncan DT, Park SH, Schneider JA, et al. Financial hardship, condomless anal intercourse and HIV risk among men who have sex with men. *AIDS Behav.* 2017; 21(12):3478–3485.

14. Duncan DT, Goedel WC, Stults CB, et al. A study of intimate partner violence, substance abuse, and sexual risk behaviors among gay, bisexual, and other men who have sex with men in a sample of geosocial-networking smartphone application users. *Am J Mens Health.* 2018; 12(2):292–301.

15. Al-Ajlouni YA, Park SH, Schneider JA, et al. Partner meeting venue typology and sexual risk behaviors among French men who have sex with men. *Int J STD AIDS.* 2018. doi:10.1177/0956462418775524.

16. Eritsyan K, Heimer R, Barbour R, et al. Individual-level, network-level and city-level factors associated with HIV prevalence among people who inject drugs in eight Russian cities: a cross-sectional study. *BMJ Open.* 2013; 3(6): e002645. doi:10.1136/bmjopen-2013-002645.

17. Grandner MA, Petrov MER, Rattanaumpawan P, Jackson N, Platt A, Patel NP. Sleep symptoms, race/ethnicity, and socioeconomic position. *J Clin Sleep Med.* 2013; 9(09):897–905.

18. Alcántara C, Patel SR, Carnethon M, et al. Stress and sleep: results from the Hispanic Community Health Study/Study of Latinos Sociocultural Ancillary Study. *SSM-Popul Health.* 2017; 3:713–721.

19. Hill TD, Trinh HN, Wen M, Hale L. Perceived neighborhood safety and sleep quality: a global analysis of six countries. *Sleep Med.* 2016; 18:56–60.

20. Oksanen T, Kawachi I, Subramanian S, et al. Do obesity and sleep problems cluster in the workplace? A multivariate, multilevel study. *Scand J Work Environ Health.* 2013; 39(3):276–283.

21. Lippman SA, Chinaglia M, Donini AA, Diaz J, Reingold A, Kerrigan DL. Findings from Encontros: a multilevel STI/HIV intervention to increase condom use, reduce STI, and change the social environment among sex workers in Brazil. *Sex Transm Dis.* 2012; 39(3):209.

22. Bonuck KA, Blank A, True-Felt B, Chervin R. Promoting sleep health among families of young children in Head Start: protocol for a social-ecological approach. *Prev Chronic Dis.* 2016; 13:E121. doi: 10.5888/pcd13.160144.

23. Christakis NA, Fowler JH. The spread of obesity in a large social network over 32 years. *N Engl J Med.* 2007; 357(4):370–379.

24. Johnson DA, Hirsch JA, Moore KA, Redline S, Diez Roux AV. Associations between the built environment and objective measures of sleep: the multi-ethnic study of atherosclerosis. *Am J Epidemiol.* 2018; 187(5):941–950.

25. Mellman TA, Bell KA, Abu-Bader SH, Kobayashi I. Neighborhood stress and autonomic nervous system activity during sleep. *Sleep.* 2018; 41(6):zsy059. doi: 10.1093/sleep/zsy059.

26. DeSantis A, Troxel WM, Beckman R, et al. Is the association between neighborhood characteristics and sleep quality mediated by psychological distress? An analysis of perceived and objective measures of 2 Pittsburgh neighborhoods. *Sleep health.* 2016; 2(4):277–282.

25

Cells-to-Society Approaches

GUIA GUFFANTI

1 Introduction

Urbanization is on the rise on a global scale; more than 70% of the world's population will live in cities by 2050. Along with opportunities, living in cities brings new challenges for the health of the individuals and their communities. The role of the environment in shaping our future development as well as our susceptibility to disease is indubitable. We are a product of our genetic makeup and environmental surroundings. A careful accounting of the empiric phenomena through which the environment influences our biology is important to define the most appropriate measures to control health and disease of urban populations. Cells-to-society approaches provide unique insights into how individual biology interacts with the urban environment to shape health. A cells-to-society framework begins at smaller units, at the personal level, with the identification of specific individual genetic risk factors then builds outward to the investigation of macro levels of the physical environment and social organization. In this chapter, I consider how new technological advancements in the field of molecular biology modified and improved our understanding of the mechanisms by which social and physical environments "get under the skin."

2 Epigenetic Vulnerability

Environmental exposure, such as nutrition, exposure to chemical compounds, physical exercise, physical and psychological stress, trauma, and many other factors, affects the way genes (DNA sequences) are ultimately expressed into a protein. The discipline that seeks to identify the mechanisms by which the environment induces alterations that change how genes function is called *epigenetics*. This emerging branch of biomedical science attempts to answer the question of how exposure to environmental stimuli may induce enduring alterations that were not genetically programmed. Such modifications arise at the molecular level without changing the genetic code of an individual, and new molecular technologies can easily quantify them.

The environmental exposure that occurs early in our lives, during embryonic development or early in the postnatal period, has the potential to mold our future growth and change how we respond to the environment or our susceptibility to disease later in life. The high sensitivity to epigenetic modification triggered by external stimuli early in our lives seems to be due to the substantial epigenetic changes naturally programmed during early development to initiate critical processes such as gametogenesis and early embryogenesis.[1] A growing body of evidence has shown an association between exposure to environmental changes early in life and the origin of late-onset disease, including metabolic, immune, cardiovascular, and behavioral complex disorders.[2,3] Although the epigenome seems to be mainly receptive to external stimuli during early development, its plasticity persists throughout the entire life course, albeit to a lesser degree. It can even leave a lasting signature that is passed on across generations. For example, clinical research in the context of war-related violence and natural disasters shows how traumatic stress may permanently alter the physiology of survivors in ways that are reflected in behavioral changes that are passed on to their descendants. Epigenetic factors can be inherited from environmentally exposed parents in the absence of further environmental influences (transgenerational effect, via the germline) or may involve a direct environmental exposure during in utero development (epigenetic inheritance, via cell-to-cell transfer). Of note, there has been increased interest in noncoding RNAs (ncRNAs) and long noncoding RNAs (lncRNAs) as mediators of gene regulation and transgenerational epigenetic inheritance. Transcriptome studies have also demonstrated the presence of ncRNAs in gametes, thus supporting the possible explanation of epigenetic transfer across generations.

This evidence all suggests an overall epigenetic vulnerability possibly interacting with the more traditionally acknowledged genetic one. Environment-induced epigenetic modification in genetically susceptible individuals may persist across the lifespan and exacerbate health outcomes, particularly during the so-called *sensitive periods*.

3 How Urban Stressors Can Get Under the Skin

As discussed elsewhere in this book, urban environments engender both physical and social stressors. Physical factors include, for example, chemical pollution, noise pollution, artificial night light pollution, infectious disease, and diet quality. Social factors include, for example, concentrated disadvantage, racial segregation, a dilapidated built environment, and crime. All of these factors are associated with some form of physiological (e.g., oxidative stress) and psychological stress.[4,5] It is evident that stressors do not act in isolation, but rather in synergy. To be able to comprehend the impact of urbanization on the biology of human populations, studies that explore the relation between each of these factors and biological changes are needed, but these remain relatively few.

Importantly, scientific advances in understanding *cells-to-society* mechanisms pave the way for newer and better science in this area. The mechanisms that mediate epigenetic regulation, including DNA methylation, the posttranslational modifications of histones, chromatin remodeling, and regulation by ncRNAs, are presented in Figure 25.1.

To date, the majority of studies implicating epigenetic phenomena as the molecular bridge that allows the environment to modify individual biology focused on DNA methylation. Epigenome association studies (EWAS) have been used consistently as

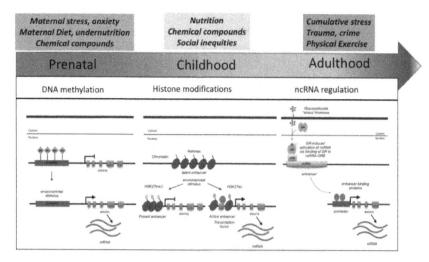

Figure 25.1 **Mechanisms underlying epigenetic vulnerability and environmental stressors across the lifespan.** The figure shows a list of the most common environmental stressors whose influence might be particularly relevant during the prenatal period, childhood, and adulthood, respectively. Also presented is a schematic of the three primary mechanisms of epigenetic effects, including DNA methylation, histone modifications, and ncRNA regulation and their activation upon exposure to an environmental stimulus.

a method to survey the epigenome of hundreds or thousands of subjects, leading to the identification of epigenetic risk factors in the etiology of several diseases, including cancer and psychiatric disorders.

Over the past two decades, unprecedented technological advances have raised new opportunities to understand the mechanisms underlying the complex machinery that determines the impact of genetic risk factors on health. International consortia such as the Human Genome Project (HGP) first and more recently the Encyclopedia of DNA Elements (ENCODE) Consortium, have revolutionized our understanding of the genome, both concerning its structure and function. Findings that genes only represent 2% of the entire human genome supported notions that other biological processes driven by the remaining 98% might influence gene expression and the observed variations in health outcomes. These discoveries empowered discussion about epigenetic effects.

New species of genes that do not produce proteins but rather transcriptional units lacking protein-coding potential with regulatory properties, commonly referred to as ncRNAs, are continually being discovered. In this context, an important class of ncRNAs remains largely understudied—that of human transposable elements (TEs), which include three major classes: long interspersed elements (LINE1), human endogenous retroviruses (HERVs), and short interspersed elements (SINE). Overall, TEs populate almost two-thirds of the human genome but are usually kept inactivated by epigenetic mechanisms, such as methylation and "silencing" histone modifications.[6] All of these ncRNAs are characterized by the presence of transcriptional regulatory elements present within their so-called promoter regions that can be bound by specific transcription factors to enhance the transcriptional regulation of neighboring target genes. The entire set of possible interactions of transcription factors with these regulatory elements has not been fully characterized, yet corticosteroid receptors/transcription factors functional elements, such as the glucocorticoid response elements (GRE), have been identified in TE sequences. This evidence opens up the hypothesis that glucocorticoid receptor (GR)-mediated mechanisms modulate the function of these regulatory elements. The primary function of ncRNAs is supposed to be the regulation of gene expression by acting as enhancers or repressors of the transcriptional activity of target genes. These recent developments are destined to revamp the traditional concept of gene-by-environment interactions, shedding light on the underlying biological mechanisms that fill the gap between the environment and the way our biology responds to it.

4 The Lifetime Temporal Aspects of Epigenetic Changes

One key feature of our emerging understanding of how environmental changes have the potential to modulate biology is that epigenetic patterns change throughout the entire lifespan. Emerging evidence of epigenetic changes over time introduced a new avenue for preventive medicine, along with the development of novel strategies for reversing the effects of this type of alteration. This provides important insights into how cells-to-society mechanisms can explain how the urban environment gets under the skin.

4.1 Prenatal Period

Exposure to environmental pollutants hazardous to human health is among the most critical risk factors in urban settings for the development of adult-onset pathologies, such as asthma and other allergic conditions later in life. These contaminants can cross the placenta during pregnancy and induce epigenetic alterations that alter the course of healthy development and set the stage for disease pathogenesis. The DNA of umbilical cord white blood cells of neonates whose mothers were exposed to airborne traffic-related polycyclic aromatic hydrocarbons (PAHs) during pregnancy revealed hypermethylation of the acyl-CoA synthetase long-chain family member 3 (ACSL3) gene, which is involved in asthma pathogenesis.[7]

Exposure to heavy metals such as cadmium early in life leads to epigenetic alterations that may persist over time into adulthood, leading to a higher risk of developing cardiovascular disease (CVD) and cancer. Cadmium intake during the periconceptional period was associated with LINE-1 hypomethylation in cord blood DNA, thereby increasing the transposable activity of this element, which has been associated with cancer.[8] LINE-1 is a transposable repetitive sequence which is normally highly methylated in normal tissues to prevent its expression; it has been found in a state of hypomethylation in cancerous tissues.

Specific groups, such as pregnant women and their young children, are particularly vulnerable to stressful and traumatic events and their consequences. Several prospective, longitudinal, mother–child cohort studies have found that children exposed to maternal psychological stress, depression, or anxiety during the prenatal period have a higher risk for behavioral and emotional problems later in life, including increased fearfulness, anxiety, and depression. Most of these studies focus on the GR and its stress-induced changes in DNA methylation, which, by alterations of the neuroendocrine system, lead to increased cortisol production. Promoter and exon 1 of GR revealed a profile of increased methylation in the cord blood and T lymphocytes of neonates of mothers exposed to maternal depression in the third trimester, with behavioral and epigenetic memory consequences that persisted to adolescence and adulthood in the hippocampal tissue of the brain.[9,10]

4.2 Childhood

Poverty, which is more frequent in urban settings than in rural areas, brings with it different stressors both physical, such as unhealthy diet habits, and social, such as increased prevalence of smoking. Both low socioeconomic status (SES) and social disadvantage influence a child's development even after the prenatal and postnatal phases, especially in those areas of the brain that are involved in response to stress and decision-making. In the past several years, several studies identified epigenetic mechanisms mediating the effect of continued exposure to stressors on the biology of childhood development. African American boys who grow up in highly disadvantaged environments display shorter telomeres (at age 9) than boys who grow up in highly advantaged environments. The association between the social environment and telomere length (TL) is moderated by genetic variation within the serotonin and dopamine pathways.[11] On the same line, lower SES during adolescence is associated with an increase in methylation of the proximal promoter of the serotonin transporter gene, which predicts more significant increases in threat-related amygdala reactivity.[12]

4.3 Adulthood

Cumulative lifetime stress was found to be associated with accelerated aging in an urban population of African Americans living in Atlanta, thereby potentially increasing the risk of developing aging-related diseases such as coronary artery disease, arteriosclerosis, and leukemias.[13] The authors of the study found that epigenetic changes induced by the stress hormone cortisol mediated the effect of cumulative lifetime stress on aging, but not childhood maltreatment or current stress alone. The study revealed that cortisol-induced methylation and consequent gene expression changes in genes harboring epigenetic marks were implicated in the regulation of the so-called *epigenetic clock*, which is commonly referred to as the comprehensive set of DNA methylation biomarkers that enable accurate age estimates for any tissue across the life course. Forms of stress exposure exacerbated in the urban setting include racial discrimination and segregation. Although these kinds of experiences have always been associated with poor health outcomes, the specific mechanisms about how perceived social inequities influence DNA methylation among minorities remain largely understudied. A large study of two longitudinal cohorts of African Americans revealed that youth exposed to high levels of racial discrimination forecast faster epigenetic aging in family environments that were less supportive than among youth in supportive family environments.[14] Another study reported on the significant epigenetic association between psychiatric disease-associated genes and perceived discrimination in African American women and their children. Although compelling, these findings warrant further investigations in high-risk populations.[15]

The evidence is accumulating that an increasing array of pollutants and toxins have an influence that extends beyond embryogenesis. The exposure to synthetic hormones and heavy metals such as nickel and benzo-a-pyrene, a pollutant resulting from residential wood burning, automobile exhausts, and cigarette smoke, induces increased expression of LINE-1 in the human transcriptome, eventually leading to increase the LINE-1 copy number in the genome, a phenomenon known as *retro-transposition*.[16–18] This phenomenon has recently been implicated in the mechanisms underlying somatic brain mosaicism. It is indeed tempting to imagine that environmental factors' effects on somatic diversity by means of stimuli-induced retrotransposition contribute to the overall genomic plasticity in the brain. Along with its importance for making up the ability to process complex information, it is possible that this source of genetic variation introduces a different layer of risk to develop brain-related disorders.[19]

Finally, densely populated urban areas often lack facilities and outdoor spaces for exercise and recreation available to the vast majority of their inhabitants. Also, the hectic lifestyle characteristic of urban living often leads to decreased time for physical activity. Exercise is widely and commonly acknowledged to have a positive impact on health and general well-being. Epigenetic alterations induced by aerobic training mediate the mechanisms through which exercise is beneficial to our health. These epigenetic changes modulate immune-related inflammatory processes as well as adipogenesis. An essential element in these processes is the regulation of metabolism. Exercise reduces promoter methylation of some genes involved in metabolic processes including PGC1-alpha in humans, thus leading to increasing upregulation of the gene relative to the amount of activity performed.[20]

5 Adaptions and Coping Mechanisms

In the previous section, we discussed how urban living contributes to epigenetic changes that influence susceptibility to a vast array of pathological outcomes. Although sporadic, research studies have started taking advantage of the technological advances in the field of epigenetics to investigate the potential of urban living to induce changes that provide a benefit to human health. Environmental factors might drive epigenetic alterations reflecting an adaptive mechanism, by which the organism can adjust its metabolism and homeostatic systems to increase survival or reproductive success in adulthood in a specific urban setting. In this context, disease development represents a form of inappropriate adaptation or maladaptation. A recent study examined how habitat and lifestyle mold the epigenetic profiles of African rainforest hunter-gatherers compared to populations that occupy primarily rural and urban deforested areas.[21] The analyses showed that DNA methylation, through its association with genetic variants, influenced the emergence of adaptive phenotypes, such as body size, conferring a better fitness to individuals in their specific habitats. Another example derived from the analysis of environmentally induced epigenetic changes that are inherited from one generation to the next. The offspring can inherit a wide array of methylation marks from both the mother and the father. We previously discussed the influence of these phenomena during perinatal life. Research revealed that a father's diet could influence the adaptation of his child to be better suited to the dietary conditions he lived in by transmitting epigenetic changes affecting the digestive systems of the child.[22] Overall, these examples demonstrate how biological insights provide a window into our understanding of how humans can be resilient to urban stressors.

6 Reversibility of Epigenetic Changes

Epigenetic changes represent an exciting area of research also because of their potential to be reversible, thus making cells adaptable to ever-changing environments and open to a wide range of possible interventions. Epigenetic changes do not affect the DNA sequence, but rather build on it through chemical reactions induced by specific enzymes, such as DNA methyltransferases (DNMTs) or histone deacetylases (HDACs), which determine the profiles of methylation and histone marks, respectively.[23] Therefore, inhibitors to specific target cells for these enzymes can reverse these epigenetic changes. Although some examples of epigenetic therapies based on these epigenetic inhibitors were successful in cancer treatment, these remain sporadic examples and many challenges remain. Concerns are raised because, by targeting an epigenetic mark, drugs might lead to large-scale epigenetic deregulation, rather than target specific candidate epigenomic elements. Research to refine these processes is still in its early stages. Another promising path to reverse changes includes the epigenomic modifiers encoded by ncRNA and microRNAs. These targets are used to modify their posttranscriptional effects, influencing the gene expression in their regulatory network. Epigenetic-modifying drugs to change cells, such as induced pluripotent stem cells (iPSCs), can be used for directing reprogramming of stem cells and, ultimately, the regeneration of tissues as a component of epigenetic medical therapy. All of these approaches highlight the key role of the manipulation of the plasticity of our epigenome to respond to a constantly changing environment, such as that presented by urban settings. Restoring the impaired epigenetic patterns is not only relevant in the context of curing diseases, but also in terms of prevention. For example, as described earlier, physical exercise is known to induce epigenetic changes that are able to influence metabolism. It is conceivable that by simply modifying physical exercise habits it is possible to manipulate metabolic rebooting, supported either via the development of pharmaceuticals, nutraceuticals, or even light-activated implants, with an overall benefit for human health.[24]

7 Future Prospects

Several findings suggest that epigenetic alterations induced by the urban environment play a significant role in health and disease, and further research is therefore warranted. This chapter reports emerging evidence of how health is influenced over the lifespan by epigenetic changes induced by the exposure to urban stressors and points out that it is necessary to carry out further studies that focus on the global effect of environment on human health in urban settings. These should include a thorough assessment of physical and social stressors, which should be studied not just in their singular repercussions, but also and most importantly in synergy. I also highlighted the sophisticated modulation of the environment during different phases of life, from prenatal to postnatal, from childhood to adulthood, and how understanding epigenomic responsiveness to temporally specific environmentally induced changes can be leveraged as an alternative tool for the prevention of diseases. Expectant mothers are an essential group to target with preventive and interventional measures. But since the delay between exposure during embryogenesis and the onset of disease in adults suggests that the environment induces stable changes, it is equally critical to investigate which genes and pathways are altered by the environment early in life that can leave a permanent signature that increases the risk of disease later in life. Furthermore, stressful exposures in adult life may trigger persistent epigenetic modifications that may interact with those involved in the process of developmental programming since the epigenome remains sensitive throughout adulthood.

Another critical issue that remains to be clarified refers to the maintenance and inheritance of environmentally induced epigenetic changes and how they can shape adaptations to increase individual fitness to the environment. Finally, we discussed the opportunities provided by the essential reversibility of epigenetic changes both regarding therapeutic and preventive interventions.

In the future, single-cell transcriptomics might prove critical for understanding the complex dynamics of gene regulation programs influenced by the environment and could be used to reveal differences among different cells to further exploit their target reversibility. As in other fields, the potential of studying molecular processes such as those characterizing epigenetic marks can be improved by considering these in the broader context of cell function. Overlapping multiple layers of information, spanning from genetic through epigenetics to transcriptomics and proteomics, is becoming the most robust approach to understanding the biology underlying molecular changes. The effect of epigenetic marks variation might be in fact associated with genetic variants and gene expression patterns or protein levels that can only be captured in a multi-omic investigation.

Studying epigenetic vulnerability and sensitivity to the environment in urban settings might open new avenues for a better understating of epigenetic changes and may play a key role in the future of interventional health programs that take into account the effect of the environment on health.

References

1. Hochberg Z, Feil R, Constancia M, et al. Child health, developmental plasticity, and epigenetic programming. *Endocr Rev.* 2011; 32:159–224.
2. Skinner MK, Manikkam M, Guerrero-Bosagna C. Epigenetic transgenerational actions of environmental factors in disease etiology. *Trends Endocrinol Metab.* 2010; 21:214–222.
3. Kubota T. Epigenetic alterations induced by environmental stress associated with metabolic and neurodevelopmental disorders. *Environ Epigenet.* 2016; 2(3):dvw017. doi:10.1093/eep/dvw017

4. Galea S, Freudenberg N, Vlahov D. Cities and population health. *Soc Sci Med.* 2005; 60: 1017–1033.

5. Galea S, Uddin M, Koenen K. The urban environment and mental disorders: epigenetic links. *Epigenetics.* 2011; 6:400–404.

6. Guffanti G, Gaudi S, Fallon JH, et al. Transposable elements and psychiatric disorders. *Am J Med Genet B Neuropsychiatr Genet.* 2014; 165B(3):201–216.

7. Perera F, Tang WY, Herbstman J, et al. Relation of DNA methylation of 5'-CpG island of ACSL3 to transplacental exposure to airborne polycyclic aromatic hydrocarbons and child-hood asthma. *PLoS One.* 2009; 4:e4488. doi:10.1371/journal.pone.0004488

8. Hossain MB, Vahter M, Concha G, Broberg K. Low-level environmental cadmium exposure is associated with DNA hypomethylation in Argentinean women. *Environ Health Perspect.* 2012; 120:879–884.

9. Oberlander TF, Weinberg J, Papsdorf M, Grunau R, Misri S, Devlin AM. Prenatal exposure to maternal depression, neonatal methylation of human glucocorticoid receptor gene (NR3C1) and infant cortisol stress responses. *Epigenetics.* 2008; 3:97–106.

10. Nemoda Z, Massart R, Suderman M, et al. Maternal depression is associated with DNA meth-ylation changes in cord blood T lymphocytes and adult hippocampi. *Transl Psychiatry.* 2015; 5:e545. doi:10.1038/tp.2015.32

11. Mitchell C, Hobcraft J, McLanahan SS, et al. Social disadvantage, genetic sensitivity, and children's telomere length. *Proc Natl Acad Sci U S A.* 2014; 111:5944–5949.

12. Swartz JR, Hariri AR, Williamson DE. An epigenetic mechanism links socioeconomic status to changes in depression-related brain function in high-risk adolescents. *Mol Psychiatry.* 2017; 22:209–214.

13. Zannas AS, Arloth J, Carrillo-Roa T, et al. Lifetime stress accelerates epigenetic aging in an urban, African American cohort: relevance of glucocorticoid signaling. *Genome Biol.* 2015;16:266.

14. Brody GH, Miller GE, Yu T, Beach SR, Chen E. Supportive family environments ameliorate the link between racial discrimination and epigenetic aging: a replication across two longitu-dinal cohorts. *Psychol Sci.* 2016; 27:530–541.

15. de Mendoza VB, Huang Y, Crusto CA, Sun YV, Taylor JY. Perceived racial discrimination and DNA Methylation among African American women in the InterGEN Study. *Biol Res Nurs.* 2018; 20:145–152.

16. Morales JF, Snow ET, Murnane JP. Environmental factors affecting transcription of the human L1 retrotransposon. I. Steroid hormone-like agents. *Mutagenesis.* 2002; 17:193–200.

17. El-Sawy M, Kale SP, Dugan C, et al. Nickel stimulates L1 retrotransposition by a post-transcriptional mechanism. *J Mol Biol.* 2005; 354:246–257.

18. Stribinskis V, Ramos KS. Activation of human long interspersed nuclear element 1 retrotransposition by benzo(a)pyrene, an ubiquitous environmental carcinogen. *Cancer Res.* 2006; 66:2616–2620.

19. Bedrosian TA, Linker S, & Gage FH. Environment-driven somatic mosaicism in brain disorders. *Genome Med.* 2016; 8:58.

20. Bajpeyi S, Covington JD, Taylor EM, Stewart LK, Galgani JE, Henagan TM. Skeletal muscle PGC1alpha -1 nucleosome position and -260nt DNA methylation determine exercise response and prevent ectopic lipid accumulation in men. *Endocrinology.* 2017; 158:2190–2199.

21. Fagny M, Patin E, MacIsaac JL, et al. The epigenomic landscape of African rainforest hunter-gatherers and farmers. *Nat Commun.* 2015; 6:10047.

22. Soubry A. Epigenetic inheritance and evolution: a paternal perspective on dietary influences. *Prog Biophys Mol Biol.* 2015; 118: 79–85.

23. Hamm CA, Costa FF. Epigenomes as therapeutic targets. *Pharmacol Ther.* 2015; 151:72–86.

24. Folcher M, Oesterle S, Zwicky K, et al. Mind-controlled transgene expression by a wireless-powered optogenetic designer cell implant. *Nat Commun.* 2014; 5: 5392.

26

Social Networks

ABBY E. RUDOLPH

1 Background

Traditionally, research in the social sciences focuses on understanding the relationship between individual-level outcomes and exposures. Social network analysis (SNA) focuses instead on the relationships between entities (e.g., people, places, organizations, etc.) and aims to understand how these relations influence attitudes, beliefs, and behaviors; the spread of infectious diseases; and the diffusion of ideas and behaviors, among other things.

SNA provides a set of tools and approaches for measuring (1) an individual's exposure to resources, information, diseases, and behaviors from his or her network members; (2) the association between individual attributes and those of network members (e.g., social norms, homophily, selection, peer influence); (3) individual positions within a network that make some more influential or susceptible than others; and (4) network-level characteristics that affect diffusion of resources, information, diseases, and behaviors. Different analytic approaches are used to address different research questions and include personal (or "egocentric"), dyadic, sociometric, and two-mode network analyses.

1.1 Egocentric

Egocentric network analyses focus on individuals and aim to understand how individuals are influenced by their network members. Variables of interest include the number of network members, personal network density (e.g., the extent to which one's network members are connected to one another), and the number (or proportion) of network members with a particular attribute.

1.2 Dyadic

Dyadic analyses focus on relationship-level characteristics, including the frequency of interaction, duration, strength, relationship type, and ego–alter similarities/differences. Relationship types can include drug use partner, sexual partner, relative, and provision of social support, among others. Dyadic analyses aim to understand whether (1) some

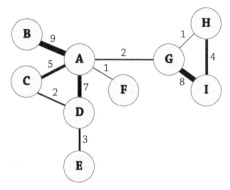

Figure 26.1 **Sociometric network with relationships of varying strength.** Circles represent individuals, lines represent relationships between individuals, and the thickness of each line and its corresponding weight indicate the strength of each relationship.

relationships are more influential than others, (2) one type of relationship predicts another, and (3) associations identified in egocentric network analyses are modified by relationship-level characteristics. Relationship-level information can also be used to create weights for other network analyses (see Figure 26.1).

1.3 Sociometric

Sociometric networks consist of all ties that exist between members of a target population. Sociometric network analyses can focus on (1) network-level measures that characterize the overall network structure; (2) individual-level measures, which characterize individuals' positions within the larger network; and (3) diffusion or contagion. For example, the overall network *density* (i.e., the number of connections in the network divided by the total number possible) can influence how quickly diseases, behaviors, and information flow through a network. Sociometric network analyses can also identify *subgroups* and *microstructures* that influence how quickly diseases, attitudes, and behaviors can spread/diffuse across the network. Individual-level network measures can identify members of the network who may be more influential due to their role as a broker (i.e., *betweenness centrality*) between distinct subgroups or their popularity (i.e., *degree centrality*), for example. *Geodesic distance* (i.e., number of relationships in the shortest path between any two network members) is also commonly used in studies that measure diffusion and contagion.

1.4 Two-Mode

Two-mode network analyses focus on relationships between two sets of entities (e.g., $mode_1$ = people and $mode_2$ = venues). Two-mode data can be converted into two one-mode network datasets representing, for example, people connected to people through shared venues and venues connected to other venues by shared patrons.

This chapter will provide an overview of how SNA has been used to advance research on gun violence and infectious disease transmission, two major public health concerns in urban settings, and will suggest directions for future research.

2 Gun Violence

Although the highest rates of gun-related homicide are in Central and South America, they were 25.2 times higher in the United States than in other high-income countries.[1] Within the United States, many studies have demonstrated that gun-related homicide is more concentrated in socioeconomically disadvantaged and minority neighborhoods.[2–4] More recent work has shed light on the fact that (1) a majority of fatal and nonfatal gunshot injuries and gun-related homicides cluster within networks and (2) interneighborhood co-offending networks may help to explain why crime rates are higher in some neighborhoods than in others.[5–8] Although risk factor approaches can determine individual-level characteristics that increase one's risk of gunshot victimization, social network approaches can help us understand why some individuals with these characteristics are more likely to be victims than others and can help explain persistent inequalities in neighborhood crime rates.[6,8]

There is rationale for examining social networks based on (1) the social learning theory, which posits that deviant social norms and peers who provide information, skills, material resources, and logistical support can promote criminal deviance; (2) literature which suggests that both peer influence and socialization shape criminal and delinquent behavior; and (3) a review article noting an increased risk of victimization and perpetration among those with interpersonal relationships to others who have either been victims or perpetrators of violence.[8–12]

Much of the social network research on gun violence involves the transformation of two-mode data (i.e., $mode_1$ = individuals and $mode_2$ = arrests) into one-mode co-offending networks, where relationships are defined by an arrest for the same offense.[5,6,13–15] For example, arrest data from Chicago were used to generate a *sociometric* network of 169,725 individuals, each with at least one co-offending tie to another person in the dataset. This network represented about 6% of Chicago's total population, but 40% of those arrested and 70% of all nonfatal shootings during the study period. While 63% of individuals were located in the main component (i.e., largest group of connected individuals), shooting victims were disproportionately represented in this component (89%). Study findings suggest that one's probability of victimization increased as network exposure to nonfatal gunshot victims (through both direct and indirect ties) increased.[6] Two-mode network analysis has also been used to construct a one-mode network of neighborhoods connected through co-offending relationships. Study findings showed that neighborhoods with higher levels of social cohesion had higher crime rates.[8,15]

In another analysis, which examined both egocentric (personal network density, percent of gang members in one's personal network, and percent of personal network members who have been shot) and sociometric network (the average geodesic distance between an individual and a shooting/homicide victim) measures, researchers reported that one's probability of gunshot victimization increased as the proportion of one's network who had been shot increased and with shorter average distances to a shooting/homicide victim.[5]

Dyadic analyses looking at co-offending stability found that as the number of individual arrests increased, the likelihood of co-offending with someone with whom they were previously arrested also increased.[13]

Finally, others have examined the spread (or contagion) of violence through networks.[14,16–18] One study reported that one's probability of being shot increased immediately after a network member was shot; after ruling out competing explanations, including homophily (propensity for individuals to associate with similar others) and confounding due to shared environment, the authors concluded that social contagion accounted for 63.1% of gunshot violent occurrences.[14]

3 Infectious Diseases

Because infectious diseases are spread through person-to-person contact, social network-based approaches have been used to (1) identify previously undiagnosed cases through contact tracing (i.e., partner notification), (2) understand disease transmission dynamics, (3) provide insight into persisting racial and socioeconomic disparities in disease incidence/prevalence, and (4) inform intervention strategies to prevent transmission to susceptible others (e.g., whom to target with vaccination, quarantine, treatment, testing, or pre-exposure prophylaxis).[19–21]

Contact tracing is a public health strategy routinely used to control infectious disease outbreaks (e.g., tuberculosis, SARS, Ebola, HIV, and other sexually transmitted infections). With contact tracing, cases are asked to provide the names and contact information for relevant contacts (e.g., determined based on the route of disease transmission). Healthcare workers then contact named individuals for further testing and questioning. This process continues until those approached and tested are no longer identified as cases. Mapping contact networks can reveal transmission patterns and network structures that facilitate/inhibit transmission.[22,23] Contact networks have also identified geographic bridges and venues which play key roles in disease transmission.[24–27]

Because network characteristics, structures, and norms influence individual-level behaviors and disease transmission, SNA has played a prominent role in HIV prevention and intervention research. To date, HIV-related egocentric network analyses have focused on the relationships (1) between network norms and drug/sex-related risk behaviors and (2) between personal network characteristics and HIV status or risk/health-seeking behaviors. While many studies find that individuals with a greater number and proportion of risk network members have higher risk sexual and drug use behaviors, the presence of multiplex relationships (e.g., multidimensional relationships) may also influence risk and health-seeking behaviors, potentially by making risk behaviors more difficult to modify when risk behaviors occur with partners who also provide social support.[28] HIV/HCV prevention interventions based on social network theory have historically leveraged existing relationships among the target population to reduce sex/drug-related risk behaviors and promote drug treatment enrollment.[29,30]

Sociometric network analyses have identified network-level (i.e., more dense networks and cohesive microstructures) facilitators of disease transmission and have determined that those in more central locations of the network are at increased risk for HIV, HCV, and STIs.[31-37] Sociometric network analyses have also highlighted targets (i.e., individuals with higher betweenness centrality) for network-based interventions.[32,36,38-42]

Two-mode network analyses, or "affiliation networks" (i.e., $mode_1$ = venues and $mode_2$ = people) have been used to identify partner meeting locations associated with riskier behaviors and which could be targeted for future prevention interventions based on their network positions.[27,43,44]

Because HIV-1 *pol* gene sequences obtained from routine genotypic tests of drug resistance encode sufficient viral variation to infer putative HIV transmission linkages,[45] researchers are increasingly using phylogenetic analysis and whole-genome sequencing for disease surveillance and prevention.[46,47] One limitation of this work is that analyses that use viral sequence information only include those with the disease; analyses that combine phylogenetic and social network data (including risk partners who do not have the disease) can identify uninfected individuals at increased risk for infection due to their contact with others who are infected.[48-54]

4 Future Directions

A common limitation of many SNAs, including many of those referenced earlier, is that sociometric network datasets may not consist of all members of the target population. The extent to which missing data or selection into the sample may influence inference is one area that requires further research and discussion. It is also frequently difficult to distinguish between influence (i.e., individuals are influenced by their peers' behaviors) and selection (i.e., individuals select peers with similar behaviors). Related to this limitation is the fact that many researchers focus on identifying social network factors associated with risk behaviors or outcomes. It is unknown, however, whether the same processes driving risk behaviors and transmission work similarly in the opposite direction. For example, would altering the network structure of co-offenders reduce gun violence? If network members start engaging in lower risk drug use practices, will an individual's drug use risk behaviors also reduce, or will they select new peers with behaviors more similar to theirs? While social network research has made important contributions to understanding urban health issues, more work is needed to develop methods to account for selection and missing data and to distinguish between peer influence and selection to better understand the social processes driving both risk and health-seeking behaviors and to inform the development of more effective health-promoting interventions.

References

1. Grinshteyn E, Hemenway D. Violent death rates: the US compared with other high-income OECD countries, 2010. *Am J Med.* 2016; 129(3):266–273.

2. Morenoff JD, Sampson RJ, Raudenbush SW. Neighborhood inequality, collective efficacy, and the spatial dynamics of urban violence. *Criminology.* 2001; 39(3):517–558.
3. Peterson RD, Krivo LJ. *Divergent social worlds: neighborhood crime and the racial-spatial divide.* New York: Russell Sage Foundation; 2010.
4. Jones-Webb R, Wall M. Neighborhood racial/ethnic concentration, social disadvantage, and homicide risk: an ecological analysis of 10 US cities. *J Urban Health.* 2008; 85(5):662.
5. Papachristos AV, Braga AA, Hureau DM. Social networks and the risk of gunshot injury. *J Urban Health.* 2012; 89(6):992–1003.
6. Papachristos AV, Wildeman C, Roberto E. Tragic, but not random: the social contagion of nonfatal gunshot injuries. *Soc Sci Med.* 2015; 125:139–150.
7. Papachristos AV, Wildeman C. Network exposure and homicide victimization in an African American community. *Am J Public Health.* 2014; 104(1):143–150.
8. Bastomski S, Brazil N, Papachristos AV. Neighborhood co-offending networks, structural embeddedness, and violent crime in Chicago. *Soc Networks.* 2017; 51:23–39.
9. Haynie DL, Osgood DW. Reconsidering peers and delinquency: how do peers matter? *Soc Forces.* 2005; 84(2):1109–1130.
10. Haynie DL. Friendship networks and delinquency: The relative nature of peer delinquency. *J Quant Criminol.* 2002; 18(2):99–134.
11. Monahan KC, Steinberg L, Cauffman E. Affiliation with antisocial peers, susceptibility to peer influence, and antisocial behavior during the transition to adulthood. *Dev Psychol.* 2009; 45(6):1520.
12. Tracy M, Braga AA, Papachristos AV. The transmission of gun and other weapon-involved violence within social networks. *Epidemiol Rev.* 2016; 38(1):70–86.
13. Grund T, Morselli C. Overlapping crime: stability and specialization of co-offending relationships. *Soc Networks.* 2017; 5(1):14–22.
14. Green B, Horel T, Papachristos AV. Modeling contagion through social networks to explain and predict gunshot violence in Chicago, 2006 to 2014. *JAMA Intern Med.* 2017; 177(3):326–333.
15. Schaefer DR. Youth co-offending networks: an investigation of social and spatial effects. *Soc Networks.* 2012; 34(1):141–149.
16. Fagan J, Wilkinson DL, Davies G. Social contagion of violence. 2007. In Flannery D, Vazsonyi A, Waldman I, eds. *The Cambridge handbook of violent behavior and aggression.* Cambridge: Cambridge University Press; 2007.
17. Topalli V, Wright R, Fornango R. Drug dealers, robbery and retaliation. Vulnerability, deterrence and the contagion of violence. *Br J Criminol.* 2002; 42(2):337–351.
18. Huesmann LR. The contagion of violence: the extent, the processes and the outcomes. Paper presented at the Institute of Medicine and National Research Council *Contagion of violence: workshop.* Washington, DC: National Academies Press; 2012.
19. Sullivan PS, Peterson J, Rosenberg ES, et al. Understanding racial HIV/STI disparities in black and white men who have sex with men: a multilevel approach. *PloS One.* 2014; 9(3):e90514. doi:10.1371/journal.pone.0090514
20. Williams KM, Prather CM. Racism, poverty and HIV/AIDS among African Americans. In McCree DH, Jones KT, O'Leary A, eds. *African Americans and HIV/AIDS.* New York: Springer; 2010: 31–51.
21. Denning P, DiNenno E. Communities in crisis: is there a generalized HIV epidemic in impoverished urban areas of the United States? Poster for the Centers for Disease Control and Prevention, National Center for HIV Viral Hepatitis STD and TB Prevention. 2010.
22. Klovdahl AS. Social networks and the spread of infectious diseases: the AIDS example. *Soc Sci Med.* 1985; 21(11):1203–1216.
23. Potterat JJ, Muth S, Rothenberg R, et al. Sexual network structure as an indicator of epidemic phase. *Sex Transm Infect.* 2002; 78(S1):i152–i158.
24. D'Angelo-Scott H, Cutler J, Friedman D, Hendriks A, Jolly A. Social network investigation of a syphilis outbreak in Ottawa, Ontario. *Can J Infect Dis Med Microbiol.* 2015; 26(5):268–272.

25. Nordvik MK, Liljeros F, Österlund A, Herrmann B. Spatial bridges and the spread of Chlamydia: the case of a county in Sweden. *Sex Transm Dis.* 2007; 34(1):47–53.

26. Kerani RP, Golden MR, Whittington WL, Handsfield HH, Hogben M, Holmes KK. Spatial bridges for the importation of gonorrhea and chlamydial infection. *Sex Transm Dis.* 2003; 30(10):742–749.

27. Oster AM, Wejnert C, Mena LA, Elmore K, Fisher H, Heffelfinger JD. Network analysis among HIV-infected young black men who have sex with men demonstrates high connectedness around few venues. *Sex Transm Dis.* 2013; 40(3):206.

28. Rudolph AE, Crawford ND, Latkin C, Lewis CF. Multiplex relationships and HIV: implications for network-based interventions. *AIDS Behav.* 2017; 21(4):1219–1227.

29. Latkin CA, Mandell W, Vlahov D, Oziemkowska M, Celentano DD. The long-term outcome of a personal network-oriented HIV prevention intervention for injection drug users: the SAFE study. *Am J Community Psychol.* 1996; 24(3):341–364.

30. Latkin CA, Sherman S, Knowlton A. HIV prevention among drug users: outcome of a network-oriented peer outreach intervention. *Health Psychol.* 2003; 22(4):332.

31. Liljeros F, Edling CR, Nunes Amaral LA. Sexual networks: implications for the transmission of sexually transmitted infections. *Microbes Infect.* 2003; 5(2):189–196.

32. Friedman SR, Neaigus A, Jose B, et al. Sociometric risk networks and risk for HIV infection. *Am J Public Health.* 1997; 87(8):1289–1296.

33. Rothenberg RB, Potterat JJ, Woodhouse DE, Muth SQ, Darrow WW, Klovdahl AS. Social network dynamics and HIV transmission. *AIDS.* 1998; 12(12):1529–1536.

34. Rothenberg RB, Potterat JJ, Woodhouse DE, Darrow WW, Muth SQ, Klovdahl AS. Choosing a centrality measure—epidemiologic correlates in the Colorado-Springs study of social networks. *Soc Networks.* 1995; 17(3-4):273–297.

35. Rothenberg RB, Sterk C, Toomey KE, et al. Using social network and ethnographic tools to evaluate syphilis transmission. *Sex Transm Dis.* 1998; 25(3):154–160.

36. De P, Singh AE, Wong T, Yacoub W, Jolly AM. Sexual network analysis of a gonorrhoea outbreak. *Sex Transm Infect.* 2004; 80(4):280–285.

37. Bell DC, Atkinson JS, Carlson JW. Centrality measures for disease transmission networks. *Soc Networks.* 1999; 21(1):1–21.

38. Shah NS, Iveniuk J, Muth SQ, et al. Structural bridging network position is associated with HIV status in a younger Black men who have sex with men epidemic. *AIDS Behav.* 2014; 18(2):335–345.

39. Neaigus A. The network approach and interventions to prevent HIV among injection drug users. *Public Health Rep.* 1998; 113:140–150.

40. Schneider JA, Zhou AN, Laumann EO. A new HIV prevention network approach: sociometric peer change agent selection. *Soc Sci Med.* 2015; 125:192–202.

41. Wang K, Brown K, Shen SY, Tucker J. Social network-based interventions to promote condom use: a systematic review. *AIDS Behav.* 2011; 15(7):1298–1308.

42. Rolls DA, Sacks-Davis R, Jenkinson R, et al. Hepatitis C transmission and treatment in contact networks of people who inject drugs. *PLoS One.* 2013; 8(11):e78286. doi: 10.1371/journal.pone.0078286

43. Fujimoto K, Williams ML, Ross MW. Venue-based affiliation networks and HIV risk-taking behavior among male sex workers. *Sex Transm Dis.* 2013; 40(6):453.

44. Brantley M, Schumacher C, Fields EL, et al. The network structure of sex partner meeting places reported by HIV-infected MSM: opportunities for HIV targeted control. *Soc Sci Med.* 2017; 182:20–29.

45. Hué S, Clewley JP, Cane PA, Pillay D. HIV-1 pol gene variation is sufficient for reconstruction of transmissions in the era of antiretroviral therapy. *AIDS.* 2004; 18(5):719–728.

46. Grabowski MK, Redd AD. Molecular tools for studying HIV transmission in sexual networks. *Curr Opin HIV AIDS.* 2014; 9(2):126.

47. Grabowski MK, Herbeck JT, Poon AF. Genetic cluster analysis for HIV prevention. *Curr HIV/AIDS Rep.* 2018; 1–8.

48. Smith DM, May S, Tweeten S, et al. A public health model for the molecular surveillance of HIV transmission in San Diego, California. *AIDS*. 2009; 23(2):225.
49. Dennis AM, Murillo W, de Maria Hernandez F, et al. Social network based recruitment successfully reveals HIV-1 transmission networks among high risk individuals in El Salvador. *J Acquir Immune Defic Syndr*. 2013; 63(1):135.
50. Lepej SZ, Vrakela IB, Poljak M, Bozicevic I, Begovac J. Phylogenetic analysis of HIV sequences obtained in a respondent-driven sampling study of men who have sex with men. *AIDS Res Human Retroviruses*. 2009; 25(12):1335–1338.
51. Pilon R, Leonard L, Kim J, et al. Transmission patterns of HIV and hepatitis C virus among networks of people who inject drugs. *PLoS One*. 2011; 6(7):e22245. doi:10.1371/journal.pone.0022245
52. Sacks-Davis R, Daraganova G, Aitken C, et al. Hepatitis C virus phylogenetic clustering is associated with the social-injecting network in a cohort of people who inject drugs. *PloS one*. 2012; 7(10):e47335. doi:10.1371/journal.pone.0047335
53. Aitken CK, McCaw RF, Bowden DS, et al. Molecular epidemiology of hepatitis C virus in a social network of injection drug users. *J Infect Dis*. 2004; 190(9):1586–1595.
54. Paintsil E, Verevochkin SV, Dukhovlinova E, et al. Hepatitis C virus infection among drug injectors in St Petersburg, Russia: social and molecular epidemiology of an endemic infection. *Addiction*. 2009; 104(11):1881–1890.

27

Urban Design

OLIVER GRUEBNER AND LAYLA MCCAY

1 Background

The relationship between urban design and urban population health has been increasingly studied over the past decades. We now understand how the features of the urban built environment can influence the daily activities and health behaviors of the people living in cities.[1-4] Consequently, there is much room for designing cities in ways that can reduce poor health and support the well-being of urban residents. Here, we aim to give a concise overview of current research on this topic and provide recommendations for urban planners and policymakers to help improve the health and well-being of urban populations. We do this by first giving a definition on what we regard as urban design and then introducing the so-called *Mind the GAPS framework*, laying out evidence-based connections between urban design and urban population health.

1.1 Conceptualizing Urban Design in Health Promotion

Urban design includes the urban physical environment: for example, *public spaces*, including the urban green, blue, and gray; *infrastructure,* including streets and transportation networks; and *building blocks,* including residences, retail outlets, and industrial facilities. In this way, urban design provides the context in which social activities may or may not happen. For example, public spaces may provide opportunities to relax, to exercise, or to interact with neighbors. Urban infrastructure may motivate the mode of transport that we choose—active versus passive—and define how well we may be able to access relevant facilities (e.g., children's playgrounds, sports fields), healthy food (e.g., farmers' markets, well-stocked supermarkets), community resources (e.g., places of worship, youth centers), or healthcare. Finally, building blocks constitute different types of land use and often impose physical barriers not only to local residents in their daily routines but also to local air circulation. All of these factors demonstrate various ways in which urban design influences the way we grow up in the city, how we behave, what we eat and drink, and how we feel. Therefore, urban design plays an ineluctable role as a determinant in the health of the urban population.

2 Extended "Mind the GAPS" Framework

In this section, we discuss evidence-based features of urban design (i.e., urban spaces, infrastructure, and building blocks) that have implications for the health and well-being of urban populations. We use the "Mind the GAPS" framework, which was originally introduced by the Center for Urban Design and Mental Health and that refers to *Green, Active, Pro-social, and Safe Places*.[1] Since this framework was originally introduced for the context of urban design and mental health, we will extend it also to a more general urban health context so that it can be more widely used by urban planners and designers in their aim to design healthy environments in our cities.

2.1 Green and Ecologically Targeted Design

Urban green and blue spaces include the vegetated land and the bodies of water within urban environments in the form of street canopy, parks, gardens, urban forestry, streams, rivers, and lakes. The literature on the urban green (i.e., vegetation) and blue (i.e., water) has documented positive associations with the health and well-being of city populations.[2,4] For example, urban trees have been found to reduce the oppressive effects of tall buildings.[5] Studies in the United Kingdom have shown that people living in greener urban neighborhoods exhibited fewer mental health problems than those living in less green neighborhoods, independent from individual and community-level socioeconomic deviation.[6] Green and blue spaces that citizens encounter in the course of their daily commute or those that provide easy access from home or work, such as parks, greenways, and river promenades, may exert their greatest positive impact when they offer safe transit ways and the possibilities for exercise, solitude, relaxation, or natural, positive social interactions. Furthermore, urban community gardens provide multiple positive health effects because they constitute social spaces where people can meet and engage in physical activities, undertake educational opportunities, and access locally grown fresh produce.[7]

An ecologically targeted urban design further acknowledges the linkages between urban features (e.g., urban spaces, infrastructure, and building blocks) and urban health. For example, urban green and blue spaces contribute to the regulation of urban climate and air quality.[8] Green and blue spaces increase evaporative cooling, while street canopy and urban forestry provide shade. Both can contribute to reducing the urban heat island, in which densely built inner-urban areas experience higher mean temperatures compared to other, less densely built areas.[9] Reducing urban gray areas (i.e., impermeable areas composed of cement, concrete, or tarmac such as building facades, streets, and parking lots) and imposing more green and blue areas instead will therefore help reduce inner-urban temperatures. Urban flooding prevention design may also include basins demarcated as safe inundation zones that can be used as sports or play fields otherwise. If vegetated, these zones will further help to reduce inner urban temperatures through evaporative cooling and shade provision. Furthermore, features of the urban infrastructure can be built to link urban parks by creating a network of greenways through the city on which people can navigate on their daily commute, thus introducing shaded bike paths for commuters and cool air corridors. In addition, building block design can further aid in reducing the urban heat island by introducing rooftop greenery or green facades. Building blocks can also be designed in a way that acknowledges regional wind patterns—versus imposing physical barriers that cause unwanted turbulence and turbine effects—and can reduce air pollution.[10]

2.2 Active Spaces Design

Cities should be designed to facilitate physical activity.[3] For example, well-designed and managed parks, urban forestry, sport fields, playgrounds, and other areas within the urban green and blue are well suited for physical exercises that have positive health effects. However, these features will only be used by people who have access to and who actually want to access these facilities. As such, urban design may intervene in people's daily practices with, for example, the provision of active transportation options to integrate exercise opportunities on people's daily commute. There is an opportunity to rethink the urban transport infrastructure in such a way that prioritizes bike and pedestrian ways: a greenway network linking public urban parks would allow citizens to navigate safely through the city while being in the green. This will have several health advantages. First, connecting available green and blue spaces increases the opportunities for walking, skating, or cycling and thereby increases the possibilities for active transport. Second, implementing and prioritizing a greenway infrastructure will decrease the dominance of car infrastructure (i.e., passive transport), thereby reducing significant health risks introduced by noise, pollution, physical danger, and prolonged sitting. Third, linking up green and blue spaces in a greenway network will provide better and easier access to facilities in neighboring communities, thus increasing the overall access to, for example, playgrounds, sports fields, farmers' markets, places of worship, youth centers, or healthcare. Finally, greenways bring opportunities to socialize naturally and to feel part of a community, inclusive of those who are unable to drive, such as older people, those with certain illnesses, or those who cannot afford a car. In addition, active urban transport options that integrate exercise opportunities into people's daily practices may include designing building blocks that motivate active choices, such as walking instead of taking the elevator, and may make rooftops accessible to building users including residents, visitors, and employees, thus providing further convenient settings to engage in sports activities.

2.3 Pro-Social Design

Positive social interaction helps promote belongingness and place attachment, social cohesion, and social capital.[11] As such, positive social interaction contributes to health and well-being in the urban population and strengthens community resilience. Moving to or within the city often results in people leaving behind crucial elements of their social support systems. An urban design that facilitates positive social interaction may help to create new social support systems. For example, public open spaces may be designed in a way that can host farmers' markets or community festivals to facilitate safe and positive social interactions. The street infrastructure can be designed to host sports events such as long-distance running throughout a city, bringing together active participants, supporters of the participants, and visitors. These events further create opportunities for volunteer activities that may deliver the health benefits of altruistic donation of time and skills. Pro-social design can be extended to street furniture, bus shelters, benches, and flower pots encouraging local residents to stop and chat. Building blocks with mixed land use, such as diverse, vital stores and cafes as well as residences and offices, allow citizens to walk between their daily routines, increase the likelihood to project positive perceptions of a neighborhood, and facilitate spontaneous social interactions. Furthermore, they facilitate feelings of community and belonging by providing settings for the neighborhood to get together.

Pro-social design can also be implemented to address the needs of specific sociodemographic groups. For example, public spaces can be designed for children to play, socialize, and explore, so that they can develop social behavior and cognitive skills. Public spaces can contribute to the development of social support, peer competence, and social capital for adolescents.[12] Public spaces, infrastructure, and building entrances should also be designed to facilitate access for people with disabilities so that they are integrated into the activities of daily life. Older persons who are socially integrated and who have feelings of social connection are less likely to have cognitive decline.[13] By providing settings for social interaction and activities of daily live, urban design may contribute to the autonomy, self-esteem, and physical and mental well-being of urban populations.

2.4 Safe, Integrative, Resilient, and Sustainable Design

Urban design should also deliver safety, preventing traumatic experiences and accidents and improving overall feelings of security. *Safe urban design* may include means of surveillance, access control, and maintenance. For example, if people think they are being observed, they are less likely to commit crimes. An urban design that creates the feeling of being watched will therefore provide powerful means for crime prevention. Buildings with windows toward pedestrian areas, sufficient lighting that illuminates faces, and walls that do not limit sightlines may be examples of built-in surveillance in urban design. Furthermore, access control measures in urban design help to make explicit whether the public is welcome in a particular space or not. Examples include clear delineations using impediments like thorny plants, reducing entry possibilities, limiting public-facing access to upper levels, or using lighting and signs to clearly discourage intrusion by public space users onto private space. In addition, good maintenance is essential to sustain the health benefits of good urban design. For example, if public spaces, infrastructure, or buildings are poorly managed, there is the risk that features fall into disrepair (e.g., damaged street lighting, waste, or demolished street furniture, and thus increase overall neighborhood disorder. Consequences may include the reduction of self-esteem and physical activity of local residents.[14]

Integrative urban design includes providing access to public spaces, infrastructure, and buildings, inclusive of those with a disability and other potentially marginalized groups. It is essential that public spaces, infrastructure, and building entries are fitted with ramps that limit obstacles to the mobility disabled. It also includes demarcations on the floor that guide visually impaired persons, ensuring that audio signals at traffic lights are well functioning, and that signposting is comprehensible to people who have dementia.

Resilient urban design requires public spaces, infrastructure, and building blocks to meet certain standards so that they will resist a minimum of extraordinary shocks associated with, for example, a natural disaster. Depending on the geographic location, extreme flood events, earthquakes, or hurricanes may occur; adequate urban design will include features such as flood overflow basins or dikes, as well as improved building structures to resist earthquakes, hurricanes, or landslides, and demarcated evacuation routes and community centers where evacuees can find shelter.

Urban design should protect both ecological and social sustainability. While an ecologically driven urban design may promote urban green and blue spaces across the city to reduce urban temperatures in the summer, a socially *sustainable urban design* may further aim to reduce environmental injustice—the phenomenon in which lower socio-economic status neighborhoods have lower access to resources such as well-maintained green spaces.[15] This would include securing equity in at least four dimensions of access: *availability, accessibility, affordability,* and *acceptability* of green and blue spaces in inner-urban areas.[16] Availability refers to the physical presence of a green or blue space in a predefined urban neighborhood, whereas the effort that it takes to get to these spaces is referred to as accessibility. For example, although a green or blue space might be available in a neighborhood, it may not be open to the public or its entrance gates may be on the opposite site of these spaces and therefore present obstacles for accessibility. Affordability may refer to green or blue spaces that are cost-prohibitive (e.g., botanical gardens), and acceptability may refer to the maintenance of these spaces, with better maintained spaces attracting more people versus poorly maintained spaces that may not be as attractive to a wider public. However, the literature on environmental justice has also reminded us that improving overall access to new green and blue spaces, especially in the park-poor areas of socioeconomically deprived urban neighborhoods, can lead to gentrification processes.[15] An urban design that acknowledges both ecological and social sustainability will increase the likelihood that most people will experience health benefits.

3 Conclusion

Designing cities in a way that can reduce poor health and support the well-being of urban residents provides many opportunities. We introduce the Mind the GAPS framework and provide recommendations for urban planners and policymakers, incorporating both ecological and social sustainability, to help improve the health and well-being of urban populations.

References

1. McCay L. Designing mental health into cities. *Urban Design Group Journal.* 2017; 142:25–27.
2. Lee ACK, Maheswaran R. The health benefits of urban green spaces: a review of the evidence. *J Public Health.* 2011; 33(2):212–222.

3. *Toward more physical activity in cities: transforming public spaces to promote physical activity—a key contributor to achieving the Sustainable Development Goals in Europe.* Copenhagen, Denmark: World Health Organization; 2017.
4. Völker S, Kistemann T. "I'm always entirely happy when I'm here!" Urban blue enhancing human health and well-being in Cologne and Düsseldorf, Germany. *Soc Sci Med.* 2013; 78:113–124.
5. Asgarzadeh M, Koga T, Yoshizawa N, Munakata J, Hirate K. Investigating green urbanism; building oppressiveness. *J Asian Architecture Building Engineering.* 2010; 9(2):555–562.
6. White MP, Alcock I, Wheeler BW, Depledge MH. Would you be happier living in a greener urban area? A fixed-effects analysis of panel data. *Psychol Sci.* 2013; 24(6):920–928.
7. Buck D. *Gardens and health: implications for policy and practice.* London: The King's Fund; 2016: 1–65.
8. Salmond JA, Tadaki M, Vardoulakis S, et al. Health and climate related ecosystem services provided by street trees in the urban environment. *Environ Health.* 2016; 15(S1):36.
9. Bowler DE, Buyung-Ali L, Knight TM, Pullin AS. Urban greening to cool towns and cities: A systematic review of the empirical evidence. *Landsc Urban Plan.* 2010; 97(3):147–155.
10. Abhijith KV, Kumar P, Gallagher J, et al. Air pollution abatement performances of green infrastructure in open road and built-up street canyon environments: a review. *Atmospheric Environ.* 2017; 162:71–86.
11. Paranagamage P, Austin S, Price A, Khandokar F. Social capital in action in urban environments: an intersection of theory, research and practice literature. *J Urban.* 2010; 3(3):231–252.
12. Aneshensel CS, Sucoff CA. The neighborhood context of adolescent mental health. *J Health Soc Behav.* 1996; 37(4):293.
13. Mitchell L, Burton E. Neighbourhoods for life: designing dementia-friendly outdoor environments. *Qual in Ageing Older Adults.* 2006; 7(1):26–33.
14. Mooney SJ, Joshi S, Cerdá M, Kennedy GJ, Beard JR, Rundle AG. Neighborhood disorder and physical activity among older adults: a longitudinal study. *J Urban Health.* 2017; 94(1):30–42.
15. Wolch JR, Byrne J, Newell JP. Urban green space, public health, and environmental justice: the challenge of making cities "just green enough." *Landsc Urban Plan.* 2014; 125:234–244.
16. Penchansky R, Thomas JW. The concept of access: definition and relationship to consumer satisfaction. *Med Care.* 1981; 19(2):127–140.

28

Urban Land Use and Health

ROHAN SIMKIN AND KAREN C. SETO

1 Urban Land, the Environment, and Health

It is well established that local environmental conditions directly impact human health.[1,2] Environmental influences on health include but are not limited to air pollution and asthma, access to green space and mental and physical health, and water pollution and water-borne disease. However, it is not only the local environment that affects health; the regional and global environments also contribute to health outcomes. This chapter explores the interdependencies between regional and global environments and human health, using urban land use as an analytical lens.

1.1 Multiscalar Environmental Impacts of Urban Land Use

First, it is important to distinguish between land cover and land use. *Land cover* refers to the physical attributes and condition of the Earth's surface, whereas *land use* emphasizes the functional role of land in human activities and how the land is utilized.[3] Forests, concrete, buildings, and shrubs describe land cover; agriculture, streets, and factories describe land uses. The two categories are not binaries but rather fall on a continuum. Sometimes the two concepts are interchangeable—pastures refer to both land cover and land use. Urban land use is highly heterogeneous and is characterized by a high degree of built-up space, often with impervious surfaces.[4] In this chapter, we use *urban land use* to also include the concept of *urban form*, which refers to the physical extent, spatial configuration, and internal patterns of human settlements, including the layout of streets and buildings.

The influence of urban land use and land cover on local environments can be illustrated with several well-studied examples. Cities with highly separated, single-use land uses (e.g., residential areas separated from commercial areas) are more likely to have high levels of motorized transport and hence air pollution than are cities with highly mixed land uses. The process of creating the built environment and urban land use results in land cover change, such as the conversion of forests, agricultural land, or wildlife habitat to human use. Urban land cover change also affects hydrological systems through altering the absorptive capacity of the surface, leading to stormwater runoff that consequently pollutes waterways.[5] Artificial surfaces dominated by materials such as concrete and bitumen absorb solar radiation and radiate it as heat more strongly than do natural surfaces, resulting in increased local temperatures.[6] The warmer temperatures can cause air to rise, driving convection currents that change local precipitation patterns.[7,8]

The multitude of impacts to local environments amalgamate to produce impacts that can be observed at global scales. The impact of urban land on ecosystems contributes to global declines in biodiversity, with global rates of extinction estimated to be as much as 1,000 times greater than the likely background level.[9] The global climate is changing due to the continued emission of greenhouse gasses, of which urban areas contribute as much as 70%.[10] Urban emissions of chemicals including gases such as carbon dioxide (CO_2) and other trace gases (e.g., nitrous oxide [NO], nitrogen dioxide [NO_2], ozone [O_3], sulfur dioxide [SO_2], nitric acid [HNO_3], and various organic acids) and urban inputs of phosphorus and nitrogen to waterways contribute to human alteration of global nutrient cycles.[5,11]

1.2 Influence of Environmental Change on Urban Health

These impacts to the physical environment degrade the quality of resources, such as air and water, that we rely directly on for basic health.[12] Changes in climate (temperature, rainfall, etc.) alter the emergence and spread of infectious disease and affect our ability to produce food to meet basic nutritional needs.[13] An increase in extreme weather events that is predicted to occur because of climate change may expose urban populations to health risks through risk of physical harm incurred during the event itself, by creating conditions that support disease transmission, by damaging health infrastructure, and by affecting long-term mental health.[13,14]

It is beyond the scope of this chapter to provide a detailed description of the multiple pathways by which environmental change driven by urban land use affects the health of urban populations. Rather, our goal is to use several illustrative examples to highlight some of the key pathways. First, we examine how urban land use can affect biodiversity, which in turn can influence the likelihood of infectious disease. Second, we describe how urban land use affects climate, on local to global scales, with wide ranging implications for urban health These interactions are summarized diagrammatically in Figure 28.1 which illustrates how the continued expansion of urban land, its configuration and composition, produce environmental changes that drive urban health outcomes.

2 Urban Land Use, Biodiversity, and Infectious Disease

Zoonotic pathogens, pathogens with a nonhuman animal source, play an important role in human health, with around 60% of emerging infectious diseases in humans originating in animals and around 70% of these originating in nondomesticated

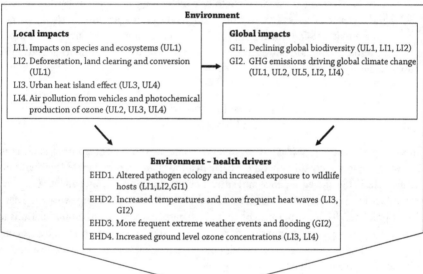

Urban land drivers of environmental change

Expansion

UL1. Converts non-urban lands to urban land use

Configuration

UL2. Influences GHG emissions from transport by determining driving behaviors

UL3. Changes the surface energy budget and urban albedo

Composition (i.e. materials)

UL4. Determines the surface energy budget and urban albedo

UL5. Determines embedded energy and GHG emissions

Environment

Local impacts

LI1. Impacts on species and ecosystems (UL1)

LI2. Deforestation, land clearing and conversion (UL1)

LI3. Urban heat island effect (UL3, UL4)

LI4. Air pollution from vehicles and photochemical production of ozone (UL2, UL3, UL4)

Global impacts

GI1. Declining global biodiversity (UL1, LI1, LI2)

GI2. GHG emissions driving global climate change (UL1, UL2, UL5, LI2, LI4)

Environment – health drivers

EHD1. Altered pathogen ecology and increased exposure to wildlife hosts (LI1, LI2, GI1)

EHD2. Increased temperatures and more frequent heat waves (LI3, GI2)

EHD3. More frequent extreme weather events and flooding (GI2)

EHD4. Increased ground level ozone concentrations (LI3, LI4)

Urban health outcomes

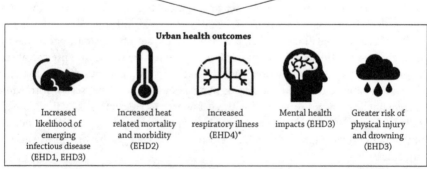

Increased likelihood of emerging infectious disease (EHD1, EHD3)

Increased heat related mortality and morbidity (EHD2)

Increased respiratory illness (EHD4)*

Mental health impacts (EHD3)

Greater risk of physical injury and drowning (EHD3)

Figure 28.1 **Urban land drivers of environmental change.** Urban land characteristics relating to urban expansion, urban configuration, and composition shape urban impacts on the environment. Urban environmental impacts can occur at local scales that aggregate to produce impacts at global scales. These environmental changes result in environmental health drivers that influence urban health. Numbers in parentheses indicate factors contributing to a given outcome. GHG, greenhouse gas. Source: *Lungs by Linseed Studio from The Noun Project licensed under CC BY 3.0, Lungs. Available at https://creativecommons.org/licenses/by/3.0/.

wildlife.[15] Modification of ecosystems can alter the pathogen dynamics of an ecosystem by changing the host species composition and abundance and species interactions (e.g., predation and competition) in ways that change the type and abundance of pathogens.[16] There is a growing body of evidence showing that land use change that modifies ecosystems and alters human–wildlife interactions can alter the likelihood of disease emergence.[16–18] As land transitions from natural to urban, the modifications to ecosystems and human–wildlife interactions that take place change the nature and likelihood of disease emergence in urban populations.

On the urban periphery, "peri-urban" areas represent sites of rapid land use change and associated impacts on biodiversity.[4] These transitional zones are characterized by juxtaposed urban and rural land uses intermixed with natural habitats where human–wildlife interactions are common, thus increasing the opportunities for pathogen transmission.[19] In these areas, the high degree of habitat fragmentation creates significant transitional (ecotonal) areas between remnant habitats and human-dominated land uses. Anthropogenic pressures within ecotonal areas create unique ecological and environmental conditions that are thought to be particularly important for disease emergence, such as enhanced biological productivity, genetic diversification, evolutionary adaptation, interspecific interactions, and the aggregation and movement of organisms, nutrients, and other materials.[20,21] A well-documented example is yellow fever in which expansion of peri-urban land into remnant forest facilitates interaction between humans, forest-dwelling primate disease hosts and mosquito vectors. This creates an opportunity for the infection of human populations on the urban fringe who are exposed to mosquitoes that have fed on infected primates.[22] The disease can then be sustained in urban populations through human to human transmission via the widespread urban mosquito species *Aedes aegypti*. At these human–wildland interfaces, livestock can act as intermediaries, allowing zoonotic pathogens to make the jump to human urban populations.[19] For example, Nipah virus, which exists in host populations of fruit bats (*Pteropus* spp.), spilled over to peri-urban human populations in Malaysia via farmed pigs in 1999.[23] The subsequent outbreak infected 265 and caused the deaths of 105 people.[24]

Within the urban core, long-established urban areas represent an example of extreme habitat modification in which natural ecosystems are largely replaced by the built environment. This results in changes to the quality and availability of resources such as nesting structures, shelter, water, and food.[25] For most species, this high degree of modification removes the resources required for persistence in urban habitats resulting in a general reduction in the diversity of wildlife.[26] However, some generalist species thrive in urban spaces in response to abundant novel resources that urban land use creates, particularly food.[25] For example, an abundance of food offered by the buildup of refuse due to poor rubbish collection services and open sewer systems in the slums of Salvador, Brazil, creates ideal habitat for the Norway rat (*Rattus norvegicus*). In these environments, the Norway rat is a carrier of *Leptospira interrogans*, a pathogenic spirochete causing leptospirosis in humans who come into contact with water contaminated by the rat's urine.[27,28] Another example is in eastern Australia, where urban fruit tree plantings attract large populations of fruit bats (*Pteropus* spp.) carrying Hendra virus.[19]

Urban ecosystems can also provide favorable habitats for invertebrate disease vectors. For example accumulated rubbish provides a breeding ground for Phlebotomine sandflies, the main vector for leishmanial parasites.[29] The mosquito *Aedes aegypti*, mentioned previously as a vector for urban yellow fever is also a vector for dengue fever, with a global burden of more than 390 million cases each year; these mosquitos have become increasingly common in urban areas, in part because of the abundance of standing water, such as in bottles, tires, and road depressions, which in turn become ideal breeding sites.[30]

A simplified interpretation of this evidence might conclude that there are benefits in separating humans from wildlife populations that harbor disease. However, separating urban populations from nature would eliminate the many health benefits of interacting with nature, such as improved mental health and increased physical activity, or the cooling influence of urban vegetation during extreme heat events.[31,32] Eliminating nature from urban areas would also fail to recognize the many services that nature provides, such as wetlands that provide storm water management and ecosystems such as mangroves that protect urban areas during extreme weather events.[32,33] Instead, understanding the mechanisms by which urban land influences the likelihood of disease outbreaks can help inform populations in ways that allow them to minimize risks. Understanding the unique role of urban land on the risk of wildlife disease in urban populations will be an important part of determining the design of programs to monitor for, respond to, and ultimately prevent disease outbreaks in the future.

3 Regional and Global Climate

This section describes the primary mechanisms by which urban land use affects regional and global climate and how they in turn affect human health. There is now unequivocal evidence that climate change is occurring and that human activities are the primary cause.[34] Urban land use is an important contributor to climate change. At local scales, the increase in urban built form changes the degree to which the surface reflects, absorbs, and/or radiates heat, and the presence of urban structures changes local wind patterns. Furthermore, the spatial structure and pattern of urban land use affects global climate change through shaping the energy used for transport, buildings, and other urban activities. The health impacts of these changes for urban populations are wide-ranging and can occur as a direct result of changed climatic conditions, such as increased mortality and morbidity associated with increased temperature or more frequent extreme weather events, or it can be indirect, where climate influences other processes related to health, such as the distribution of vectors for infectious disease. Here, we illustrate the influence of urban land on climate and health by examining the climatic influences of urban land use at different scales.

3.1 Urban Heat Island

At local to regional scales, urban land use has a direct influence on temperature through the urban heat island (UHI) effect. The UHI is the observed temperature difference between urban and adjacent non-urban areas.[6] It is caused by several key differences between rural and urban land uses that can result in temperatures 5°–11°C hotter than surrounding non-urban areas.[35] First, the way that energy is absorbed and stored by urban land and exchanged with the atmosphere, known as the *surface energy budget*, is different for urban and non-urban lands. Urban surfaces comprised of dark materials with low albedo (i.e., reflectivity) have a greater capacity to absorb and store solar radiation and convert it to sensible heat.[6,36] Energy stored during the day is released as heat primarily at night, with the result that the UHI is most acute after dark.[36] The ability of urban materials to absorb and reemit solar energy is augmented by the three-dimensional urban structure. This structure creates greater active surface area available for energy exchange and allows for reflection of radiation between buildings and ground surfaces, thus increasing the absorption of incoming radiation.[36] Decreased skyview caused by urban buildings results in less radiation being lost to the sky.[36]

Water and urban vegetation also play an important role in the surface energy budget. Urban surfaces such as concrete and bitumen are largely impervious and do not retain water, meaning that urban land is typically drier than rural land.[36] Urban land is also less vegetated. The result is a combined decrease in the amount of evaporation from soils and transpiration from vegetation (known as *evapotranspiration*) which would otherwise provide evaporative cooling in urban areas.[36,37]

Aside from changes in the surface energy budget, the other key contributor to the UHI is heat emitted from anthropogenic sources.[36] Urban anthropogenic heat sources arise through use of energy such as the combustion of fossil fuels in cars; electric heating and air conditioning in buildings; energy used for lighting and cooking; and energy used in industrial processes.[6,36] Heat is also emitted during human and animal metabolism.[36] The degree to which anthropogenic heat sources contribute to the UHI depends on the strength of demand for heating and cooling of buildings, which is greater in colder and hotter climates, respectively, and the density of urban populations, with higher density populations representing concentrated sources of energy use and therefore heat.[36]

The most immediate impact of the UHI on health is the direct impact of exposure to high temperatures, which can affect health in ways ranging from exacerbation of minor conditions to increased risk of hospitalization and death.[37] Those most at risk are older adults, young children, and infants, who have a limited ability to thermoregulate, and those with cardiovascular and cardiopulmonary disease.[38] While heat stroke as the result of UHI can cause death, heat is more often a contributory factor to deaths and morbidity from other causes, such as respiratory illness.[37]

The impact of the UHI on health is most pronounced during extreme events. During extreme heat, the UHI magnifies the temperature increase within cities, further increasing the risk of heat-related death.[39] This effect is particularly relevant during the night, when increased temperature has been epidemiologically associated with excess mortality.[39]

A second pathway by which UHI affects health is through the formation of air pollution. Ozone is formed in urban areas via a chemical reaction involving volatile organic compounds (VOC) in the presence of nitrous oxides (NOx) and sunlight.[40,41] This chemical reaction is enhanced by temperature, with higher temperatures resulting in greater ozone formation.[41]

The primary components of this reaction VOC and NOx are emitted through anthropogenic combustion of fossil fuels, and concentrations may be elevated in urban areas from vehicle emissions and other sources.[40] When combined with UHI-induced temperature increases and the reduced dispersion effects of wind in urban areas due to the influence of buildings, ozone concentrations in urban areas may become elevated at ground level.[40,42]

Ground-level ozone produced in urban areas also presents a significant health risk. Repeated exposure to ozone can cause permanent lung damage and can worsen heart disease, bronchitis, emphysema, and asthma.[40] At the global scale, anthropogenic emissions of ozone are thought to result in 700,000 (±300,000) respiratory mortalities annually, so the potential enhancement of ozone levels via the UHI represents a significant urban health challenge.[43]

3.2 Global Climate Change

Urban land use is also a significant source of greenhouse gas emissions, the dominant cause of global climate change. It is estimated that urban land use contributes up to 70% of global CO_2 emissions from global final energy use.[10] Three major pathways by which urban areas contribute to global emissions of greenhouse gasses have been identified.[40] First, the arrangement of urban land use shapes the way that people travel within urban areas, which is a major determinant of the amount of vehicle emissions.[44] Low-density, single-use development, sometimes known as "urban sprawl," increases driving distances and reliance on cars, resulting in overall higher emissions.[45,46] Second, the composition of the urban built environment affects the emissions embodied in building materials (i.e., emissions associated with the manufacture of materials such as cement and steel) and those produced during their ongoing use.[44] Finally, the transformation of natural land to urban use involves alterations in vegetation and wildlands that produce emissions.[44] This impact is particularly relevant in pan-tropical regions, where emissions associated with projected urban growth between 2000 and 2030 are estimated to make up approximately 5% of the total emissions associated with tropical deforestation and land use change.[47]

The emissions from urban land use contribute to global climate change that can influence the health of urban populations. Under climate change scenarios, the frequency and severity of extreme heat events is predicted to increase, which, when combined with the amplifying effects of the UHI, may increase the impacts of heat-related mortality and morbidity.[39] The potential for heat to cause significant mortality can already be observed. In the United States, heatwaves are the most prominent cause of weather-related mortality, responsible for more deaths annually than hurricanes, tornadoes, floods, and lightning combined.[39] Heatwaves in Europe in 2003 caused approximately 22,000–45,000 heat-related deaths.[35]

In some areas, climate change will increase the frequency of storms, heavy precipitation events, and sea level rise, increasing the risk of flooding.[48] Urban areas are at particular risk of flooding due to the high degree of impermeable surfaces that increase runoff, inadequate drainage systems that are quickly overloaded during heavy rain events, and modification of wetlands and other natural buffers to flooding.[38] This risk is particularly high for the urban poor who are more likely to live in flood-prone areas.[49]

In the short term, mortality due to drowning or acute trauma is a serious health risk. Floods are estimated to have killed 53,000 people over the period 2002–2011, with the ratio of deaths in resource-poor countries to high-income countries a staggering

23:1.[49] Flooding may also increase the risk of infectious diseases such as hepatitis E, leptospirosis, and gastrointestinal (GI) diseases, which are particularly prevalent in regions with inadequate hygiene and clean drinking water.[49] Vector-borne diseases may be enhanced where floodwaters act as suitable breeding grounds for disease vectors, such as mosquitoes.[49] Over longer timeframes, flooding may exacerbate the impact of noncommunicable diseases by interrupting treatment or making it difficult for patients to access medication; cause mental health disorders such as posttraumatic stress disorder, depression, and anxiety; or affect birth outcomes by affecting the physical and mental health of mothers.[49]

4 Conclusion

Urban land use change contributes in a substantial way to altering the biophysical environment at local to global scales. At local scales, the influence of urban land use is evident in local environments including ecosystems, waterways, and air quality. At global scales, urban land use change influences the environment both through the aggregate effect of local impacts and by influencing global systems such as global atmospheric processes. These environmental changes link urban land use to the health of urban populations.

Here we demonstrate this link by showing that urban land use drives changes in ecosystems that decrease biodiversity and modulate the risk of outbreaks of infectious disease from wildlife populations. We also show the influence of urban land on climate where, at local scales, the impact of UHI increases heat-related illness and respiratory illness through the formation of ozone, and at global scales increases the risk of extreme heat and flooding events.

As the world population and land surface both become increasingly urban, understanding the health consequences of urban land use–driven environmental change becomes critically important. Understanding these relationships is a necessary condition to planning urban development in ways that may be co-beneficial for both the environment and human health.

References

1. Klitzman S, Matte TD, Kass DE. The urban physical environment and its effects on health, in cities and the health of the public. In Freudenberg N, Galea S, Vlahov D, eds. *Cities and the health of the public*. Nashville, TN: Vanderbilt University Press; 2006.
2. Prüss-Üstün A, Wolf J, Corvalán CF, Bos R, Neira MP. *Preventing disease through healthy environments: a global assessment of the burden of disease from environmental risks*. Geneva, Switzerland: World Health Organization. 2016.
3. Seto KC, Woodcock CE, Song C, Huang X, Lu J, Kaufmann RK. Monitoring land-use change in the Pearl River Delta using Landsat TM. *Int J Remote Sens*. 2002; 23(10): 1985–2004.
4. Hasse D. How is urban land use unique? In Seto KC, Reenberg A, eds. *Rethinking global land use in an urban era*. Cambridge, MA: MIT Press; 2014.
5. Grimm NB, Faeth SH, Golubiewski NE, et al. Global change and the ecology of cities. *Science*. 2008; 319: 756–760.
6. Rizwan AM, Dennis LYC, Liu C. A review on the generation, determination and mitigation of urban heat island. *J Environ Sci*. 2008; 20(1): 120–128.

7. Hasse D, Schwarz N. Urban land use in the global context. In Seto KC, Solecki WD, Griffith CA, eds. *The Routledge handbook of urbanization and global environmental change.* New York: Routledge; 2016.

8. Shepherd JM. A review of current investigations of urban-induced rainfall and recommendations for the future. *Earth Interact.* 2005; 9(12): 1.

9. Pimm SL, Jenkins CN, Abell R, et al. The biodiversity of species and their rates of extinction, distribution, and protection. *Science.* 2014; 344(6187): 1246752.

10. Seto KC, Dhakal S, Bigio A, et al. Human settlements, infrastructure and spatial planning. In: Edenhofer O, Pichs-Madruga R, Sokona Y, et al., eds. *Climate change 2014: mitigation of climate change. contribution of working group III to the fifth assessment report of the intergovernmental panel on climate change.* Cambridge: Cambridge University Press. 2014.

11. Hobbie SE, Finlay JC, Janke BD, Nidzgorski DA, Millet DB, Baker LA. Contrasting nitrogen and phosphorus budgets in urban watersheds and implications for managing urban water pollution. *Proc Natl Acad Sci U S A.* 2017; 114(16): 4177–4182.

12. Myers SS. Planetary health: protecting human health on a rapidly changing planet. *Lancet.* 2017; 390(10114): 2860–2868.

13. Costello A, Abbas M, Allen A, et al. Managing the health effects of climate change: *Lancet* and University College London Institute for Global Health Commission. *Lancet.* 2009; 373(9676): 1693–1733.

14. Ebi KL, Frumkin H, Hess JJ. Protecting and promoting population health in the context of climate and other global environmental changes. *Anthropocene.* 2017; 19: 1–12.

15. Jones KE, Patel NG, Levy MA, et al. Global trends in emerging infectious diseases. *Nature.* 2008; 451(7181): 990–993.

16. Myers SS, Gaffikin L, Golden C, et al. Human health impacts of ecosystem alteration. *Proc Natl Acad Sci U S A.* 2013; 110(47): 18753–18760.

17. Keesing F, Belden LK, Daszak P, et al. Impacts of biodiversity on the emergence and transmission of infectious diseases. *Nature.* 2010; 468(7324): 647–652.

18. Jones BA, Grace D, Kock R, et al. Zoonosis emergence linked to agricultural intensification and environmental change. *Proc Natl Acad Sci U S A.* 2013; 110(21): 8399–8404.

19. Hassell JM, Begon M, Ward M, et al., Urbanization and disease emergence: dynamics at the wildlife-livestock-human Interface. *Trends Ecol Evol.* 2017; 32(1): 55–67.

20. Despommier D, Ellis BR, Wilcox BA. The role of ecotones in emerging infectious diseases. *Ecohealth.* 2006; 3(4): 281–289.

21. Lambin EF, Tran A, Vanwambeke S, et al. Pathogenic landscapes: interactions between land, people, disease vectors, and their animal hosts. *Int J Health Geogr.* 2010; 9:13.

22. Barrett, ADT, Monath TP. Epidemiology and ecology of yellow fever virus. In Chambers TJ, Monath, TP, eds. *Adv Virus Res.* 2003; 61:291–315.

23. Chua KB. Nipah virus outbreak in Malaysia. *J Clin Virol.* 2003; 26(3):265–275.

24. Daszak P, Plowright RK, Epstein JH, et al. The emergence of Nipah and Hendra virus: pathogen dynamics across a wildlife-livestock-human continuum. In Collinge SK, Ray C, eds. *Disease ecology: community structure and pathogen dynamics.* Cary, NC: Oxford University Press; 2006.

25. Becker DJ, Streicker DG, Altizer S. Linking anthropogenic resources to wildlife-pathogen dynamics: a review and meta-analysis. *Ecol Lett.* 2015; 18(5):483–495.

26. McKinney M.L. Urbanization, biodiversity, and conservation. *BioScience.* 2002; 52: 883–890.

27. de Faria MT, Calderwood MS, Athanazio DA, et al. Carriage of Leptospira interrogans among domestic rats from an urban setting highly endemic for leptospirosis in Brazil. *Acta Trop.* 2008; 108(1):1–5.

28. Costa F, Ribeiro GS, Felzemburgh RDM, et al. Influence of household rat infestation on Leptospira transmission in the urban slum environment. *PLoS Negl Trop Dis.* 2014; 8(12) e3338. doi:10.1371/journal.pntd.0003338

29. Alirol E, Getaz L, Stoll B, Chappuis F, Loutan L. Urbanisation and infectious diseases in a globalised world. *Lancet Infect Dis.* 2011; 11(2): 131–141.

30. Neiderud C-J. How urbanization affects the epidemiology of emerging infectious diseases. *Infect Ecol Epidemiol.* 2015;5. doi:10.3402/iee.v5.27060

31. Braubach M, Egorov A, Mudu P, Wolf T, Thompson CW, Martuzzi M. Effects of urban green space on environmental health, equity and resilience. In Kabisch N, Korn H, Stadler J, Bonn A, eds. *Nature-based solutions to climate change adaptation in urban areas: linkages between science, policy and practice.* Dordrecht, Netherlands: Springer; 2017.

32. Elmqvist T, Fragkias M, Goodness J, et al. *Urbanization, biodiversity and ecosystem services: challenges and opportunities a global assessment.* Dordrecht, Netherlands: Springer; 2013.

33. Gómez-Baggethun, E, Barton DN. Classifying and valuing ecosystem services for urban planning. *Ecol Econ.* 2013; 86:235–245.

34. Intergovernmental Panel on Climate Change. *Climate change 2013: the physical science basis. Contribution of working group I to the fifth assessment report of the intergovernmental panel on climate change.* Stockholm, Sweden: Intergovernmental Panel on Climate Change; 2013.

35. Patz JA, Campbell-Lendrum D, Holloway T, Foley JA. Impact of regional climate change on human health. *Nature.* 2005; 438(7066):310–317.

36. Oke TR, Mills G, Christen A, Voogt JA. *Urban climates.* Cambridge: Cambridge University Press; 2017.

37. Heaviside C, Macintyre H, Vardoulakis S. The urban heat island: implications for health in a changing environment. *Curr Environ Health Rep.* 2017; 4(3):296–305.

38. *Global report on urban health: equitable, healthier cities for sustainable development.* Geneva, Switzerland: World Health Organization; 2016.

39. Luber G, McGeehin, M. Climate change and extreme heat events. *Am J Prev Med.* 2008; 35(5):429–435.

40. Lo CP, Quattrochi DA. Land-use and land-cover change, urban heat island phenomenon, and health implications. *Photogramm Eng Remote Sensing.* 2003; 69(9):1053–1063.

41. Cardelino CA, Chameides WL. Natural hydrocarbons, urbanization, and urban ozone. *J Geophys Res Atmos.* 1990; 95(D9): 13971–13979.

42. Lai LW, Cheng WL. Air quality influenced by urban heat island coupled with synoptic weather patterns. *Sci Total Environ.* 2009; 407(8): 2724–2733.

43. Anenberg SC, Horowitz LW, Tong DQ, West JJ. An estimate of the global burden of anthropogenic ozone and fine particulate matter on premature human mortality using atmospheric modeling. *Environ Health Perspect.* 2010; 118(9):1189–1195.

44. Stokes EC, Seto KC. Climate change and urban land systems: bridging the gaps between urbanism and land science. *J Land Use Sci.* 2016; 11(6) 698–708.

45. Transportation Research Board and National Research Council. *Driving and the built environment: the effects of compact development on motorized travel, energy sse, and CO2 emissions— Special Report 298.*Washington, DC: National Academies Press; 2009:256.

46. Anderson WP, Kanaroglou PS, Miller EJ. Urban form, energy and the environment: a review of issues, evidence and policy. *Urban Studies.* 1996; 33(1):7–35.

47. Seto KC, Güneralp B, Hutyra LR. Global forecasts of urban expansion to 2030 and direct impacts on biodiversity and carbon pools. *Proc Natl Acad Sci U S A.* 2012; 109(40): 16083–16088.

48. Intergovernmental Panel on Climate Change. *Climate change 2014: synthesis report. Contribution of working groups I, II and III to the fifth assessment report of the intergovernmental panel on climate change.* Stockholm, Sweden: Intergovernmental Panel on Climate Change; 2014.

49. Alderman K, Turner LR, Tong S. Floods and human health: a systematic review. *Environ Int.* 2012; 47:37–47.

29

Community-Based Participatory Research

An Approach to Research in the Urban Context

BARBARA A. ISRAEL, AMY J. SCHULZ, CHRIS M. COOMBE, EDITH A. PARKER,
ANGELA G. REYES, ZACHARY ROWE, AND RICHARD L. LICHTENSTEIN

1 Background and Rationale for a Community-Based Participatory Research Approach

Health inequities are reflected in differential rates of morbidity and mortality based on socioeconomic position (SEP), as well as on racial or ethnic status, with an excess burden of morbidity and mortality occurring for conditions as diverse as asthma, heart disease, cancer, and stroke.[1] Excess burden of disease is greatest among Americans with low SEP and ethnic minority status living in areas of concentrated urban poverty.[2,3] Health inequities derive from the uneven distribution of resources (e.g., income, housing, education) as well as from exposures that may harm health (e.g., air pollutants, discrimination, and other stressors) and that disproportionately affect these urban areas. These social, economic, and environmental conditions have been termed the *social determinants of health*.[4] There is a continuing need for basic etiologic research that integrates these multiple dimensions of health inequities (e.g., biomedical, social, behavioral, environmental). Furthermore, there is an urgent need to examine how these interconnecting factors and forces can be addressed through interventions at multiple levels (e.g., individual, family, community, societal) and through policy change to reduce and ultimately eliminate health inequities. Such research requires a commitment to creating opportunities for multiple perspectives and insights to be part of the knowledge-building process, with explicit attention paid to eliminating inequities in influence and power between academic researchers and those most adversely affected by social inequalities.[5-7] Community-based participatory research (CBPR) approaches focus on reducing these inequities.

Specifically, CBPR approaches engage community members and researchers as equal partners in all aspects of the research process to both increase knowledge and understanding and to integrate knowledge gained with interventions and policy change to improve community health and well-being.[5,6,8] These approaches seek to address some of the historic exclusion and disenfranchisement in research and practice experienced by low-income communities and communities of color, integrating local knowledge and community strengths with technical expertise to conduct relevant and culturally appropriate research.[5-8]

In this chapter, we consider the substantial value of CBPR to address health inequities within the context of urban communities. Specifically, we (1) define and describe key principles of CBPR; (2) discuss its applicability to multiple types of research, study designs, and research methods; and (3) offer case examples of the use of CBPR to conduct both basic etiologic research to inform change and intervention research, grounded in our work in Detroit, Michigan. We conclude with a discussion of the benefits, challenges, and lessons learned using CBPR in urban communities.

2 Definition of Community-Based Participatory Research

CBPR draws on two historical traditions of collaborative approaches to research from multiple disciplines both domestically and globally, including "action research," often referred to as the "Northern tradition" or a "problem-solving utilitarian approach," and "participatory research" and "participatory action research," often referred to as the "Southern tradition" or an "emancipatory approach."[7,9-12] These approaches have in common research that is conducted in partnership between academic researchers and members of the group or community at the center of the research questions or challenges to be addressed. While a wide range of terms are used to refer to such research approaches globally, within public health in the United States, such approaches have increasingly been described as CBPR.[13,14] While there is no one definition of CBPR, in our work, we have defined it as a partnership approach to research that equitably involves diverse partners (e.g., academic researchers, health professionals, community members) in all phases of the research process, with all partners contributing their expertise and with shared influence, decision-making, and ownership.[5,6,8] The overall goal of CBPR is to increase both knowledge and understanding of a given phenomenon (i.e., address basic etiologic research questions) *and* to apply the knowledge gained to inform the development of interventions, policy, and social change to promote health equity.[5,6,8] While recognizing and building on the important global body of work, the focus of this chapter is on case examples in the United States, given the importance of the context within which CBPR is conducted.[14]

3 CBPR Principles

The process of determining core values and principles to guide collaborative efforts is critical to the development of individual CBPR partnerships. Recognizing that there is no one set of principles applicable for all partnerships, we present nine guiding CBPR principles (Box 29.1) grounded in our experience.[5,6,8] These principles are presented as ideals to strive for and are offered to help inform other partnerships as they develop principles that are relevant for their own purpose, context, and partners involved.

Box 29.1 **Principles of Community-Based Participatory Research**

1. CBPR recognizes community as a unit of identity.[5,6,8,15]
2. CBPR builds on strengths and resources within the community.[5,6,8]
3. CBPR facilitates a collaborative, equitable partnership in all phases of research, involving an empowering and power-sharing process that attends to social inequalities.[5,6,8,16,17]
4. CBPR promotes co-learning and capacity-building among all partners.[5,6,8]
5. CBPR integrates and achieves a balance between research and action for the mutual benefit of all partners.[5,6,8]
6. CBPR emphasizes the local relevance of public health problems and ecological perspectives that attend to the multiple determinants of health inequities.[5,6,8]
7. CBPR disseminates findings to all partners and involves them in the dissemination process.[5,6,8]
8. CBPR requires a long-term process and commitment to sustainability.[5,6,8]
9. CBPR addresses issues of race, ethnicity, racism, and social class and embraces cultural humility.[5,6,18]

---

4 Overview of CBPR as an Approach to Research, Not a Method

CBPR is not a research "method"; rather it is an approach to research for which multiple research types, study designs, and methods are applicable.[5] Specifically, CBPR approaches can be used to conduct basic etiologic or intervention research using multiple study designs (e.g., cross-sectional, longitudinal, staggered intervention trial), and it can include the use of qualitative, quantitative, and mixed methods. For the purpose of this chapter, we will discuss the applicability of a CBPR approach to understand and address urban health inequities, drawing on case studies from Detroit and illustrating a wide range of objectives, study designs, and methodological approaches.

5 Overview of Detroit URC and Two Affiliated Partnerships

The Detroit Urban Research Center (Detroit URC) was established in 1995 with initial funding from the US Centers for Disease Control and Prevention's (CDC) Urban Research Centers Initiative. The Detroit URC involves partners from nine community-based organizations, the local health department, a managed care organization, and an academic institution (see Acknowledgments). These organizations comprise the Board, which oversees all activities, including adherence to CBPR principles and development of new, affiliated partnerships.[15] The overarching goal of the Detroit URC is to foster and support the development of CBPR partnerships aimed at addressing social and physical environmental determinants of health to reduce and ultimately eliminate health inequities in Detroit communities. The Board has identified priority health issues of the communities involved and established several affiliated partnerships to address these issues.[15] Case examples from two of these affiliated partnerships, the Healthy Environments Partnership (HEP) and Community Action Against Asthma (CAAA), are provided later.

6 Basic Etiologic Research to Inform Action and Change

The aim of many CBPR studies is to gain knowledge of a given phenomenon to both contribute to a body of science (i.e., basic etiologic research) and translate that knowledge into interventions and policy change strategies.[5,6,8] The commitment to knowledge transfer and social change is a fundamental difference between CBPR and some other approaches to research, such as basic etiologic research. Achieving this end requires active engagement of all partners in the interpretation of data, action planning, and implementation processes, as described here.

6.1 Healthy Environments Partnership: Basic Etiologic Research Case Example

The HEP was established in 2000 with funding for a basic etiologic study to assess social, physical, and environmental determinants of cardiovascular health disparities, as part of the National Institute of Environmental Health Sciences' (NIEHS) Health Disparities initiative. The Detroit URC Board supported the development of the HEP study design and assisted in the identification of several new organizations from areas of the city involved in the study to join the HEP Steering Committee (SC). Members of the HEP SC worked together to design specific components of the initial study, which included the development of a conceptual model, a stratified random sample community survey with biomarker data collection from a subset of survey respondents, a neighborhood observational checklist, and focus groups.[16] In addition, the SC played a critical role in interpreting and disseminating the results and deciding how the results would be applied to improve heart health in Detroit.[17] The SC carries out these roles through a combination of monthly meetings of the entire SC, more frequent meetings of time-limited subcommittees (e.g., a Survey Subcommittee responsible for survey design), and regular email communication as needed.[18] In keeping with the focus of this chapter, we provide a brief elaboration of some of the different study designs and research methods used by HEP in the conduct of these etiologic studies.

The initial HEP basic etiologic research funded by NIEHS was designed as a cross-sectional study involving qualitative, quantitative, and mixed methods. The mixed-method study design that was used has been described by Creswell and colleagues as *exploratory sequential*, in which qualitative data collection and analysis are used to inform questionnaire construction (e.g., quantitative variables, instruments).[19] It consisted of focus groups conducted in three focal neighborhoods to gain a more in-depth understanding of the nature and types of stressors and protective factors experienced by community members and their perceived relationships with health.[20] The HEP SC was instrumental in designing the interview protocol, recruiting focus group sites and participants, and collecting and interpreting the data.[20] Focus group results were used by the HEP Survey Subcommittee to guide development of a closed-ended survey questionnaire, with constructs including stressors, neighborhood characteristics, health-related behaviors, social integration, responses to stressors, and self-reported health.[18] In addition to the survey questionnaire, anthropometric indicators of cardiovascular risk were assessed (e.g., blood pressure, body mass index, blood glucose).

The survey questionnaire was administered to 919 respondents in the same three neighborhoods using a stratified sampling design.[18] Data were used to examine a number of basic etiologic research questions, including relationships between stress and cardiovascular risk, built environments (e.g., neighborhood walkability) and cardiovascular risk, food environments (e.g., location of grocery stores, access to healthy foods) and risk factors for cardiovascular disease (CVD), and air quality (e.g., exposure to airborne particulate matter) and blood pressure.[21–25] In 2005, HEP received another grant from NIEHS; this work included a follow-up survey ($N = 460$) using a similar closed-ended questionnaire.[18] Using these two waves of data, HEP has examined change over time in social and physical environmental contexts and implications for change over time in physical activity, dietary practices, and related cardiovascular risk factors.[18]

The HEP SC used the data gathered through these etiologic research efforts to engage in a multiyear participatory planning process resulting in the development, implementation, and evaluation of a multilevel intervention.[17] This intervention, supported by the National Institute of Minority Health and Health Disparities, was effective in reducing cardiovascular risk among participants with excess cardiovascular risk living in Detroit communities.[26]

7 Intervention Research

CBPR strives to reach a balance between research and action for the mutual benefit of all partners involved. This may take the form of beginning with a basic etiologic study that ultimately informs action (see the preceding HEP example), or the work may begin with an intervention research study.[5,6,8] Here again, such studies may use different research designs and different research methods, in all instances actively involving all partners in the design, implementation, and evaluation of the intervention, as described here.

7.1 Community Action Against Asthma: Intervention Research Case Example

In 1998, in response to one of the priority areas identified by the Detroit URC Board, the CAAA partnership was established to understand and address environmental triggers of childhood asthma; it was funded by the NIEHS and the US Environmental Protection Agency.[15] While CAAA also included several basic etiologic research studies, here we focus on the study design and data collection methods used in the initial household intervention study. CAAA is guided by a SC that met monthly, consisting of representatives from community-based organizations, the local health department, an academic institution, and an integrated healthcare system (see Acknowledgments). The CAAA SC, in keeping with the CBPR principles it adopted, has been responsible for all major decisions regarding study design as well as decisions concerning, for example, recruitment strategies, development and administration of data collection instruments, hiring of personnel, determining incentives, interpretation of data, development of feedback materials to intervention participants, and establishment of dissemination guidelines and disseminating study findings.[27-30]

This household intervention study utilized a community health worker (CHW) model to assist caregivers of children with asthma in identifying and reducing environmental triggers and in the concomitant management and reduction of their child's asthma symptoms. The CAAA intervention consisted of a planned minimum of nine household visits over a 1-year period by CHWs called *community environmental specialists* (CESs). The CESs, residents of the communities in which they worked, were hired by a subcommittee of the CAAA SC. They worked with families to make home environmental changes to reduce the child's exposure to multiple common asthma triggers. Topics addressed, as needed, included clinical aspects of asthma, allergens, and asthma; strategies for reducing environmental asthma triggers; and accessing the medical care system. At the suggestion of community partners on the SC, the CESs provided referrals for a range of issues, such as housing needs, lack of health insurance, food banks, and help with paying electricity bills, recognizing that these challenges, faced by many families, affected their ability to manage their child's asthma.

Households in the CAAA intervention were randomly assigned to one of two waves in a staggered intervention research design.[30] Wave 1 households received an intensive household intervention averaging nine visits the first year and three support visits the second year. Wave 2 households began the same intervention one year after the Wave 1 families, thus initially serving as a control group and subsequently receiving the intervention. This study design assured that all enrolled in the study would receive the intervention and its potential benefits.[6] The main study comparison was for Year 1 between Wave 1 (intervention) and Wave 2 (control).

Data collected for this study included both quantitative and qualitative data. Quantitative data included survey questionnaires with caregivers and children with asthma, allergy skin testing, assessment of household characteristics, dust sampling in the child's bedroom, air quality monitoring, and lung function assessment.[27,30] Qualitative data included written case notes completed by the CESs following each home visit documenting the content of their discussions, provision of education and supplies, non–asthma-related activities (e.g., food referrals), subsequent actions to be taken, and general observations made during the visit.[31] The qualitative data were analyzed on a regular basis, discussed by the CESs with their field supervisor, and used to enhance the activities undertaken during their home visits. For example, over time, the role of the CESs expanded beyond providing contact information and referrals to include social support, connecting families to human service agencies to ensure that they received the assistance they needed, and offering assistance to other family members.[31] The intervention was shown to be effective in increasing some measures of lung function, reducing the frequency of some asthma symptoms, reducing the proportion of children requiring unscheduled medical visits and reporting inadequate use of asthma controller medication, reducing caregiver depressive symptoms, reducing

concentrations in the dust of dog allergen, and increasing some behaviors related to reducing indoor environmental triggers.[27,30]

8 Benefits, Challenges, and Lessons Learned Using a CBPR Approach in Urban Communities

There are benefits and challenges associated with using a CBPR approach in urban
areas; the following sections reflect on the benefits, challenges, and lessons learned from
conducting this type of research.

8.1 Benefits of Using a CBPR Approach in Urban Communities

There are a number of benefits of using CBPR to conduct research to examine and address
health inequities in urban areas. These include ensuring that the focus and type of research
comes from, or reflects, the strengths and concerns of the communities involved; enhancing
the relevance and applicability of the research findings by all partners; recognizing the
complex set of determinants of health inequities and bringing together partners with
diverse skills, knowledge, and expertise to address these factors; enhancing the quality,
validity, cultural appropriateness, and applicability of research and interventions by including the local knowledge and expertise of the participants; strengthening confidence
in the research results; and increasing the likelihood of overcoming the distrust of research
by communities that traditionally have neither benefitted from nor had input into—and
sometimes been harmed by—such research.[5,6,8]

8.2 Challenges of Using a CBPR Approach in Urban Communities

The challenges specific to research type, design, and methods when using a CBPR
approach in an urban context include balancing active involvement and shared
decision-making power on the part of all partners with the burden on partner time and
resources[18,32,33]; managing and synthesizing the decision-making process in the context
of the diverse ideas, preferences, and insights of multiple partners[18]; creating mutually
agreed upon strategies for conducting, interpreting, and disseminating the results of
different data collection methods[18]; identifying and training community members as
data collectors, interpreters, and disseminators[33]; developing dissemination and feedback materials that are appropriate for the local community context[33]; ensuring the
credibility of the data collected for both the immediate purpose and context and more
broadly[33]; balancing the time needed to analyze the data with the sometimes more immediate needs of the project[32]; and ensuring that the research design and data collection
methods are adequate for addressing the research questions being asked.[32]

8.3 Lessons Learned Using a CBPR Approach in Urban Communities

There are a number of lessons to be learned in using CBPR within the context of
urban communities, particularly regarding research, research designs, and research

methods. Five broad areas are presented here. First is the importance of engaging respected community organizations as partners,[15,33] budgeting adequate resources and support for those partners to engage in the research process,[33] and demonstrating the value placed on their contributions as well as study participants' contributions through, for example, funding, stipends, feedback of results, and commitment to co-presentations of study findings.[18] Second is a dedication to developing multiple strategies and mechanisms that enable diverse groups to participate in and influence all aspects of the research and action planning process,[32] and ensuring maximum use of everyone's time[18] including procedures for determining when input is needed and from whom.[18,32] Third is a clear commitment to identifying and incorporating multiple methods to address complex research questions,[19,32,34] including providing the time needed for the iterative process of drafting and revising measurement instruments and protocols tailored to the local community context.[32] Fourth is the value of hiring and training local community members (e.g., as data collectors, project coordinators), building on and strengthening capacity within the involved communities.[18,33] Fifth is developing and sustaining a mutual commitment among both community and academic partners to balancing research and action over the long term.[18]

9 Conclusion

This chapter described the rationale for, definition of, and key principles of CBPR specifically in urban contexts in the United States and offered case examples of its application in multiple types of research, research designs, and research methods. Benefits, challenges, and lessons learned in using CBPR are described briefly. Many other viable approaches to research within urban communities are presented throughout this book. While our focus has been on the application of CBPR within a US context, as presented here, this approach is in keeping with the emancipatory approach emanating from the Southern tradition of participatory research originating in and continuing to be embraced globally, as, for example, in Asia, Latin America, and Africa. Within a global context, a potential limitation in bringing about change within local communities is that local change may or may not result in broader social change. However, we suggest that CBPR and global approaches to participatory research are particularly salient for both contributing to a body of knowledge and bringing about community and social change, especially in communities that have historically been excluded from and lacked power and influence over the process of examining and addressing widespread health inequities.

Acknowledgments

The authors would like to acknowledge the invaluable contributions of the partner organizations involved in the community-based participatory research partnerships described here. The following lists the names of the partners of each of these three partnerships.

The Detroit URC Board involves the following partner organizations: Detroit community-based organizations—Community Health and Social Services, Inc., Communities In Schools, Detroit Hispanic Development Corporation, Detroiters Working for Environmental Justice, Eastside Community Network, Friends of Parkside, Institute for Population Health, Latino Family Services, and Neighborhood Service Organization; local public health agency (Detroit Health Department); health service organization (Henry Ford Health System); and academic institution (the University of Michigan Schools of Public Health, Nursing and Social Work).

HEP Steering Committee Partners have included: Detroit-based community organizations—Brightmoor Community Center, Butzel Family Center, Chandler Park Conservancy, Detroit Hispanic Development Corporation, Eastside Community Network, Friends of Parkside, Institute for Population Health, and Southwest Detroit Environmental Vision; community members; local public health agency (Detroit Health Department); health service organization (Henry Ford Health System); and academic institution (the University of Michigan School of Public Health).

CAAA Steering Committee Partners have included: Arab Community Center for Economic and Social Services (ACCESS); Butzel Family Center; Community Health and Social Services Center; Inc. (CHASS); Communities In Schools; Detroit Health Department; Detroit Hispanic Development Corporation; Detroiters Working for Environmental Justice; Eastside Community Network; Friends of Parkside; Henry Ford Health System; Kettering/Butzel Health Initiative; Latino Family Services, Michigan Department of Agriculture, Plant, and Pest Management Division; University of Michigan-Michigan Medicine; University of Michigan-School of Public Health; United Community Housing Coalition; and a community member at large.

References

1. Schiller JS, Lucas JW, Peregoy JA. Summary health statistics for US adults: national health interview survey, 2011. Centers for Disease Control and Prevention website. Published 2012. Available at https://stacks.cdc.gov/view/cdc/21423. Accessed May 1, 2018.
2. Bishaw A. *Areas with concentrated poverty: 2006-2010.* Vol 9. US Department of Commerce, Economics and Statistics Administration, US Census Bureau website. Published 2011. Available at: https://ok.gov/odmhsas/documents/Areas%20with%20Concentrated%20 Poverty.pdf. Accessed May 1, 2018.
3. McCord C, Freeman HP. Excess mortality in Harlem. *N Engl J Med.* 1990; 322(3):173–177.
4. World Health Organization. *Closing the gap in a generation: health equity through action on the social determinants of health: Commission on Social Determinants of Health final report.* Geneva, Switzerland: World Health Organization; 2008.
5. Israel BA, Eng E, Schulz AJ, Parker E. Introduction to methods for CBPR for health. In Israel B, Eng E, Schulz AJ, Parker E, eds. *Methods for community-based participatory research for health.* 2nd ed. San Francisco, CA: Jossey-Bass; 2013:3–38.
6. Israel B, Schulz A, Parker E, et al. Critical issues in developing and following CBPR principles. In Wallerstein N, Duran B, Oetzel J, Minkler M, eds. *Community-based participatory research for health: advancing social and health equity.* 3rd ed. San Francisco, CA: Jossey-Bass; 2018:31–46.

7. Wallerstein N, Duran B. Theoretical, historical, and practice roots of CBPR. In Wallerstein N, Duran B, Oetzel J, Minkler M, eds. *Community-based participatory research for health: advancing social and health equity.* 3rd ed. San Francisco, CA: Jossey-Bass; 2018:17–29.

8. Israel BA, Schulz AJ, Parker EA, Becker AB. Review of community-based research: assessing partnership approaches to improve public health. *Annu Rev Public Health.* 1998; 19(1):173–202.

9. Reason P, Bradbury H, eds. *The SAGE handbook of action research: participative inquiry and practice.* 2nd ed. London: SAGE; 2013.

10. Hall BL, Tandon R, Tremblay C, eds. *Strengthening community university research partnerships: global perspectives.* Victoria, Canada: University of Victoria; 2015.

11. Hall BL, Tandon R. Decolonization of knowledge, epistemicide, participatory research and higher education. *Res All.* 2017; 1(1):6–19.

12. Fals Borda O. Participatory (action) research in social theory: origins and challenges. In Reason P, Bradbury H, eds. *Handbook of action research: participative inquiry and practice.* Thousand Oaks, CA: Sage; 2006:27–37.

13. Israel B, Eng E, Schulz A, Parker E, eds. *Methods for community-based participatory research for health.* 2nd ed. San Francisco, CA: Jossey-Bass; 2013.

14. Wallerstein N, Duran B, Oetzel J, Minkler M, eds. *Community- based participatory research for health: advancing social and health equity.* 3rd ed. San Francisco, CA: Jossey-Bass; 2018.

15. Israel BA, Lichtenstein R, Lantz P, et al. The Detroit Community-Academic Urban Research Center: development, implementation, and evaluation. *J Public Health Manag Pract.* 2001; 7(5):1–19.

16. Schulz AJ, Kannan S, Dvonch JT, et al. Social and physical environments and disparities in risk for cardiovascular disease: the Healthy Environments Partnership conceptual model. *Environ Health Perspect.* 2005; 113(12):1817–1825.

17. Schulz AJ, Israel BA, Coombe CM, et al. A community-based participatory planning process and multilevel intervention design: toward eliminating cardiovascular health inequities. *Health Promot Pract.* 2011; 12(6):900–911.

18. Schulz AJ, Zenk SN, Kannan S, Israel BA, Stokes CA. CBPR in survey design and implementation: the Healthy Environments Partnership survey. In Israel BA, Eng E, Schulz AJ, Parker EA, eds. *Methods in community-based participatory research for health.* 2nd ed. San Francisco, CA: Jossey-Bass; 2013:197–224.

19. Creswell JW, Creswell JD. *Research design: qualitative, quantitative, and mixed methods approaches.* 5th ed. Thousand Oaks, CA: SAGE Publications; 2018.

20. Israel BA, Schulz AJ, Estrada-Martinez L, et al. Engaging urban residents in assessing neighborhood environments and their implications for health. *J Urban Health.* 2006; 83(3):523–539.

21. Schulz AJ, Zenk SN, Israel BA, Mentz G, Stokes C, Galea S. Do neighborhood economic characteristics, racial composition, and residential stability predict perceptions of stress associated with the physical and social environment? Findings from a multilevel analysis in Detroit. *J Urban Health.* 2008; 85(5):642–661.

22. Schulz AJ, Mentz GB, Sampson N, et al. Race and the distribution of social and physical environmental risk: a case example from the Detroit metropolitan area. *Bois Rev Soc Sci Res Race.* 2016; 13(2):285–304.

23. Schulz A, Mentz G, Johnson-Lawrence V, et al. Independent and joint associations between multiple measures of the built and social environment and physical activity in a multi-ethnic urban community. *J Urban Health.* 2013; 90(5):872–887.

24. Zenk SN, Schulz AJ, Izumi BT, Mentz G, Israel BA, Lockett M. Neighborhood food environment role in modifying psychosocial stress–diet relationships. *Appetite.* 2013; 65(SC):170–177.

25. Dvonch JT, Kannan SS, Schulz AJ, et al. Acute effects of ambient particulate matter on blood pressure: differential effects across urban communities. *Hypertension.* 2009; 53(5):853–859.

26. Schulz AJ, Israel BA, Mentz GB, et al. Effectiveness of a walking group intervention to promote physical activity and cardiovascular health in predominantly non-hispanic black and hispanic

urban neighborhoods: findings from the walk your heart to health intervention. *Health Educ Behav Off Publ Soc Public Health Educ.* 2015; 42(3):380–392.

27. Edgren KK, Parker EA, Israel BA, et al. Community involvement in the conduct of a health education intervention and research project: Community Action Against Asthma. *Health Promot Pract.* 2005; 6(3):263–269.

28. Parker E, Israel B, Williams M, et al. Community Action Against Asthma: examining the partnership process of a community-based participatory research project. *J Gen Intern Med.* 2003; 18(7):558–567.

29. Parker EA, Robins TG, Israel BA, Brakefield-Caldwell W, Edgren K, Wilkins DJ. Developing and implementing guidelines for dissemination: the experience of the Community Action Against Asthma project. In Israel BA, Eng E, Schulz AJ, Parker EA, eds. *Methods for community-based participatory research for health.* 2nd ed. San Francisco, CA: Jossey-Bass; 2013:405–434.

30. Parker EA, Israel BA, Robins TG, et al. Evaluation of Community Action Against Asthma: a community health worker intervention to improve children's asthma-related health by reducing household environmental triggers for asthma. *Health Educ Behav.* 2008; 35(3):376–395.

31. Chung Densen LK. *An examination of life stressors experienced by families of children with asthma in low-income communities of color.* [Dissertation]. Ann Arbor: The University of Michigan; 2012.

32. Israel BA, Lantz PM, McGranaghan RJ, Guzman JR, Lichtenstein R, Rowe Z. Documentation and evaluation of community-based participatory research partnerships: the use of in-depth interviews and closed-ended questionnaires. In Israel BA, Eng E, Schulz AJ, Parker EA, eds. *Methods for community-based participatory research for health.* 2nd ed. San Francisco, CA: John Wiley and Sons, Ltd; 2012:369–403.

33. Kieffer E, Salabarría-Peña Y, Odoms-Young A, Willis S, Palmisano G, Guzman J. The application of focus group methodologies to community-based participatory research. In Israel B, Eng E, Schulz A, Parker E, eds. *Methods for community-based participatory research for health.* 2nd ed. San Francisco, CA: Jossey-Bass; 2013:249–276.

34. Creswell JW. *A concise introduction to mixed methods research.* Los Angeles, CA: Sage; 2014.

CASE STUDIES IN URBAN HEALTH

30

The Healthy Cities Movement

AGIS D. TSOUROS

1 Introduction

There is no shortage of literature on the history and diverse features and activities of the Healthy Cities movement around the world.[1,2] This chapter addresses the key conceptual and strategic features of Healthy Cities in the context of today's urban health challenges. I will argue that the Healthy Cities approach is more relevant than ever and that this thriving global movement can be an effective vehicle for change and innovation. Most global public health, social, and environmental challenges, as well as the implementation of the new Sustainable Development Goals (SDGs) for the planet, require local action and strong local leadership.

The Healthy Cities movement was launched at the peak of the new public health era in the 1980s, very much inspired by the strategy Health for All and the Ottawa Charter for Health Promotion.[3,4] It proved very attractive to local political and community leaders: it has inspired a wide range of professionals and actors from different sectors, and it spread quickly to different parts of the world. It emerged as a dynamic global movement in the form of city projects and initiatives as well as national and international Healthy Cities networks and alliances.

There are a host of initiatives in different regions that come under the Healthy Cities "umbrella," including healthy municipalities, healthy villages, health islands, and healthy communities. Very often, healthy settings projects, such as healthy schools, healthy workplaces, and healthy markets, are locally supported by or linked with Healthy Cities projects.

2 Healthy Cities Is a Political Project that Became a Movement

Jo Asvall, the director of the World Health Organization (WHO) Regional Office for Europe, introduced Healthy Cities in his speech at the European Congress on Healthy Cities in 1987. He said, "Building a healthy city becomes first and foremost a formidable challenge on how to create a movement for health where many players can be inspired and motivated for taking actions to think new and better solutions and to work together in new partnerships for health."[5]

Healthy Cities was launched as a value-based, political, and intersectoral project, with the aim to put health high on the social and political agendas of cities. Its creation was based on the recognition of the importance of urban health, action at the local level, and the key role of local governments in health and sustainable development.

Healthy Cities embodies a number of key features (constants) that proved, over the past three decades, crucial in its success, including its strong emphasis on values and principles (the right to health and well-being, equity and social justice, gender equality, solidarity and social inclusion, universal coverage, and sustainable development), the prerequisite for strong political commitment and partnership-based approaches, and the emphasis on democratic governance, strategic thinking, and networking.

It should be stressed that Healthy Cities is strongly underpinned by enduring classic health promotion concepts based on the Ottawa Charter for Health Promotion: creating supportive environments for health, making the healthy choices the easy choices, creating health-promoting settings, and empowering individuals and communities as a prerequisite for success.

3 Healthy Cities Is a Dynamic and Continuously Evolving Concept

The specific agenda, themes, and goals of Healthy Cities projects locally, nationally, and regionally are generally shaped by three elements: the constant Healthy Cities values and principles, local urban health priorities and concerns, and WHO regional priorities and strategies and global strategies and priorities that are relevant to urban development.

A Healthy City has been described in terms of 11 qualities (Box 30.1).[6]

A Healthy City is a city for all. Its main attributes reflect its values and principles. A Healthy City is caring, inclusive, supportive, and equitable; it invests in human and social capital; it shapes its physical and built environments to promote well-being; it is open, smart, and creative; and it sees health and sustainable development as a precondition for a successful future.[7]

Healthy Cities has continuously evolved over the past 30 years, integrating new global developments (such as the sustainable development agenda), new WHO and UN strategies and goals (such as the noncommunicable diseases action plans and global goals), new evidence (e.g., the social determinants of health), new concepts (such as the Health in All Policies [HiAP] concept), emerging concerns and priorities (such as those related to preparedness to address public health emergencies related to climate change and migration and health), and, last, new knowledge from experience and practice. Box 30.2 outlines key concepts and issues that should be integrated in a twenty-first-century Healthy Cities approach.

The Healthy Cities agenda should be meaningful not only to politicians and academics but also, very importantly, to citizens and communities and a wide range of local stakeholders. Constantly deepening the community and intersectoral roots of Healthy Cities as well as enriching its agenda with new ideas and concepts are prerequisites for its success and sustainable future.

Box 30.1 **Eleven Qualities of a Healthy City**

1. A clean, safe, high-quality environment including affordable housing
2. A stable ecosystem
3. A strong, mutually supportive, and nonexploitative community
4. Much public participation in and control over decisions affecting life, health, and well-being
5. The provision of basic needs (food, water, shelter, income, safety, and work) for all people
6. Access to a wide range of experiences and resources with the possibility of multiple contacts, interaction, and communication
7. A diverse, vital, and innovative economy
8. Encouragement of connections with the past, with the varied cultural and biological heritage, and with other groups and individuals
9. A city form (design) that is compatible with and enhances the preceding characteristics
10. An optimum level of appropriate public health and care services accessible to all
11. A high health status (both a high positive health status and low disease status)

From Tsouros AD, ed. *World Health Organization Healthy Cities project: a project becomes a movement, a review of progress 1987 to 1990.* Copenhagen, Denmark: World Health Organization; 1991.

---

4 Healthy Cities Action Domains and Potential to Make a Difference in People's Health and Well-Being

Healthy Cities is active in six main domains. These are (1) politics and governance; (2) community level; (3) policies, regulations, planning processes, and city development strategies; (4) local services and programs; (5) people and their needs: whole populations, different social groups, families, and individuals; and (6) the social, built, and physical environments.[7]

Healthy Cities can exert their influence on health and equity through a wide range of mechanisms and processes. First, through regulation. For example, cities are well-positioned to influence land use, building standards, and water and sanitation systems and to enact and enforce occupational health and safety regulations and restrictions on tobacco use. Second, through integration. Local governments can develop and implement integrated policies and strategies for health promotion and social and sustainable development. Third, through intersectoral governance. Cities' democratic mandates convey authority and the power to convene partnerships and encourage contributions from many sectors and stakeholders from the private and voluntary domains. Fourth,

---

Box 30.2 **Modern Public Health Concepts and Approaches**

The right to health and equity
Health and well-being
The determinants of health and upstream interventions
Health in all policies
Health, sustainable development, and the Sustainable Development Goals (SDGs)
Universal coverage and patient-centered services
Public health systems, prevention, and health promotion
Population-based approaches
Whole-of-(local)-government, Whole-of-society approaches
Life-course approach
Health literacy
Urban planning and health
Environmental health and climate change
Community resilience
Community action and empowerment
Urban governance and governance for health
Leadership for health and city diplomacy

---

through community engagement. Local governments have everyday contact with citizens and are closest to their concerns and priorities. They present unique opportunities for partnering with civic society and citizens' groups. Fifth through an equity focus. Local governments can mobilize local resources and deploy them to create more opportunities for poor and vulnerable population groups and to protect and promote the rights of all urban residents.

5 Designing and Implementing Healthy Cities Projects

The implementation of Healthy Cities projects requires several factors. It requires explicit political commitment and partnership agreements at the highest level in the city to make health, equity, and sustainable development core values in the city's vision and strategies. Organizational structures and processes are needed to manage, coordinate, and support change and facilitate national-local cooperation, local partnerships, and action across sectors, along with active citizen participation and community empowerment. Promotion of health in all policies, setting common goals and priorities, and developing a strategy or plan for health, equity, and well-being in the city are central to the Healthy Cities projects.

Systematically monitoring the health of the population and the determinants of health in the city is also required, including the production of a comprehensive city health profile as a sine qua non for understanding the health conditions in the city and for setting priorities and accountability mechanisms. And, finally, implementation of Healthy Cities projects requires formal and informal networking and platforms for dialogue and cooperation with different partners from the public, private, voluntary, and community domains.

Deciding the priorities, the agenda, and the methods to be employed as well as how to position the Healthy Cities project in the city is a crucial first step. The use of traditional methods to address the complex urban health priorities of our time will have limited effect. In addition, it would be a waste of the prestigious Healthy Cities brand to exert energy on trivial or low-impact projects or to spend a disproportionate amount of time organizing health education events and celebrating the various world health days.

In fact, what matters is not *what* priorities a city wishes to address, but *how* that city plans to address those priorities in order to achieve maximum impact. Comprehensive city health profiles (which include social and environmental conditions and measure health inequalities) and integrated health plans that draw on the contributions of different sectors and stakeholders are essential.

A comprehensive Healthy Cities strategy and plan should ideally include the following broad areas of action: equity, HiAP, healthy people (e.g., giving every child a healthy start in life, promoting healthy aging, and addressing the health needs of migrants), community development and empowerment, health literacy, healthy urban planning, expanding green and smoke free spaces and cycling lanes, introducing systematic prevention programs addressing obesity and noncommunicable diseases, and offering health and social care to all.

Because Healthy Cities is value-based, it encourages local leaders and communities to reflect on what society they wish to have. Strong leadership must be complemented by the capacity to manage a multifaceted strategic project that covers most domains of city activity. A key to the success of Healthy Cities is also how well it is connected with other local agendas and strategies. Last, a good way to bring different sectors around the table is by identifying goals that would require the contribution of many stakeholders to be reached.

6 A Diverse Global Movement

The Healthy Cities movement is not uniform in its operational modalities and priorities across regions and individual countries.[8] Five different types of organizational entities can be identified.[9] These are:

1. Healthy Cities projects in cities, municipalities, provinces, territories, islands, or other administrative entities;
2. National or subnational Healthy Cities networks most often run as nongovernmental organizations (NGOs) with or without the support or involvement of ministries of health and/or national associations of local authorities. National Networks provide strategic and technical support to their member cities and provide links with national ministries and other entities;[10]

3. Regional networks of national networks (e.g., the WHO European Network of National Networks) or multistakeholder partnerships (e.g., the Alliance of Healthy Cities in Western Asian region whose members include municipal governments, national governments, NGOs, private sectors, academic institutions, and international agencies. The Alliance has a close collaboration with WHO);
4. Linguistic networks, as is the case of the francophone Healthy Cities network;
5. Leadership and support structures: most WHO Regional Offices run Healthy Cities programs and have designated focal points. The European Region runs a network of approximately 100 cities from across the Region that are designated on the basis of specific requirements, and the network is also supported by an external secretariat. Other regions limit their role to providing guidance tools, standards, and evaluation schemes as well as capacity-building support to needy cities and national networks. A number of WHO collaborating centers provide analytical support. For many years, there have been very few (mostly bilateral) interregional exchanges between Healthy Cities and no focal point at the heart of WHO in Geneva. In 2016, the Shanghai Consensus on Healthy Cities (adopted at the International Mayors Forum, on the occasion of the 9th Global Conference of Health Promotion) provided a political boost to the global Healthy Cities movement.[11] The Americas Region of WHO did the same also in 2016, with the Santiago Declaration, and the European Region in 2018, with the Copenhagen Statement. This new impetus has been tremendously reinforced by the new UN 2030 sustainable development agenda, which is highly relevant to cities.

However, the global Healthy Cities movement lacks a common agenda. Its regional diversity is a definitive strength and a source of creative thinking and rich experiences, but the lack of a minimal common strategic frame hinders the fulfilment of its immense potential. Healthy Cities involves thousands of cities around the world, but many countries remain still beyond its reach and their inclusion requires a concerted global effort.

Healthy Cities is adaptable to local political and organizational contexts and thus it can overcome potential obstacles in pursuing its ambitious agenda. For example, obstacles in establishing mechanisms, platforms, and processes to cooperate closely with statutory and nonstatutory partners exist. For this reason, some cities found it easier or more effective to create project offices outside formal municipal structures in the form of nonprofit organizations.

Experience with the European movement has shown that creating and sustaining Healthy Cities depends on three critical factors: first, protecting Healthy Cities from political changes through consensus, ownership-building, and broad partnerships across sectors and political parties; second, passing the national network leadership baton to committed Healthy Cities champions; and third, making sure that Healthy Cities maintains its relevance and credibility by constantly working on local public health priorities and upholding its values and principles.

7 Epilogue and the Way Forward

Mayors are emerging as powerful and influential agents for change locally, nationally, and internationally. The Healthy Cities movement, with its modern and evidence-informed approach, its political legitimacy, and global recognition as well as its considerable experience can make a difference in all parts of the world.

The Healthy Cities movement represents a unique and powerful platform for innovation and change. Its potential for impact can be significantly enhanced through integrated global leadership, increased interregional coherence, and strategic thinking.

The Healthy Cities movement would benefit from a global strategic framework that should identify common principles and priorities as well as performance and accountability standards and indicators in key areas of action. This framework will promote coherence and synergies between regional Healthy Cities initiatives.

Regularly renewing political commitment is valuable, but the impact of mayors' conferences and their statements will be short-lived unless they are combined with well-thought-out plans. Examples include expanding the movement to new countries and cities or committing to address childhood obesity by agreeing on a plan of action.

Creating platforms for interregional dialogue is a must. Such platforms will enable mutual learning and sharing of experiences and also offer opportunities for enhancing city diplomacy at the global level.

National governments should do more to support and use national Healthy Cities networks and also strengthen the national-local cooperation for health and well-being. National legislation can empower cities to lead in health promotion and recognize their key role in the implementation of the SDG agenda.

The local voice must be represented and heard in international fora such as the World Health Assembly, and this could be done by including mayors in country delegations. Furthermore, scaling up and strengthening the global Healthy Cities movement should also involve forging new and widening existing partnerships with agencies concerned with urban human, social, and sustainable development.

Urban health should be recognized as an important cross-cutting domain of the WHO's work, and the urban dimension should be systematically explored in all its technical work. The time is right to create a strong global Healthy Cities movement. The new sustainable development agenda provides a new opportunity to strengthen health and equity in our cities and communities. Healthy Cities and the SDGs are mutually reinforcing and provide enormous legitimacy for strong leadership and action.

References

1. Tsouros AD. Twenty-seven years of the WHO European Healthy Cities movement: a sustainable movement for change and innovation at the local level. *Health Promo Int.* 2015; 30(S1): i3–i7.
2. de Leeuw E, Simos J, eds. *Healthy cities: the theory, policy, and practice of value-based urban planning.* New York: Springer; 2017.
3. World Health Organization. *Health for all targets.* Copenhagen, Denmark: World Health Organization; 1984.
4. Ottawa Charter for Health Promotion, 1986. *Health Promot Int.* 1986; 1(4):405.
5. Asvall J. Presentation at the European Congress on Healthy Cities. Dusseldorf, Germany: World Health Organization Europe; 1987.
6. Tsouros AD, ed. World Health Organization Healthy Cities project: a project becomes a movement, a review of progress 1987 to 1990. Copenhagen, Denmark: World Health Organization; 1991.

7. Tsouros AD. *City leadership for health and sustainable development–critical issues for successful Healthy Cities projects.* Kuwait City, Kuwait: Global Healthy Cities; 2017.

8. de Leeuw E. Evaluating WHO Healthy Cities in Europe: issues and perspectives. *J Urban Health.* 2013; 90(S1):14–22.

9. Tsouros AD, de Leeuw E, Green G. Evaluation of the fifth phase (2009–2013) of the WHO European Healthy Cities Network: further sophistication and challenges. *Health Promot Int.* 2015; 30(S):i1–i2. doi:10.1093/heapro/dav045

10. World Health Organization. *National healthy cities networks in the WHO European Region. Promoting health and well-being throughout Europe (2015).* Copenhagen, Denmark: World Health Organization; 2015.

11. Healthy Cities Mayors Forum. *Shanghai Consensus on Healthy Cities 2016.* Geneva, Switzerland: World Health Organization; 2016.

31

The Partnership for Healthy Cities

*Activating Urban Governments as Engines of Public
Health Practice*

ARIELLA ROJHANI, CHARITY HUNG, SALLY CHEW, CHRISTINA HONEYSETT,
SANDRA MULLIN, AND ADAM KARPATI

1 Background

In September 2011, representatives from countries and organizations around the world
assembled at the United Nations for the first UN high-level meeting on the Prevention
and Control of Noncommunicable Diseases (NCDs). It was in the Political Declaration
adopted at this meeting that heads of state finally acknowledged what epidemiologists
and a small but vocal number of advocates had long contended: "The global burden and
threat of noncommunicable diseases constitutes one of the major challenges for development in the twenty-first century."[1]

City health departments—mirroring their national and state/regional
counterparts—have been ill-equipped to handle the challenges of addressing NCDs
and injuries. City health departments typically are organized around traditional public
health functions, such as outbreak investigations and other infectious disease control
activities, food safety, and other regulatory activities. Funding streams for NCD and
injury prevention are extremely limited, and relevant workforce skills, such as legislative
development, strategic communications, and behavioral epidemiology are not widely
available, especially in low- and middle-income countries (LMICs).

NCDs (cancer, cardiovascular diseases, diabetes, and chronic respiratory diseases)
account for 39.5 million deaths annually, or 70% of global mortality. About 30.7 million
of these deaths, or 78%, occur in LMICs. Nearly 17 million of these deaths are premature (i.e., occurring before the age of 70).[2]

Alongside the devastating increase of NCDs has been a rise in disability and deaths
from injuries. Nearly 5 million people die every year from injuries, representing 9% of
all global deaths. Approximately 1.3 million of these deaths are caused by road traffic
crashes, with 93% of all fatalities occurring in LMICs. More than half of these deaths
are pedestrians, cyclists, and motorcyclists. Road traffic crashes are the leading cause of
death in persons 15–29 years of age.[3]

Global epidemiologic data on NCDs and injuries of these types are typically available only at national levels. City-level information is scarce, and there is no global compilation and comparison. In most countries, behavioral risk factor surveys are not sampled and powered for city-level estimates. In LMICs, the absence of high-functioning civil registration and vital statistics systems makes robust city-level mortality information nearly impossible to obtain.

Major commercial determinants of NCDs include tobacco, unhealthy food, and alcohol. Important environmental exposures include unsafe street design and poor indoor and ambient air quality. Nowhere is the intersection of these exposures as pronounced as it is in cities. In 2016, more than half the world's population lived in urban settlements.[4] This number will rise to nearly 60% by 2030, with one in three people on Earth living in a city with more than half a million people.[5] Cities are the economic hubs for many countries, attracting formerly rural populations with the promise of greater economic prosperity, particularly as climate change renders prosperity from agrarian livelihoods increasingly unsustainable. Unfortunately, the urban population boom is, in most cases, preempting planned urban development, resulting in rapid growth of urban areas without the necessary concurrent adjustments to laws and regulations, infrastructure, and services. Put in the context of public health and NCD and injury prevention, more people are living in urban environments that are both unable to protect people from exposure to risk factors and to provide necessary health services to cope with the rising morbidity and injury impacts. Aware of the growth but unprepared or ill-equipped to implement necessary changes, many city governments are now recognizing the need to reform their policies, plans, and programs to address NCD and injury prevention.

2 Partnership for Healthy Cities

In August 2016, former New York City mayor, entrepreneur, and philanthropist Michael R. Bloomberg was appointed the World Health Organization (WHO) Global Ambassador for NCDs.[6] For more than a decade, his charitable foundation, Bloomberg Philanthropies, has supported countries around the world to implement population-level policies in tobacco control, obesity prevention, road safety, public health data systems, and other domains. As Mayor of New York City, Bloomberg supported rigorous chronic disease prevention legislation and regulation, including a landmark ban on smoking indoors, later extended to include outdoor public places; taxation of cigarettes; a ban on industrial trans fats in commercially prepared food; and nutrition standards for schools, daycares, hospitals, and other public institutions.[7]

The global initiatives supported by Bloomberg Philanthropies all entail the application of a focused set of evidence-informed interventions, typically codified in guidance from the WHO. These include the MPOWER and Save LIVES technical packages for tobacco control and road safety, respectively. Such technical packages are useful to governments for policy and planning because they distill complex evidence and diverse intervention options into a short set of the most impactful and robust actions.[8]

Bloomberg Philanthropies created the Partnership for Healthy Cities (PHC) to translate its successful model of country-level NCD and injury prevention activities to cities. Formally launched in May 2017 in partnership with WHO and Vital Strategies, PHC provides catalytic support to mayors and their departments of health or transportation to accelerate progress in one high-impact, evidence-based NCD or injury-prevention intervention by December 2018. The single activity and short timeline were designed to demonstrate rapid success and create positive momentum toward more substantial local attention and investment in the future.

The initiative extended invitations to participate to mayors in large (>1.5M population) cities in all regions of the world; no more than four cities were approached in any one country. Invited cities were selected based on population, length of term of the mayor, prior demonstrated innovative public health actions, and favorable national context, such as newly established laws or regulations.

By October 2017, 54 cities across the globe had enrolled in the Partnership.[9] Three-quarters of the cities are in LMICs.[10] Each of the cities was presented with a menu of policy and program intervention options upon enrollment in the Partnership, from which they selected one to implement. Several were cost-effective practices from WHO's technical packages. The list comprised two actions to address tobacco control: smoke-free public places and advertising bans (both referenced in the MPOWER technical package); two food policy activities: sugar sweetened beverage taxation and sodium reduction/institutional food policies; three road safety strategies: speed reduction, drink driving prevention, and seat belt/motorcycle helmet use (all referenced in the Save LIVES technical package); two environmental interventions: urban design for physical activity promotion and improving air quality; and one surveillance activity: NCD risk factor surveys (such as WHO's STEPS surveys).[11-13] As a participant in the initiative, each city would receive technical assistance, as needed, to guide implementation of its chosen activity; a $US100,000 seed grant; and strategic communication technical support for both mass media campaigns in support of behavior change and to promote awareness of the issue and its intervention progress locally.

Cities were encouraged to select interventions that responded to local priorities, that leveraged existing or planned commitments by city government, and that built on activities already under way. The distribution of chosen intervention topics was generally even, with 12 cities pursuing tobacco control activities, 12 cities selecting interventions to improve food policy, 10 cities pursuing road safety, 13 cities electing to make their cities more walkable or bikeable, and 7 cities choosing to improve NCD risk factor surveillance. Few cities selected taxation of sugary beverages, reflecting the limitations of such authority at the city level. Air quality improvement was another area with limited uptake, reflecting a general perception that such work was outside the remit of health authorities or that local action would be insufficient in the absence of strong national efforts.

Within the cities' chosen topical areas, the actual intervention activities that cities are implementing is quite varied, with many cities implementing multiple intervention types: 20 cities are pursuing some form of policy change (drafting new or amending current legislation, regulations, or protocols); 21 are conducting specific projects, such as road design; 28 are strengthening enforcement of an existing regulation; and 43 cities are designing and implementing a communication or mass media campaign.

3 Results to Date

While still early in the implementation process, a number of cities can already claim success in their initiatives. Such results are testament to the agility of local governments, particularly when in receipt of targeted support. Early success was found in Bengaluru, India, where the municipal government embarked on a multipronged strategy to improve enforcement of the smoke-free law while publicly communicating the harms of second-hand smoke exposure via media campaigns. Also pursuing an initiative to enhance enforcement of an existing law, Quito, Ecuador, is implementing and enforcing national food marketing standards in local schools. Melbourne, Australia, and Fortaleza, Brazil, each improved the walkability and bikeability of their cities: Melbourne developed a mobile app to promote more regular physical activity via incentives, and Fortaleza expanded its bike sharing program. Montevideo, Uruguay, which was already quite advanced in its approach to reducing salt consumption, has required restaurants previously mandated to remove high-sodium condiments from tabletops to also make 10% of all menu items with no added salt.

Each city that finds success in this targeted approach to accelerating local policy action shares common factors for that success. To start, a motivated technical lead within the appropriate municipal department is indispensable. This devolution of the day-to-day work seldom compromises the political support already committed by the mayor in joining the network, while allowing for the more quotidian tasks of intervention implementation to proceed without political overhead. Another factor for success has been the intensive provision of technical assistance to all cities in the network, including high-income cities. Even cities with more advanced systems and policies in place found benefit in receiving regular, high-quality technical assistance from global experts. Finally, cities with sufficient human resources to dedicate to implementation were generally more successful than those without a natural institutional "home" for programmatic activities. This situation of city governments lacking capacity to support best-practice interventions is proving to be a persistent and, in some cases insurmountable, barrier to implementation. It suggests a larger capacity gap in city health departments around chronic disease and injury prevention in spite of the present needs.

In some cities, a challenge in advancing the initiative's goals has been securing consistent high-level political support. This can be due to competing priorities on a mayor's agenda, situational demands on a mayor's time, and/or politics and calculated assessments of project impact on a politician's popularity and electability. In contrast, the presence of active mayoral engagement, while not sufficient to ensure success, is necessary and can dramatically facilitate progress.

The initiative has endeavored to create a strong network among participating cities. Strong communications support to mayoral and agency press offices has helped cities publicize their work, not only locally, but also at the national and international levels and to their peer governments. The initiative has organized a series of training workshops for technical leads to build leadership and management skills, to further familiarize them with global best practices and guidance, and to promote intercity exchange of experience and insight.

4 Looking Ahead

Few mechanisms exist to support the translation of global and national public health guidance into practical local action. The PHC, although in an incipient stage, is one such model that catalyzes local action through the targeted delivery of technical and financial resources and the visibility of participation in a global network. By the end of the initiative, dozens of cities in countries around the world, in both lower and higher resource settings, will have implemented some form of best practice NCD or injury prevention. The broader ambition is to use the examples and lessons learned from this initiative to demonstrate that the political and technical resources of cities can be powerful engines for real public health action and to show to mayors and health directors that it is both imperative and opportunistic to claim a leadership role in these domains alongside their national and regional counterparts.

References

1. United Nations. *Political declaration of the high-level meeting of the General Assembly on the prevention and control of non-communicable diseases.* New York: United Nations General Assembly; 2011.
2. World Health Organization. *NCD morbidity and mortality.* World Health Organization Global Health Observatory (GHO) data website. Available at http://www.who.int/gho/ncd/mortality_morbidity/en/. Accessed July 1, 2018.
3. World Health Organization. *Global status report on road safety 2015.* Geneva, Switzerland: World Health Organization; 2015.
4. UN-Habitat. *World cities report 2016. Urbanization and development: emerging futures.* Nairobi, Kenya: UN-Habitat; 2016.
5. United Nations. *The world's cities in 2016. Data booklet.* New York: United Nations; 2016.
6. Michael R. Bloomberg becomes WHO global ambassador for noncommunicable diseases. World Health Organization website. 2016. Available at http://www.who.int/en/newsroom/detail/17-08-2016-michael-r-bloomberg-becomes-who-global-ambassador-for-noncommunicable-diseases. Accessed July 1, 2018.
7. Frieden TR, Bassett MT, Thorpe LE, Farley TA. Public health in New York City, 2002-2007: confronting epidemics of the modern era. *Int J Epidemiol.* 2008;37(5):966–977.
8. Frieden TR. Six components necessary for effective public health program implementation. *Am J Public Health.* 2014; 104(1):17–22.
9. Partnership for Healthy Cities website. Available at https://partnershipforhealthycities.bloomberg.org/. Accessed July 1, 2018.
10. World Bank. Country and lending groups. The World Bank website. Available at https://datahelpdesk.worldbank.org/knowledgebase/articles/906519. Accessed July 1, 2018.
11. World Health Organization. Tobacco free initative. World Health Organization website. Available at http://www.who.int/tobacco/mpower/en/. Accessed July 1, 2018.
12. World Health Organization. *Save LIVES: a road safety technical package.* World Health Organization website. Available at http://www.who.int/violence_injury_prevention/publications/road_traffic/save-lives-package/en/. Accessed July 1, 2018.
13. World Health Organization. STEPwise approach to surveillance (STEPS). World Health Organization website. Available at http://www.who.int/ncds/surveillance/steps/en/. Accessed July 1, 2018.

32

CityHealth

Policies for Today's Urban Health Challenges

BRIAN C. CASTRUCCI, ELIZABETH A. CORCORAN, SHELLEY L. HEARNE,
KATIE KEITH, ELIZABETH VOYLES, AND CATHERINE PATTERSON

1 Introduction

Personal health and community health are indelibly linked. After all, the choices we make regarding food, schools, recreation, and other key health determinants depend largely on the choices available to us. While individual responsibility plays a big role in personal health outcomes, there is increasing recognition that making behavior changes is not always feasible without first changing environments and institutions. Despite the efforts of dedicated practitioners delivering cutting-edge, innovative treatments, focusing on the individual patient is no longer enough. We must increase our commitment to community health to improve individual health nationwide.

Case in point: chronic disease is the single greatest threat to America's health. The statistics tell a stark story. Chronic disease is the leading cause of premature death.[1] The proportion of mortality attributed to chronic disease has quadrupled in the past 100 years to become the leading cause of morbidity and mortality.[2] More than half of the US population has a chronic disease, and one in four adults has two or more chronic conditions.[3] Chronic disease is a major driver of increases in healthcare spending, accounting for 86% of our nation's healthcare costs.[4]

Chronic disease prevalence is often linked to geography, and experts have found that the chance of having a chronic disease is influenced more by zip code than by personal choice.[5] People who live in concentrated impoverished areas with struggling schools and unsafe neighborhoods have very different opportunities than their counterparts with stable incomes in thriving communities. Yet, instead of examining the root causes of health issues and addressing them with population-level policy changes, the United States remains overly reliant on the healthcare system to deliver solutions.

Fortunately, change is coming on a global scale. Both the United Nations Millennium Development Goals and the World Health Organization's (WHO) nine constitutional principles reflect the understanding that where people live, work, and play have the most significant impact on their health.[6] These collective visions emphasize the social determinants of health, environmental sustainability, and the basic communal necessities for healthy people and populations. Together, they mark an encouraging shift in the global conversation about health that mirrors an emerging dialogue in the United States.

2 Understanding the Role of Policy

There is no question that policy has a major influence on health. Procurement policies, for example, make healthy foods more readily available. In turn, this incentivizes people to make smarter nutritional decisions. Policies can require elementary schools to offer physical education and new infrastructure projects to include biking and walking access. Landlord and property management policies that mandate regular maintenance and building updates can reduce asthma triggers and lead sources. Policies that increase the price of cigarettes have curbed tobacco use.

Policy change played a critical role in increasing life expectancy during the twentieth century, especially in the areas of motor vehicle safety and occupational health and safety.[7] There are more cars on the road traveling more miles than ever before, but fatalities per mile traveled have steadily declined.[8] The decline resulted from policies that increased vehicle safety, required car safety seats for infants and children and seat belt use for adults, and increased penalties for drunk and impaired driving. Similarly, policy changes ushering in strong new workplace practice and safety standards have prevented tens of thousands of employee deaths each year in contrast to 1930s labor practices.[9] Just as policy worked in these arenas, it can bring about changes in our communities to reduce the burden of chronic illness and improve overall health.

3 What Is CityHealth?

In 2014, the de Beaumont Foundation, founded in 1998 to promote better health by improving the effectiveness and capacity of state and local health departments, created CityHealth to identify the most effective local policy solutions to make communities healthier, more vibrant, and more productive places to live. CityHealth identifies and promotes solutions to boost the overall vitality and safety of cities and their residents. These principles are reflected in CityHealth's package of nine policies (Figure 32.1).

CityHealth targets city-level policy change because cities are where innovative solutions are born, tested, and proved. City officials, frequently at the forefront of emerging challenges, are swift and highly skilled at adopting new policies—often despite state and federal gridlock. Sound policies can also help cities attract families who want the best opportunities, young people who expect varied transportation options, and businesses that want a healthy environment for employees. Furthermore, cities have the resources—such as talent, access to technology, critical mass of population, and strong public health department leadership—to serve as effective policy incubators. With three out of every five Americans living in cities, policy change in the nation's most populous urban areas has the most tangible opportunity to impact people's daily lives and health outcomes.

CityHealth Policies

Earned Sick Leave

Earned sick leave laws reduce the spread of contagious illnesses, increase employment and income stability, and save cities money in health care costs.

High-quality, Universal Pre-Kindergarten

Children who attend high-quality pre-k are more likely to succeed in school, go on to stable jobs and earn more as adults—all of which are linked to better health and stronger communities.

Affordable Housing / Inclusionary Zoning

As cities grow, it's important that residents of all income levels have access to affordable housing that sets them up for good health.

Complete Streets

Complete streets policies unlock opportunities by allowing city residents to safely walk, bike, drive and take public transit around their community.

Alcohol Sales Control

Neighborhoods with high concentrations of alcohol outlets are linked to more drinking and higher rates of violence and driving under the influence. Policies that control the number of alcohol sales outlets can reduce crime, increase safety, and reduce spending on health care and criminal justice.

Tobacco 21

Curbing tobacco use among young adults has been shown to decrease the number of people who start—and continue—smoking.

Smoke Free Indoor Air

Comprehensive smoke-free laws protect non-smokers from secondhand smoke and reduce smokers' consumption of tobacco—the leading cause of preventable death in the US.

Food Safety and Inspection Rating

Policies requiring food establishments to publicly post safety inspection "grades" empower consumers, reduce foodborne illness rates and cut down on health care costs.

Healthy Food Procurement

Policies that make sure healthy food options are available on public property aid city residents in making smart decisions that will help them achieve and maintain a healthy weight.

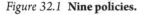

Figure 32.1 **Nine policies.**

4 Finding What Works

To identify which practical policy solutions to include in the CityHealth package for city leaders with the greatest influence on population health, we conducted a review of current laws at a municipal level in nine categories. Once the policies were identified, we assessed each one across six criteria (Figure 32.2). To vet the range of policy options, the CityHealth team assembled a policy advisory committee representing a diverse group of national thought leaders.

The committee included elected officials and leaders from the academic public health community, national health product retail chains, hospitals and healthcare systems, national membership organizations, and local chambers of commerce. To view the full list of advisors, visit http://www.cityhealth.org/advisors/. Members were instructed to offer counsel on which policies to include based on the strength of the evidence base supporting each policy's efficacy, whether the policy was typically under city jurisdiction, and the advisor's experience and judgment on how likely the policy would be to garner broad appeal. Their task was to help CityHealth identify the right mix of policies that would inspire leaders to action and improve their cities.

CityHealth combined the advisory group's input with legal analysis to determine the ideal characteristics for each policy and create criteria that would be used to award medals to cities based on the quality of their policy. The following medal categories were set: Best (Gold), Good (Silver), Passable (Bronze). Cities with no policies or policies that did not meet the minimum criteria for a quality policy were not awarded a medal.

With the policies selected and standards defined, CityHealth reviewed laws on the books in each of the nation's 40 largest cities (based on population size) to determine the

CityHealth categories and criteria

Selected policy categories

- Education
- Housing
- Employment/Income
- Food/Nutrition
- Active living/Transportation
- Mental health/Substance abuse
- Public health/Emergency preparedness
- Public safety
- Environment / Air quality

Selected assessment criteria

- Evidence of return on investment
- Impact on city revenue
- Potential to impact health disparities
- Political feasibility
- Ease of implementation

Figure 32.2 **Categories and criteria.**

City Medal Criteria

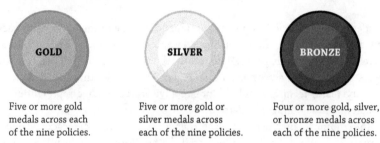

GOLD	SILVER	BRONZE
Five or more gold medals across each of the nine policies.	Five or more gold or silver medals across each of the nine policies.	Four or more gold, silver, or bronze medals across each of the nine policies.

Figure 32.3 **Definitions of Gold, Silver, and Bronze cities.**

degree to which the policies in each city met CityHealth medal standards. For example, a gold medal smoke-free indoor air policy had to specifically address non-hospitality workplaces, including workplaces, childcare, and long-term care facilities; public places; restaurants; and bars. If three of these criteria were specifically addressed, the policy received a silver medal. Two of the four criteria earned a bronze.

When possible, we shared results of this policy assessment with city health leaders to ensure the validity of the assessment. Cities earned overall medals based on the total number of medals they received for each of the nine policies (Figure 32.3).

5 Findings from Our First Assessment

After a 2-year policy assessment, CityHealth released its inaugural ratings of the nation's 40 largest cities in February 2017. Five of the cities had the number and quality of policies needed to receive overall gold medals: Boston, Chicago, Los Angeles, New York, and Washington, DC.

Five other cities received silver medals, and nine received bronze medals. Twenty-one of the 40 cities did not have enough strong policies in place to earn an overall medal (Figure 32.4).

In addition to the overall city medals, CityHealth awarded individual policy medals. Of these 360 possible medals, CityHealth awarded 171, with each city receiving at least one medal. The remaining 189 medals represent significant opportunities for city leaders to use policy as a lever to improve quality of life and well-being and to help their communities thrive.

CityHealth policies fell into two distinct groups: policies with high city penetration (more than three-quarters of all 40 cities have the policy) or policies with low city penetration (fewer than 20 cities have the policy).

Most of the cities had adopted policies regarding clean indoor air, complete streets (streets designed for the safety and mobility of all users), and high-quality, universal pre-K. Clean indoor air policies received the most medals (36), reflecting the success of a long-term, national advocacy movement to prohibit the use of tobacco in indoor spaces. The remaining policies had low penetration. Affordable housing/inclusionary zoning policies tied with paid sick leave garnered the fewest number of gold medals (2), while food safety/restaurant grading had the lowest number of medals overall (12) (Figure 32.5).

Map of CityHealth Cities with Medal Status (2017)

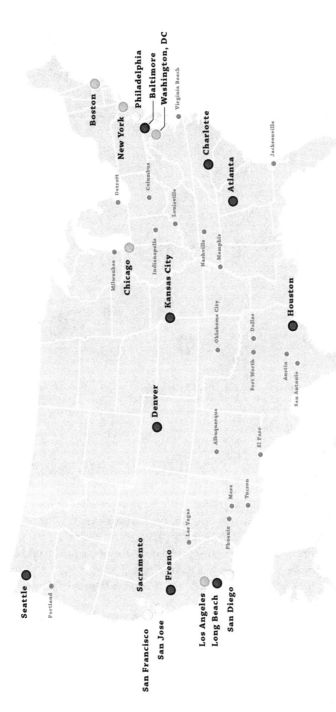

Figure 32.4 Map of CityHealth cities.

Medals by Policy (2017)

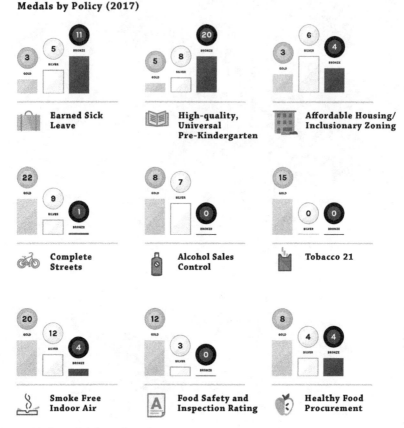

Figure 32.5 **Medals by policy.**

6 Preemption: A Caution and Consideration

Amid increasing state and federal gridlock, cities have become the primary laboratory for innovative policy solutions.[10] However, many local policies have become targets for state political leaders often aided by industry.[11] These state leaders restrict or remove local policy authority through legislative preemption. State preemption prevents local governments from adopting policies that their communities want, repeals existing laws that voters have already approved, and keeps communities from strengthening existing protections.

For example, a 2015 ordinance passed in the City of St. Louis established a minimum wage higher than Missouri's state minimum wage. After a protracted legal battle, the Missouri State Supreme Court ruled in favor of the city and allowed for the new minimum wage.[12] In response, the Missouri State Legislature crafted and passed legislation prohibiting other cities from exceeding the state minimum wage.[12] State legislatures have also used preemption to target city-level efforts on issues including fracking, nondiscrimination protections, gun control, and restaurant portion sizes.[13]

State preemption was also widely observed among CityHealth policies in the 40 largest cities. Preemptive state policies prevented cities from earning 45 of the 360 possible CityHealth medals—the most frequent targets of preemption were those involving affordable housing, paid sick leave, and alcohol control. Of the four cities without clean indoor air policies, three are preempted from adopting or strengthening such policies at the city level.

Not all statewide preemption is detrimental: state policy can have a positive impact on cities as well. States can, for instance, set strong minimum standards that apply to all cities while expressly allowing local leaders to adopt more rigorous standards. For example, all seven of California's largest cities each earned at least an overall bronze medal due in part to statewide policies that satisfied CityHealth's policy criteria.

CityHealth encourages city-level leadership and action to promote the public's health. While this can draw interest and attention that result in increased preemption, the risk of preemption should not deter cities from improving the health of their citizenry through policy. Rather, local leaders should anticipate, assess, and, if necessary, counter preemptive policy proposals.[14]

7 Communicating Clearly

Buy-in goes a long way toward ensuring that a policy makes an impact. That said, urban leaders and residents may not always recognize just how policy links to community health improvements. Effective messaging and appropriate framing could significantly boost policy adoption. Prior to releasing the CityHealth policy package, we partnered with experts in message research to explore various framing options for voters and legislators. CityHealth conducted key informant interviews with elected city leaders—such as mayors, city managers, and county executives—and commissioned a series of focus groups with registered voters in four cities. The goal was to understand how policymakers and residents view their city and its residents' health and then gauge their reactions to city-based public health policies.

These interviews and focus groups revealed that health in a traditional sense was not a key issue on policymakers' or voters' minds. The most pressing issues facing policymakers were economic development, public safety, and housing affordability. As one policymaker said:

> [Health] tends to be a chronic long-term problem as opposed to a hot-button topic. You know, crime is very immediate, so is health insurance for employees, so is zoning and all those other things. I think human beings naturally are less concerned with important but not pressing problems.

Although they did not rank health among their top issues, policymakers agreed that public policy has an essential role in making cities as healthy as possible. Similarly, residents did not view health as a top-of-mind issue, but they did raise concerns about issues related to health. Among the top issues for residents were uneven development, traffic and roads, homelessness, education, and crime.

Presenting strong evidence-based public health policies as part of a comprehensive agenda to improve the city on many levels, not just health, resonated most among residents. The most salient messages had uplifting, aspirational tones that focused on themes related to economic benefits and well-being, the significance of place and the built environment, and improved livability. Safe streets, affordable housing, and good education—all of which are touched on in the CityHealth policy package—appealed to residents in the context of making their city a more attractive place to live and work and as a driver of new economic opportunity.

Successful health policy initiatives need to leverage and communicate these themes to demonstrate how policy works as a tool for holistic improvements in cities, which will have a commensurate (though possibly unpublicized) impact on health. Shifting the conversation from the individual to the community inside of the health field is not enough; health should be a consideration in all policies and inform the decisions made in other sectors as well.

It is important to note that some focus group participants objected to what they perceived as governmental overreach into people's lives. For example, some of the comments included: "There would be too much government involvement and we would be handing over too many freedoms"; "Some of these policies would turn our city into a 'nanny state,' but on the other hand, many of these policies feel like the right way to do things"; and, "People would be imposing their views on nutrition on the public and education would be better."

Public health policy approaches that include increased taxes, bans, and other regulatory limits are often viewed as governmental overreach or disruptive in a free market economy.[15] These "nanny state" criticisms are expected, so city leaders and advocates must develop strategies to respond to them.

As part of their outreach, public health leaders should clearly communicate the potential for negative outcomes that could result from a lack of policy intervention—for example, how the absence of paid sick leave could increase the transmission of infectious diseases like the flu, which leads to increased absenteeism and reduced productivity.[15] To improve the likelihood of buy-in on the broadest scale, public health leaders should consider forging coalitions that include those with more politically moderate or conservative leanings and those who may be outside of the public health sphere, such as chambers of commerce or other business leaders.[15,16]

8　Making Progress Toward 40 Gold

One of the primary goals of CityHealth is to see each of the nation's 40 largest cities achieve an overall gold medal. To this end, we are not just an evaluator of local governments; we are a partner. Through a mix of technical assistance, policy expertise, and long-term accountability, CityHealth actively engages and supports cities that share our desire to give all residents equal opportunities to live full, healthy lives.

In 2018, CityHealth released updated medal scores. In just 1 year, 10 of the nation's 40 largest cities increased their overall medal status. Five new cities earned an overall bronze medal for the first time, four new cities earned an overall silver medal, and one new city (San Jose, California) earned an overall gold medal.

Policy changes are the driving force behind these improvements. Here are some of the most notable changes cities made since CityHealth released its first report: (1) San Antonio became the first city in Texas to adopt a Tobacco 21 ordinance, which raises the minimum legal age for tobacco and nicotine sales to 21. The policy will go into effect in October 2018. This successful effort was led by the mayor, the director of the San Antonio Metropolitan Health District, and a coalition comprising the University of Texas MD Anderson Cancer Center, the Campaign for Tobacco Free Kids, and the American Heart Association. (2) Kansas City, Missouri, updated its complete streets ordinance to help improve access to safe and accessible transportation—including walking, biking, public transit, and cars. (3) Fort Worth, Texas, and Louisville, Kentucky, strengthened their smoke-free laws by prohibiting smoking in bars and long-term care facilities. (4) In Seattle, Washington, the King County Public Health department implemented a new restaurant grading system that requires food establishments to post safety inspection grades in their window. This helps empower consumers to make informed choices about where to eat and reduces foodborne illnesses.

9   Using Policy to Promote Equity

CityHealth believes that every person, in every city, deserves to live the healthiest possible life. We also realize that not everyone has the same opportunities to thrive due to income, education, and other cultural, social, and economic factors. Policy can bridge the gaps and help erase disparities.

In 2018, Kaiser Permanente joined the de Beaumont Foundation as a national partner in the CityHealth initiative. The addition of Kaiser Permanente—recognized as one of America's leading healthcare providers and not-for-profit health plans—better positions CityHealth to catalyze meaningful change with policies that improve population health and reduce healthcare costs. Moreover, it reflects the growing understanding that the clinical environment alone does not hold all the solutions to reforming America's health system. Following the lead of Kaiser Permanente, other healthcare providers and payers across the country should consider pursuing similar alliances with advocates and city officials who share their goal of bolstering equity with policy-based solutions. Working together, we can connect the dots between health and the other issues important to policymakers and voters. Most important, we can implement policies that vastly improve the choices, institutions, and environments that affect the lives and health of millions of people across America.

References

1. Bauer UE, Briss PA, Goodman RA, Bowman BA. Prevention of chronic disease in the 21st century: elimination of the leading preventable causes of premature death and disability in the USA. *Lancet.* 2014; 384(9937):45–52.
2. Frieden TR. Asleep at the switch: local public health and chronic disease. *Am J Public Health.* 2004; 94(12):2059–2061.
3. Ward BW, Schiller JS, Goodman RA. Multiple chronic conditions among US adults: a 2012 update. *Prev Chronic Dis.* 2014;11:E62. doi:10.5888/pcd11.130389

4. Gerteis J, Izrael D, Deitz D, et al. *Multiple chronic conditions chartbook.* AHRQ Publications No, Q14-0038. Rockville, MD: Agency for Healthcare Research and Quality; 2014.

5. Graham GN. Why your zip code matters more than your genetic code: promoting healthy outcomes from mother to child. *Breastfeed Med.* 2016; 11:396–397.

6. World Health Organization. Constitution of WHO: Principles. July 22, 1946. World Health Organization website. Available at http://www.who.int/about/mission/en/. Accessed May 29, 2018.

7. US Centers for Disease Control and Prevention (CDC). Ten great public health achievements—United States, 1900-1999. *MMWR Morb Mortal Wkly Rep.* 1999; 48(12):241–243.

8. US Centers for Disease Control and Prevention (CDC). Motor-vehicle safety: a 20th century public health achievement. *MMWR Morb Mortal Wkly Rep.* 1999; 48(18):369–374.

9. US Centers for Disease Control and Prevention (CDC). Improvements in workplace safety—United States, 1900-1999. *MMWR Morb Mortal Wkly Rep.* 1999;48(22):461–469.

10. Institute of Medicine. *For the public's health: revitalizing law and policy to meet new challenges.* Washington, DC: National Academies Press; 2011.

11. Riverstone-Newell L. The rise in state preemption laws in response to local policy innovation. *Publius: The Journal of Federalism.* 2017; 47(3):403–425.

12. Wellford HW. Missouri legislature approves minimum wage preemption bill. May 15, 2017. Littler Mendelson website. Available at https://www.littler.com/publication-press/publication/missouri-legislature-approves-minimum-wage-preemption-bill. Accessed May 4, 2018.

13. Florida R. City vs. state: the story so far. City Lab website. June 13, 2017. Available at https://www.citylab.com/equity/2017/06/city-vs-state-the-story-so-far/530049/. Accessed May 4, 2018.

14. Pertschuk M, Pomeranz JL, Aoki JR, Larkin MA, Paloma M. Assessing the impact of federal and state preemption in public health: a framework for decision makers. *J Public Health Manag Pract.* 2013; 19(3):213–219.

15. Chokshi DA, Stine NW. Reconsidering the politics of public health. *JAMA.* 2013; 310(10):1025–1026.

16. Matthews G, Burris S, Ledford SL, Gunderson G, Baker EL. Crafting richer public health messages for a turbulent political environment. *J Public Health Manag Pract.* 2017;23(4):420–423.

33

New York City

The Fit City Example

KAREN LEE

1 The Growing Burden of Noncommunicable Disease Worldwide

Although infectious diseases were previously the leading causes of death, noncommunicable diseases (NCDs) such as heart disease and strokes, cancers, diabetes, and chronic lung diseases have become the world's leading causes of morbidity and mortality, in both high- and low-income countries.[1,2] Successes in infectious disease control through public health programs and policies that worked to improve sanitation infrastructure, large-scale immunization programs, food and water safety, and control of animal and insect transmission vectors, among others, have made key contributions to the declines in infectious disease mortality worldwide. Around the world today, public health organizations undertake a key set of activities aimed at controlling infectious diseases within their jurisdictions. A large number of these efforts focus on improving our environments to prevent the transmission of diseases. Although the efforts are still far from equitable and far from complete, we have seen large successes from such systematic infectious disease prevention and control efforts globally over the past century.

Unfortunately, such systemic and systematic efforts to control the current epidemics of NCDs have been slow to follow suit.[3,4] Even though NCDs have been the leading causes of death in many parts of the high-income world since the mid-twentieth century, even now, some 70 years later in the twenty-first century, systematic public health programs for NCD prevention and control remain relatively few and far between. Instead, ad hoc initiatives abound. And although extensive research has been conducted over the past several decades on interventions, including community-level interventions, the translation of this evidence into formal public health department efforts is still largely lacking.[5]

2 The Example of New York City

New York City (NYC) has been an exception to this complacency, initiating a wide-spread effort within its Department of Health and Mental Hygiene during the administration of Mayor Michael Bloomberg to tackling NCDs and their key risk factors of tobacco use, unhealthy eating, and physical inactivity.[6] NYC has been a global leader in healthy urban design and in improving the "built environment"—the human-made environment consisting of our neighborhoods, streets, buildings, and their amenities—to assist in the prevention and control of the current epidemics of NCDs and their risk factors. Through the translation of research-based health evidence into the development and implementation of user-friendly resources with and for non–health professionals involved in the planning, design, construction, maintenance, and renovation of the built environment, such as the Active Design Guidelines and its supplements, NYC pioneered formal efforts toward systematic evidence-based environmental design that can decrease physical inactivity and sedentariness, key risk factors for mortality and morbidity around the world today, while addressing other key public health issues like healthy food and beverage access, safety and equity.[7–10] According to the World Health Organization (WHO), more than 3 million deaths per year can be attributed to physical inactivity.[1,2]

The comprehensive efforts have been accompanied by unprecedented improvements in measured health outcomes, including some of the earliest reversals in the United States of childhood obesity trends, physical activity levels far exceeding the rest of the United States, and increases in life expectancy that exceed those in the rest of the country.[11–14]

3 Motivation Behind the Changes in NYC

By 2006, the research evidence had been accumulating for the important role that environmental factors play in NCD risk factors such as physical inactivity. The Task Force on Community Preventive Services convened by the US Centers for Disease Control and Prevention (CDC) of the US Department of Health and Human Services had recently published a number of systematic reviews between 2001 and 2006 on community interventions to increase physical activity. Among interventions recommended for increasing physical activity based on sufficient or strong levels of scientific evidence were using point-of-decision prompts and signage to increase stair use, enhancing access to places for physical activity, and undertaking community-level as well as street-level urban design and land-use interventions.[15,16] In addition to these interventions, emerging studies were being conducted on other environmental factors that could address physical inactivity and unhealthy diets.

In 2006, leadership at NYC's Department of Health and Mental Hygiene made a decision that the time had come to address these environmental factors that had now accumulated a sufficient evidence base to justify public health efforts and resources. A new position was created within its Bureau of Chronic Disease Prevention and Control dedicated to improving the built environment to address the risk factors of physical inactivity and unhealthy eating. A Deputy to the Assistant Commissioner for Chronic

Disease Prevention and Control, concurrently the inaugural built environment director, was hired, an individual with previous experience working on healthy built environment projects at CDC to address physical inactivity, obesity, and chronic diseases. The hired individual was given a senior title and position, as well as dedicated and protected time to working on NCD prevention and control issues, and this individual was charged with creating a new initiative to improve the built environment of NYC for obesity and chronic disease prevention and control. The individual was given permission to conduct outreach to the leadership and senior staff of other NYC government and nongovernmental agencies and departments. Soon after starting, the hired individual asked for initial staff who could assist in the work. Resources were dedicated for first one, then two, initial staff for the Inaugural Built Environment Director, and the small team began its work to build the multisectoral partnerships that would be required to improve urban design and urban planning for health in the City. The small team would garner multiple grants in the following years, expanding the staff to a total of 12.

4 The Fit City Effort

The multisectoral partnership work in NYC has been documented in several other publications.[6,14,17,18] As with the work elsewhere that has since followed suit with assistance from the NYC Built Environment Director acting as a consultant, including work in Miami; Sao Paolo, Brazil; London; and New South Wales, Australia,[19-21] the work in NYC was helped along with the creation of a forum for multisectoral dialogue, the "Fit City" conference, organized by the Built Environment Director and the then Executive Director of the American Institute of Architects New York Chapter (AIANY). Over a 6-month or so period, monthly then biweekly then weekly meetings were conducted to organize the first Fit City conference in NYC. Invitations were drafted and sent out through the NYC Health Commissioner's office to a broad array of departments in the City of New York, including City Planning, Transportation, Buildings, Design and Construction, Parks and Recreation, Housing Preservation and Development, the Mayor's Office of Sustainability, and the Mayor's Office of People with Disabilities, among others. AIANY sent out invitations to its several thousand members in the NYC area. The Planning Committee of the AIANY also sent out invitations to the New York Chapter of the American Planning Association. The new Built Environment Director reached out to other Healthy Built Environment experts at the CDC to serve as potential health keynote speakers. Local speakers from built environment and design disciplines were also asked to speak, to share projects that could serve as good case studies for active-living and health-promoting design locally.

The first Fit City conference in NYC was held at AIANY's Center for Architecture and attracted approximately 150 participants from a broad array of fields. This conference was used to launch the Healthy Built Environment and Healthy Urban Design and Planning work for Active Living and Healthy Eating in NYC. Over the years, the annual Fit City conferences in NYC would fill the 500-person capacity of the AIANY space to standing room only. Eventually, the ninth Fit City conference had to be moved to the auditorium of the New School campus to address the conference space overcrowding that was occurring in the years prior.

5 Other Components of New York City's NCD Reduction Efforts

Although the Fit City conferences were effective in generating excitement and buzz and created an opportunity for professionals from different sectors to meet each other, they were in themselves likely insufficient to make the progress needed on improving the urban built environment for health. Also critical were the initiatives created *between* the conferences each year. The Built Environment team at the NYC Department of Health and Mental Hygiene undertook active outreach after each year's conference to meet with the most interested non–health professionals, departments, and organizations who proposed ideas of initiatives that could be feasibly started after the conference and that also aligned with the scientific evidence for promoting active living and healthy eating.

Perhaps the most famous initiative that NYC is known for in the field combining urban design and active living is its development and implementation of the Active Design Guidelines (ADGs) and its supplements.[7-10] The ADGs were created through the joint leadership efforts of four city departments and with participation from eight more as well as inputs from the private and nongovernmental sectors.

For some years, the Department of Design and Construction (DDC) in NYC had already routinely created guidelines to promote best practices in design and construction in NYC. Previous guidelines had focused on such issues as high-performance buildings and environmental sustainability. Such guidelines were used in government design and construction projects and were also promoted for voluntary use among private sector projects. At the second Fit City conference in 2007, it became known that the DDC was looking for a new topic on which to focus the next set of NYC's design and construction guidelines. Thus, the idea was born that the next set of such guidelines could focus on the promotion of physical activity and health, using the available health evidence.

At the time, the Built Environment Director at NYC's health department was already working with the health department's own architects and facility managers on a set of healthy guidelines for the construction and renovation of the health department's own clinic facilities. The Built Environment Director was also working with architects at the Department of Buildings, the Mayor's Office of Management and Budget, and the Mayor's Office of Sustainability on a new Leadership in Energy and Environmental Design (LEED) green building rating system, Innovation Credit on Design for Active Occupants.[22,23] These initiatives had resulted from the Built Environment Director's follow-up with interested architects who had proposed these ideas at or after the first Fit City conference. So, immediately after the second Fit City conference, the health department's Built Environment Director followed-up with a meeting with DDC leadership.

After the second Fit City conference, a working group was assembled consisting of the NYC Departments of Design and Construction, City Planning, Transportation, and Health and Mental Hygiene, as well as the Mayor's Office of Management and Budget. Academic consultants with expertise in healthy environmental design, architecture, and planning were hired to assist in systematically identifying and reviewing the available evidence. The health department's Built Environment Director and ADG Coordinator ensured that the monthly meetings occurred and that the work done between meetings and assigned to both consultants and working group members was completed, first during the 2.5-year process to create and publish the ADGs, and then subsequently in the years following publication to disseminate and implement the ADGs within NYC. Following the publication of the guidelines, the health department's Built Environment Director and staff also wrote grant proposals to ensure that resources, including staffing, were available for implementation of the ADGs through stakeholder outreach, the development and roll-out of training programs for different sector professional groups, and policy development encompassing public policies found outside the healthcare sector.[6,14,17,18] The health department's Built Environment Team also conducted or partnered in health-related evaluations for research translation initiatives that created innovative urban design policies and programs incorporating interventions found in the ADGs.[24-28] The comprehensive efforts in environmental change for NCD prevention and control by the Built Environment and other health department teams in NYC have in turn been accompanied by some of the earliest reversals in the United States of childhood obesity trends, physical activity levels far exceeding the rest of the country, and increases in life expectancy that exceed those in the rest of the United States. [11-14]

6 Conclusion

Key lessons have been learned from NYC's successful NCD prevention initiatives, focusing on environmental change efforts to reduce barriers and improve supports for active living and healthy eating. Rather than merely focusing on health education, the NYC Department of Health and Mental Hygiene achieved improvements in health outcomes by turning its resources and focus to the creation and implementation of programs and policies that incorporated evidence-based interventions for improving the physical and food environments of our neighborhoods, streets, buildings, and their amenities, to support active transportation, active recreation, active buildings, and healthy food and beverage access. The health department went so far as to create a new program focused on improving the healthiness of our built—or human-made—environments, with its own dedicated director and staff. Silos that naturally form from busy professionals working in their own fields were transcended by the creation of regular forums for intersectoral dialogues in NYC, such as the annual Fit City conferences beginning in 2006. The excitement and buzz arising out of the conferences were channeled into real-world practice and policy change initiatives that cross-sector professionals in multiple government agencies and nongovernmental organizations could participate in between conferences. Co-benefits that were priorities for non–health sectors, such as environmental sustainability and economic development, were aligned as key intended outcomes in addition to health priorities. New urban planning and design initiatives to improve physical activity and healthy eating through non–health sector practice and policy improvements were supported by dedicating leadership and staff-level personnel at the NYC Department of Health and Mental Hygiene to these efforts. Although funding at the health department first came from city government budgets for a limited number of permanent staff positions, over time, grant funding was also garnered to grow the human and material resources available to expand the work. Throughout, the NYC Department of Health and Mental Hygiene played a critical role in supporting the initiation, implementation, and evaluation of cross-sectoral initiatives involving non–health sectors working together with health professionals to improve health outcomes. Public health departments and organizations globally need to recognize—and start to take on—the important and feasible role that they can and need to play in supporting cross-sectoral initiatives for environmental improvements for NCD prevention and control.

References

1. World Health Organization. *Global status report on non-communicable diseases 2010*. Geneva, Switzerland: World Health Organization; 2011.
2. World Health Organization. *Global report on urban health*. Geneva, Switzerland: World Health Organization; 2016.
3. Frieden TR. Asleep at the switch: local public health and chronic disease. *Am J Public Health*. 2004; 94(12):2059–2061.
4. Lee K, Rottensten K. A proposed model for the prevention and control of chronic diseases: analogies from communicable diseases. *Public Health & Epidemiology Report Ontario*. 2001; 12(9):305–313.
5. USDHHS. The guide to community preventive services. US Department of Health and Human Services website. Available at: https://www.thecommunityguide.org/. Accessed May 15, 2018.
6. Kelly PM, Davies A, Greig AJM, Lee KK. Obesity prevention in a City State: lessons from New York City during the Bloomberg administration. *Front Public Health*. 2016; 4:60. doi:10.3389/fpubh.2016.00060.
7. City of New York. *Active design guidelines: promoting physical activity and health through design*. New York: City of New York; 2010. Available at: https://www1.nyc.gov/assets/planning/download/pdf/plans-studies/active-design-guidelines/adguidelines.pdf. Accessed January 14, 2019.
8. City of New York. *Active design supplement: promoting safety*. New York: City of New York; 2012. Available at: http://www.drkarenlee.com/resources/usa. Accessed January 14, 2019.
9. City of New York. *Active design: affordable designs for affordable housing*. New York: City of New York; 2013. Available at: http://www.drkarenlee.com/resources/usa. Accessed January 14, 2019.
10. City of New York. *Active design: shaping the sidewalk experience*. New York: City of New York; 2013. Available at: https://www1.nyc.gov/assets/planning/download/pdf/plans-studies/active-design-sidewalk/active_design.pdf. Accessed January 14, 2019.
11. US Centers for Disease Control and Prevention (CDC). Obesity in K-8 students—New York City, 2006-07 to 2010-11 school years. *MMWR Morb Mortal Wkly Rep*. 2011; 60(49):1673–1678.
12. Bartley K, Eisenhower D, Harris TG, Lee KK. Patterns of physical inactivity in NYC and the US: findings from accelerometer and survey data. Under review.
13. Li W, Maduro GA, Begier EM. Increased life expectancy in New York City, 2001-2010: an exploration by cause of death and demographic characteristics. *J Public Health Manag Pract*. 2016; 22(3):255–264.
14. Designed to move. Active cities: a guide for city leaders. 2015. Available at: http://e13c7a4144957cea5013-f2f5ab26d5e83af3ea377013dd602911.r77.cf5.rackcdn.com/re-sources/pdf/en/active-cities-full-report.pdf. Accessed January 14, 2019.
15. Task Force on Community Preventive Services. Recommendations to increase physical activity in communities. *Am J Prev Med*. 2002; 22(4S):67–72.
16. Heath GW, Brownson RC, Kruger J, Miles R, Powell KE, Ramsey LT; Task Force on Community Preventive Services. The effectiveness of urban design and land use and transport

policies and practices to increase physical activity: a systematic review. *J Phys Act Health*. 2006; 3(s1): s55–s76.

17. Rube K, Veatch M, Huang K, et al. Developing built environment programs in local health departments: lessons learned from a nationwide mentoring program. *Am J Public Health*. 2014; 104(5): e10–e18. doi:10.2105/AJPH.2013.301863

18. World Health Organization. *Cities for health*. Kobe City, Japan: World Health Organization; 2014. Available at: http://www.drkarenlee.com/resources/who-citiesforhealth. Accessed January 14, 2019.

19. Miami-Dade College. Fit by design. *College Forum*. 2014; 18(2). Available at http://www.mdc.edu/main/collegeforum/archive/vol18-02/features/l0100_fitcity.aspx. Accessed January 14, 2019.

20. New South Wales. FitNSW 2014—supportive environments for active living—collective action and next steps. New South Wales Government Premier's Council for Active Living website. 2014. Available at: http://www.pcal.nsw.gov.au/fitnsw/2014. Accessed January 14, 2019.

21. New South Wales. Integrating health, active transport and land use planning. New South Wales Government Premier's Council for Active Living website. 2013. Available at: http://www.pcal.nsw.gov.au/resources/presentations/integrating_health_active_transport_and_land_use_planning. Accessed January 14, 2019.

22. US Green Building Council. Innovation: design for active occupants. LEED BD+C: New Construction/ v3—LEED 2009. US Green Building Council website. 2009. Available at: https://www.usgbc.org/node/10592095?return=/credits/new-construction/v2009/innovation-catalog. Accessed January 14, 2019.

23. Lee K. Developing an Active Design Index for LEED—assessing the physical activity promoting potential of LEED projects. GBIG Insight website. Published March 5, 2014. Available at: http://insight.gbig.org/developing-an-active-design-index-for-leed/. Accessed January 14, 2019.

24. Lee KK, Perry AS, Wolf SA, et al. Promoting routine stair use: evaluating the impact of a stair prompt across buildings. *Am J Prev Med*. 2012; 42(2):136–141.

25. Noyes P, Fung L, Lee KK, Grimshaw VE, Karpati A, Digrande L. Cycling in the city: an in-depth examination of bicycle lane use in a low-income urban neighborhood. *J Phys Act Health*. 2012; 11(1):1–9.

26. Ruff RR, Rosenblum R, Fischer S, Meghani H, Adamic J, Lee KK. Associations between building design, point-of-decision stair prompts and stair use in urban worksites. *Prev Med*. 2014; 60:60–64.

27. Day K, Loh L, Ruff R, Fischer S, Rosenblum R, Lee KK. Does bus rapid transit promote walking? An examination of New York City's Select Bus Service. *J Phys Act Health*. 2014; 11:1512–1516.

28. Wolf S, Grimshaw VE, Sacks R, Maguire T, Matera C, Lee KK. The impact of a temporary recurrent street closure on physical activity in New York City. *J Urban Health*. 2015; 92(2):230–241.

34

Boston

A Case Study

RUSS LOPEZ

1 Introduction

Understanding the history of a place is essential for incorporating local concerns and values into decision-making. Most important, history is present whether we acknowledge it or not. Mindy Fullilove, writing of the grief experienced by people displaced by urban renewal in Pittsburgh, noted that "The experience of place is encoded in our muscles and our bones."[1(p. 226)] Ignoring the past does not erase it; on the contrary, denying its existence makes the present less comprehensible. Furthermore, ignoring history burdens efforts to create positive change. Lewis Mumford, the great twentieth-century urbanist, wrote, "Without a long running start in history, we shall not have the momentum needed, in our own consciousness, to take a sufficiently bold leap into the future."[2(p. 3)] Creating change and improving the lives and health of the public demands effective public policies. These policies must rest on the foundation of a city's or neighborhood's history. We will discuss Boston as a case study, aiming to understand how history shapes cities and creates health in urban populations.

Boston, Massachusetts, is one of the oldest cities in the United States and one where history is embedded deep in its neighborhoods. From the Battle of Bunker Hill, which took place in Charlestown, north of downtown, to the site where the famous 54th Regiment of African American soldiers was mobilized in Hyde Park at the southern tip of the city, to live, work, or visit the city is to walk arm in arm with the past.

Boston also demonstrates that past events, decisions, and policies can have impacts and provide lessons for centuries after they occur. Seemingly small, inconsequential events such as filling in a small patch of marshland or creating a citizen's advisory group to oversee the cleanup of a growing city can echo for generations. Similarly, the large-scale programs that cities sometimes commit to can also prompt reactions that last much longer than the programs themselves. Though the examples here might seem parochial to Boston, they have parallels in every place; our regions, cities, and neighborhoods are each a product of a past that includes triumphs and compromises.

This chapter highlights three actions from Boston history that have affected the lives of thousands of residents and continue to have public health repercussions today. First is the extensive land filling that added more than 2 square miles of land around the edges of downtown. Prompted by the need for more space to accommodate a growing population and extreme environmental degradation caused by ill-conceived economic development projects, these areas, now home to tens of thousands yet barely above sea level, are at growing risk of flooding caused by global climate change. Second is the city's commitment to public health infrastructure that stretches from the country's first public health department, organized by Paul Revere, through a network of community health centers established in the 1960s, to its addressing some of the most important challenges of today. Boston's public health institutions have not always been benign, but even those facilities that were once the sites of bigotry were eventually repurposed to serve all without prejudice. Third is the city's traumatic urban renewal program that dominated the city's agenda in the 1950s and 1960s. It left a series of scars across the urban landscape and has continued to shape how neighborhoods react to city programs and private development proposals.

2 Land Filling

The area that became Boston had been occupied for thousands of years by prosperous native tribes that took advantage of the abundant food sources around the Shawmut Peninsula and opportunities for farming on the adjacent mainland. By the time European settlers arrived in the region in 1620, most of the natives had been killed by a horrific epidemic, and what would become the core of downtown was an abandoned core of stubby glacial hills, perhaps 400 acres in area, connected to the mainland by a narrow mile-long neck of land that was often flooded during storms and astronomical high tides.

After independence, a growing population needed more land and the city embarked on a series of projects to fill in land along the margins of the peninsula, a project that only ended in the 1960s. The two largest areas reclaimed were the neighborhoods to the north of the neck, the Back Bay and the northern half of the South End, and the neighborhoods to the south of downtown and the neck, Chinatown, the South Boston waterfront, and the southern half of the South End. In both areas, the need to control costs resulted in streets being rarely raised more than 8 feet above the low tides at the time and often the interiors of blocks were even lower.[3]

From the very beginning, these neighborhoods needed extensive infrastructure to provide drainage and to keep them from flooding. The city built large pumping stations that were engineering marvels in the early 1900s when they opened. But, by the 1990s, the limitations of these facilities were becoming clear as a series of heavy rains caused extensive flooding. At the same time, the need to keep subway and underground highway tunnels free of water caused overpumping at points along their routes, resulting in land subsidence and rotting of the wooden piles that supported nineteenth-century buildings.

The neighborhoods sitting on the filled land have become a mix of densely populated buildings and highly valued commercial properties. The Back Bay had been one of the city's most expensive residential neighborhoods from the time it was developed, for example. In the mid-twentieth century, it also saw extensive office and retail construction that attracted thousands of workers daily. The nearby South End was built to be an exclusive neighborhood as well, but it quickly failed, and, for more than a hundred years, it was a rooming house district housing many of the city's poor and working-class residents. After 1960, it began to gentrify, but neighborhood activists successfully fought for the creation of more than 6,000 subsidized and publicly owned units and helped preserve the area's extensive network of social service organizations and home-less shelters. Thus, even as the South End became more expensive, it has continued to house many of the city's most fragile residents.

Meanwhile, the South Boston waterfront was developed to help maintain Boston's maritime commerce, but the filled land was created just as port traffic was declining. By the 1970s, the area that had been reclaimed from the harbor was mostly devoid of buildings and used for cheap parking for downtown workers. Then, after 2000, the area benefited from extensive infrastructure projects, including a bus rapid transit line, a new convention center, and a newly cleaned up harbor. This investment of billions of dollars came at a time when the economy was booming, sparking the rise of new office buildings and hotels as the area grew into one of the largest employment centers in New England.

Unfortunately, global climate change is causing sea levels to rise faster along the Massachusetts coast than in other parts of the United States. Coupled with storms that are increasing in frequency and severity, flooding is becoming more common, and as-tronomical high tides can cause parts of the South Boston waterfront and downtown Boston to flood under several feet of sea water. The public first became aware of the potential for flooding when a nonprofit group published an analysis of sea level rise and coastal vulnerability in 2013.[4] Unfortunately, the first responses ranged from denial to whimsical suggestions. One early popular proposal, for example, included a canal to cut across the Back Bay, put forward by a team that was evidently unaware of how a canal led to flooding in New Orleans when it was hit by Hurricane Katrina in 2005.[5]

It was a major storm in 2018 that caused flooding along much of the South Boston waterfront as well as along the inlet that separates South Boston from Downtown that finally resulted in serious discussions regarding how to mitigate and adapt to rising sea levels.

The mechanisms to prevent flooding to these vulnerable neighborhoods, housing more than 100,000 people, including many with extreme wealth but also many who are homeless or who have limited incomes and few resources, has not yet been deter-mined. It is most likely not possible to raise the thousands of at-risk acres sufficiently to make them safe from even modest additional sea level rise, much less some of the higher forecasts for storm surges that may be experienced by the end of the century. New proposals include a barrier that extends several miles across the opening to Boston Harbor that will protect land well outside the urban core that is similarly vulnerable. With a lack of a consensus on what should be done, the costs of protection are not known and the source of funding for a flood protection system is not yet identified. And, year by year, the extent and frequency of flooding is certain to increase. Adapting to global climate change and sea level rise is essential for protecting the public's health (e.g., in addition to flood, the increased likelihood of heat waves directly threatens the health of Boston's poor and elderly). As coastal flooding increases, cities will lose affordable housing, residents will face the destruction of a lifetime of accrued assets, and much of the infrastructure that is in place to help those who are vulnerable—public transit, community health centers, neighborhood social ties, and so forth—will be destroyed.

The lesson is not that nineteenth-century civic leaders should have been able to forecast potential problems that arose 150 years later. No one then could have foreseen global warming now. However, twenty-first-century municipal governments will have to address the consequences created by their predecessors. Nineteenth-century land surveyors and engineers created an infrastructure that was sufficient to keep newly filled land from flooding for almost a century, but conditions after that time changed to render their efforts insufficient for a different set of problems. Nor is this need to address legacy threats to health and safety limited to Boston or to coastal communities. Cities and regions dependent on large-scale aqueducts in the Southwest will have to confront the challenges posed by increased frequencies and severities of droughts. The entire Pacific coast needs to assess vulnerability to earthquakes as engineering flaws are exposed and new forecasts of potential earthquake magnitudes are developed. Cities everywhere will have to address decaying infrastructure or problematic designs posed by antiquated urban development programs.

3 Public Health Infrastructure

As one of the oldest cities in the country, Boston had the first municipal health department in the United States (Figure 34.1). With founding member Paul Revere, this early commission was focused on preventing fires and controlling garbage and human and animal waste in the streets of the growing town. More than 200 years later, the city's

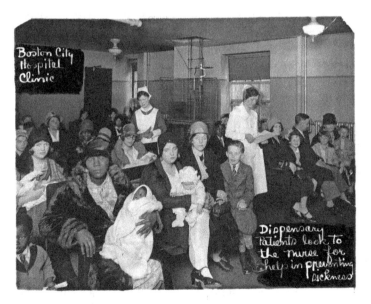

Figure 34.1 **Boston City Hospital outpatient clinic with nurses and patients, c. 1920.**
Source: Boston City Hospital collection, Collection 7020.001, City of Boston Archives, Boston, MA.

Public Health Commission administers programs ranging from infectious disease control to senior programs, and it works with other public and private agencies to coordinate responses to natural disasters, provide healthcare to the homeless, and manages many other vital programs.

This commitment to protecting the public's health has a long history. In response to a cholera epidemic and using funds donated by a private citizen, the city founded a public hospital in 1851.[6] With its primary facility in the South End, as well as operating other programs throughout the city, for nearly 150 years Boston City Hospital was the primary care provider for uninsured people in the state. Budget issues resulted in the hospital being merged with Boston University. The hospital, now known as Boston Medical Center, continues to operate and continues to be the main provider for the poor. The state has an uninsured rate of less than 2%, so most patients have some sort of insurance, but many still rely on the hospital for routine, emergency, and specialized care, and, fortunately, Boston has been able to serve its diverse population.

Like many institutions, Boston City Hospital has had problematic episodes in its history. In the nineteenth century, for example, the city prohibited priests from entering the hospital even though Irish Catholics made up one of the largest segments of its patient population, and, well into the twentieth century, racist employment policies prohibited the hiring of African Americans.[7,8] But the institution has willingly come to embrace current standards of inclusion.

Though the city is home to some of the best hospitals in the country, like many urban areas, its poor and working-class residents had a difficult time accessing healthcare not only because of insurance issues but also because of a lack of providers with the willingness and expertise to provide primary care to the poor, elderly, and non–English speaking population in the neighborhoods where they live. As a result of this problem of access coupled with a wave of activism in communities across the city, an extensive network of community health centers opened across the city beginning in the 1960s. Now mostly affiliated with two important hospitals, Boston University Medical Center and the Beth Israel—Deaconess Hospital, these health centers have continued to provide a large range of outpatient services in almost every neighborhood in the city.

Some health centers provide specialized services. For example, the Fenway Community Health Center, for example, is one of the country's leading clinics for lesbian, gay, and transgender people, and the South Cove Community Health Center has the special mandate of servicing the city's large Asian population. But all of the city's health centers provide prenatal, routine, and preventative care.

The contribution of this robust infrastructure to protecting the public's health cannot be underestimated. Although, like the rest of the country, Boston has a large disparity between black and white infant mortality rates, Boston's black infant mortality rate is among the lowest in the country, in part because of the long-standing relationship between the city's African American community and its health centers.[9] Similarly, when the HIV/AIDS crisis hit the gay male community beginning in 1981, the Fenway Health Center, founded by gay, lesbian, and other neighborhood activists, quickly became a leader in providing care and services to the ill and their families at a time when many providers failed to treat gay men because of fear. In 2018, as an opioid epidemic threatened the health of thousands, the city's network of hospitals, clinics, and public health professionals was on the front line, trying to find effective treatments and serving people in acute crisis.

No one can predict the nature of the next public health crisis while ongoing problems have reduced the life expectancy of many groups in the United States. As the work of public health is not yet complete, there remains a great need to maintain and improve its infrastructure.

4 Urban Renewal

Although Boston is now one of the most prosperous cities in the country, this is a recent development. Its economy had peaked around World War I and then went into a decline that took almost 70 years to reverse itself. The drivers of mid-twentieth-century prosperity, manufacturing and the production of raw materials, were absent here, and, as a result, in the 1940s and even as late as the late 1970s, it was one of the country's most distressed city.[10]

Boston city began to revitalize itself using the same tactics that were eventually discredited elsewhere: City Hall-led projects that demolished large sections of neighborhoods, replaced private-sector low-income housing with luxury buildings, and promoted policies that attempted to lure suburban shoppers and employers back into the center city.

Many of these urban renewal projects were failures that traumatized residents throughout the city. The destruction of two neighborhoods, the beloved West End and the densely populated New York Streets, resulted in thousands of people being displaced. The new development was sterile and out of place in the case of the West End, and a failed industrial park stood where the New York Streets once thrived (Figure 34.2).

Stung by these controversial failures, the city took a new tack in the 1960s, hiring Ed Logue from New Haven to lead a new redevelopment program. Logue promised "planning with the people," but, in reality, his program was just as disconnected from the city's poor and working-class households as his predecessors'.[11] His signature business district projects, Government Center and the Prudential Center, have been the focus of great reworking. The Prudential, which was once an isolated complex of outdoor plazas surrounded by a ring road, has been mostly rebuilt, while Government Center plaza remains a mostly unused sterile wasteland despite nearly 50 years of attempts to activate its expanse.

It was Logue's residential projects that created the most conflict, however.[12] He endorsed a policy that 20% of a neighborhood had to be demolished to create a new pro-investment atmosphere. To achieve this, he would propose demolition on the scale of 50% or more in order to make his 20% goal seem reasonable. He would also promise that no one would be displaced by the projects, a promise that residents never believed and which he never met: more than 10,000 would lose their homes and be forced out of the neighborhood by the South End Urban Renewal Project alone.[13]

Residents in the city's neighborhood urban renewal districts, which covered nearly 40% of Boston, reacted in anger to these projects. In heavily Irish Catholic Charlestown, for example, the fury over its proposed renewal program resulted in the devout hurling insults at their priests who had been appointed to a citizens' advisory board because of

322   CASE STUDIES IN URBAN HEALTH

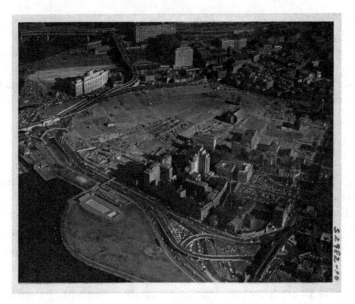

Figure 34.2 **West End project area looking northeasterly, c. 1949–1954.** Source: Urban
Redevelopment Division, Boston Housing Authority photographs in Boston Redevelopment Authority
photographs, Collection # 4010.001, City of Boston Archives, Boston, MA.

their support for renewal.[14] South Boston organized its residents to oppose any renewal,
leading to the city abandoning renewal efforts there, while in the South End, resident
opposition resulted in at least four plans being proposed before one was approved. Only
primarily African American Roxbury welcomed renewal because housing conditions
were so desperate there that any investment was welcome. Even in Roxbury, however,
residents turned on the city within a few years after new housing failed to materialize
even though the demolitions were well under way. The displacements caused by urban
renewal resulted in profound negative physical and mental health impacts. Former
residents experienced grief and a profound sense of loss, that persisted for decades after
they were displaced. Many elderly people were unable to cope with the stresses of losing
their homes, and children suffered from the tearing away of social networks that might
have nurtured them. These effects have colored the lives of generations.

In these confrontations, Boston residents learned to distrust all outsiders. Their
clergy, their elected officials, the bankers, real estate people, and their government
wanted them out of the city and threatened to destroy their way of life. The only way
to prevent displacement, residents realized, was to protest loudly and continuously.
One result was that when the courts ordered the city to desegregate its schools a few
years later, residents were well organized to fight against integration, much to the
sad legacy of the city.[15] This distrust continues to this day as nearly all large-scale
pubic improvements and private development proposals soon result in the horrors of
urban renewal being resurrected.[16] A major lesson for all from Boston's urban renewal
programs is that trust is easily lost and then takes generations to rebuild, if it ever can
be regained.

5 Conclusion

None of these examples explored here is unique to Boston. The 1960s, urban renewal programs destroyed neighborhoods in hundreds of US cities, and the dislocations caused by new development affect communities on almost every continent from the destruction of traditional neighborhoods in Beijing to the forced relocations of residents for the Olympics in Brazil. Similarly, almost no community is immune to global climate change; almost every place will have to adapt its current development patterns to a new, less forgiving environment. Few areas have the luxury of starting from a clean slate, and most will have to use their existing public health infrastructure to meet the challenges that are to come.

Channeling new development, preserving and protecting health, and meeting new challenges posed by changing environmental conditions rely on the participation and support of thousands of people. These issues are never discussed in a vacuum, and no problems are solved without regard to history and memory. The Boston experience highlights the need for careful consideration of present conditions in order to prepare for the unknown future.

References

1. Fullilove MT. *Root shock: how tearing up city neighborhoods hurts America, and what we can do about it.* New York: New Village Press; 2016.
2. Mumford L. *The city in history: its origins, its transformations, and its prospects.* New York: Mariner Press; 1968.
3. Seasholes NS. *Gaining ground: a history of landmaking in Boston.* Cambridge, MA: The MIT Press; 2003.
4. Douglas E, Kirshen P, Li V, Watson C, Wormser J. *Preparing for the rising tide.* Boston, MA: Boston Harbor Association; 2013.
5. Ross C. Report offers ideas for a Boston beset by rising seas. *Boston Globe.* September 30, 2014:1.
6. Committee of the Hospital Staff. *A history of Boston City Hospital from its founding until 1904.* Boston, MA: Boston Municipal Printing Office; 1906.
7. Ryan DP. *Beyond the ballot box: a social history of the Boston Irish, 1845–1917.* Rutherford, NJ: Fairleigh Dickinson University Press; 1983.
8. Lukas A. *Common ground: a turbulent decade in the lives of three American families.* New York: Vintage Books; 1986.
9. Rorie J-A, Richardson K, Gardner R. Public health approaches to community-based needs: Boston's infant mortality crisis as a case study. *J Midwifery Women Health.* 1997; 42(6):527–534.
10. Bradbury KL, Downs A, Small KA. *Urban decline and the future of American cities.* Washington, DC: Brookings Institution Press; 1982.
11. Kennedy L. *Planning the city upon a hill: Boston since 1630.* Boston, MA: University of Massachusetts Press; 1994.
12. O'Connor T. *Building a new Boston: politics and urban renewal 1950 to 1970.* Boston, MA: Northeastern University Press; 1993.
13. Lopez R. *Boston's South End: the clash of ideas in a historic neighborhood.* Boston, MA: Shawmut Peninsula Press; 2015.
14. Mollenkopf JH. *The contested city.* Princeton, NJ: Princeton University Press; 1983.

15. Vrable J. *People's history of the new Boston*. Amherst, MA: University of Massachusetts Press; 2014.

16. Deehan M. In a move to rebrand the BRA, Walsh renames it; protesters unimpressed. *WGBH*. September 27, 2016. Available at https://www.wgbh.org/news/2016/09/27/politics-government/move-rebrand-bra-walsh-renames-it-protesters-unimpressed. Accessed May 2, 2018.

35

Richmond, California

Health Equity in All Urban Policies

JASON CORBURN AND JOSEPH S. GRIFFIN

1 Introduction

In Richmond, California, residents, government, academics, and others have transformed the city from an unhealthy and violent place into a more equitable and healthy city. This chapter reviews some of the key practices and projects that have contributed to this transformation.

Richmond is a working-class community of color in the San Francisco Bay Area with about 115,000 residents. In the early 2000s, Richmond was one of the poorest, most violent, and, by almost every measure, unhealthiest cities in the United States. Richmond is also one of the most ethnically diverse cities in the San Francisco Bay Area, with a population comprising more than 26% African American, 40% Latino, 31% white, and 14% Asian-Pacific Islanders. In 2010, the zip code in central Richmond (94603) had a life expectancy of 71.2 years (the California state average is 78.4 years), whereas a few miles away in another zip code over the Richmond Hills life expectancy was more than 87 years (Figure 35.1). In 2007, Richmond was the ninth most violent city in the United States, with 47 gun homicides per 100,000.

Yet, by 2017, many indicators of the social determinant of health—or the life-supporting resources, living conditions, social and economic experiences, and opportunities that influence which populations get sick, suffer unnecessary disability, and die early—had turned around. Richmond residents were reporting feeling safer and healthier, and they rated their community and city positively. Unemployment and gun homicides were at historic lows (Table 35.1).

This chapter briefly reviews how Richmond turned itself around from a violent and unhealthy population into a more equitable and healthy city.

2 From Crisis to Community Innovation

In part a response to social and health inequities, community groups in Richmond mobilized to demand change. Environmental justice (EJ) groups mobilized after a

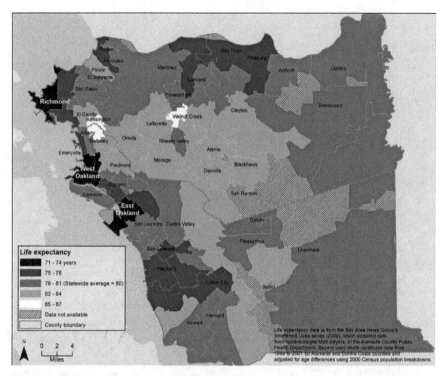

Figure 35.1 **Life expectancy in 2000 by zip code: Alameda and Contra Costa Counties, California.**

Table 35.1 **Richmond rising: indicators of healthy transformation**

Year	2007	2017
Unemployment rate	18.5%	3.7%
Self-rated health, good/excellent	36%	60%
Positive place to live	20%	47%
Experience with discrimination/racism	42%	24%
Positive place to raise children	9%	24%
Quality of city services	17%	35%
Overall image, good/excellent	4%	24%
Gun homicides per 100,000	47	15

From Community Surveys. City of Richmond, California website. 2018. Available at https://www.ci.richmond.ca.us/1871/Community-Surveys. Accessed June 10, 2018.

series of toxic releases from the city's Chevron oil refinery and formed the Richmond Equitable Development Initiative (REDI). This coalition conducted "citizen science" to survey, measure, and document the environmental, social, economic, and health issues in Richmond. Using their community-based research, the REDI demanded that EJ, gun violence, and health equity be at the center of the city's General Plan Update process that had started in 2005.[1] The General Plan is the long-range development and policy "blueprint" for the city, but neither EJ nor health had ever been considered in such a plan.

The city and community group leaders secured support from the California Endowment to integrate health into the General Plan process. What emerged was California's first ever Community Health and Wellness Element (CHWE), or chapter, as part of a General Plan.[2] Yet the community coalition demanded that the plan not "sit on a shelf" and wanted to pilot health-promoting actions. Neighborhood-specific action plans focused on three of the most polluted, impoverished, and unhealthy neighborhoods. A series of place-based, low-cost actions were recommended, such as street painting and signal timing to improve intersection safety, converting abandoned tennis courts to *futsal* courts, creating road diets to slow traffic, cleaning vacant lots, and bringing mobile clinics to local schools. Urban Tilth, a local nonprofit food security organization, was supported to develop school and community gardens to teach and employ community members to grow, distribute, cook, and consume local produce.[3]

2.1 Investing in the Heart of the Community: Pogo Park

In one neighborhood, called the Iron Triangle, residents demanded that an unsafe playground in the center of the community be improved. Resources were allocated to design improvements to an existing park, called Elm Playlot, that had been overrun with drug use and other criminal activity. Instead of hiring a design firm to do this, a nonprofit organization cooperated with residents to co-design the park. The organization, Pogo Park, worked with residents and local youth to design and build the space incrementally. Residents wanted a safe and healing space, as well as jobs, so Pogo Park worked with surrounding industries and artists to train residents in construction skills to build their own park. Pogo Park secured a long-term lease on the land from the city to create a program of park activities; these included a community meeting space, an industrial kitchen, a county food distribution program, healing gardens, exercise classes, and other activities. Notably, residents are hired to operate and maintain the park.[4]

2.2 An Office of Peace Making, Staffed by Former Felons

The number one health issue identified by residents in the CHWE was gun violence. City officials hired consultants to explore alternatives to militarized policing and incarcerating young men of color as the solution to urban gun violence. What emerged in 2008 was a new, non–law enforcement city agency called the Office of Neighborhood Safety (ONS), with the goal of reducing gun homicides by eliminating retaliatory violence and targeting the young people most likely to engage in gun violence. The ONS was staffed with former felons with gun-related charges who had the street "cred" to reach likely "trigger pullers." The former convicts are city staff called Neighborhood Change Agents, and they use daily street outreach to mediate conflicts and engage the hardest to reach likely gun offenders in an 18-month program called the Peacemaker Fellowship. Each Fellowship cohort numbers about 25 African American men between the ages of 16 and 24, and they receive intensive mental health and other counseling, positive adult mentoring, internship and employment training, and opportunities to travel outside of Richmond. If they comply with the goals created in their individual LifeMaps, they are also eligible for a stipend of up to $1,000 per month to stay engaged and avoid gun violence. Since the first cohort was enrolled in 2010, 84 fellows have participated, 94% are alive, 83% have had no gun-related injuries or hospitalizations, and 77% have had no new gun charges.

3 Health in All Policies and the Richmond Healthy Equity Partnership

Wanting to further institutionalize the health equity work, a group of community organizations, the county health department, the local school district, and city officials were organized by UC Berkeley Professor Jason Corburn into the Richmond Health Equity Partnership (RHEP). The first task of the RHEP was to engage residents and city staff to describe what they thought were the key barriers to and opportunities for being healthy in Richmond. Emerging out of these dialogues and workshops was a constant narrative about the trauma, fear, and discrimination residents experienced on a daily basis and that regularly caused them to worry and frequently engage in unhealthy behaviors, including smoking, overeating, and alcohol and drug use. The RHEP translated community narratives into a graphic of "cumulative stressors" and linked this to the biomedical research on *toxic stress*—or how prolonged adversity alters the body's cognitive and immune systems and contributes to some of the most prevalent diseases in Richmond, such as obesity, hypertension, diabetes, asthma, and poor mental health. The sources of toxic stress were identified as structural racism, and reducing stressors required addressing structural discrimination and building structural competencies within government policies and decision-making processes.

In 2012, the RHEP used the toxic stress and structural racism frameworks to draft a Health in All Policies (HiAP) strategy.[5] The HiAP strategy would identify ways to reduce or eliminate key community toxic stressors through city agency decisions, budget allocations, and through new partnerships with other institutions, according to six action areas: (1) governance and leadership, (2) economic development and education, (3) full-service and safe communities, (4) neighborhood built environments, (5) environmental health and justice, and (6) quality and accessible health homes and social services. Each action area included short-term (1–2 years) and medium-term (5-year) policy and programmatic strategies targeting one or more "toxic stressors" in Richmond and quantifiable indicators to track progress for both specific population groups (i.e., African-Americans) and neighborhoods (Table 35.2). After more than

Table 35.2 **Examples of Health in All Policies action areas in Richmond, California**

Action area	Short term	Medium term	Targeted toxic stressor(s)	Responsible agencies
Governance and leadership	Integrate health equity indicators into city's 5-year budget plan	Develop capacity within every city agency for health equity impact assessments	City responsiveness Institutional racism	Finance City Manager All
Economic development and education	Align City's YouthWorks program with high school academies	Resource high quality childcare	Economic insecurity	Employment and training West County Unified School District
Full service and safe communities	Resource and expand Office of Neighborhood Safety	Resource restorative justice and trauma-informed youth programs	Racial profiling Violence	Public Safety City Manager
Residential and built environment	Expand in-home lead abatement program	Protect low-income residents from displacement through housing program and supportive housing	Housing safety and security	Code Enforcement Housing and Community Development
Environmental health and justice	Expand community-based air pollution monitoring and industrial pollution control	Re-designate truck routes away from areas with high asthma rates and "calm" traffic to reduce pedestrian injuries	Fear of toxics Noise	Planning Bay Area Air Quality Management District
Quality and accessible health care	Increase enrollment in food stamps/EBT, WIC, and Head Start	Expand training and employment of community health workers	Economic and food insecurity Access to culturally competent care	City Manager County health department

3 years of collaborative work, the Richmond City Council passed the nation's first HiAP ordinance in 2014.

4 An Integrated Health Equity Strategy

The multiple strategies, integrated actions, and indicators within the HiAP Strategy and Ordinance provided a new health equity framework for all city agencies and demanded new partnerships between government and community-based organizations. An interdepartmental team, led by the City Manager's Office, was established to coordinate actions within and across city agencies as well as strengthen ties between the city, community groups. and county government. A series of health equity–focused policies emerged from these intracity and city–community partnerships. For example, unions, activists, and the city drafted a living wage ordinance that was adopted in June 2014 that mandated $15 per hour and adjusted the rate annually according to the regional Consumer Price Index. A city program called RichmondBUILD refocused its efforts to train young people, many formerly incarcerated, in building-trade skills. These same skills were contracted by the city in its partnership with the nonprofit Grid Alternatives to offer subsidized and free solar power and home energy efficiency upgrades to low-income residents. The solar power and housing improvement programs emerged from the Richmond Climate Action Plan, which included an "energy-poverty" reduction strategy for all low-income residents. As part of this plan, the city and EJ groups sued Chevron for failing to disclose the environmental impacts of its facility expansion. One result of the lawsuit was a $90M community benefit agreement in 2014 that directed resources to air pollution reduction, free college tuition for Richmond high school graduates, and neighborhood improvement projects.

In an attempt to stabilize neighborhoods, reduce economic stress, and promote healthy housing, in 2013, the city legislated Richmond CARES (Community Action to Restore Equity and Stability). Richmond CARES would use the power of eminent domain to "take" underwater mortgages from private banks, purchase them, restructure the loans with a nonprofit organization, and resell the mortgages back to homeowners at an affordable rate, all to eliminate evictions and displacement. While community residents and the Service Employees International Union lauded the program, the California Association of Realtors, Wells Fargo, Deutsche Bank, and BlackRock Inc. sued the city, claiming that the program was unconstitutional. The suit was dismissed in California Supreme Court as property values began to rise in the Bay Area. However, the city remained committed to healthy housing partnerships and, in 2016, worked with community-based organizations to become only the fifteenth city in California to pass a rent control, just cause for eviction, and homeowner protection ordinance. The city also launched the first Social Impact Bond program to finance the rehabilitation of abandoned and blighted housing. While once a symbol of divestment and abandonment, Richmond in 2018 had approved 2,025 new residential housing units, 50 units of supportive housing, more than 450 affordable units, and 1,300,000 square feet of new warehouse and distribution space.

5 Transforming a Sick City

This chapter has highlighted some of the processes and outcomes that have helped transform Richmond from a sick to a more equitable and healthy city. While the transformation is ongoing and incomplete, we offer the following principles that contributed to today's successes: (1) develop a long-range plan, co-drafted *with* residents not for them; (2) develop a health equity strategy explicitly framed around structural racism and toxic stress to ensure that you address the root causes of poor health; (3) put youth, undocumented residents, former felons, and other highly marginalized groups at the center, not margins, of the work; (4) ensure that residents benefit economically, such as through employment, and politically, from strategies; (5) institutionalize health equity through the law and municipal budgets to avoid overburdening nonprofits and relying on private foundations; (6) embrace *urban acupuncture*, or focused efforts to support the most vulnerable population groups and places, and ensure that strategies are not one or the other; and (7) do not expect to get it all right the first time: learn-by-doing, measure impacts along the way, and adjust interventions as new knowledge emerges.

References

1. Corburn J, Curl S, Arredondo G, et al. Making health equity planning work: a relational approach in Richmond, California. *J Plan Educ Res.* 2015; 35(3):265–281.
2. Health initiatives. City of Richmond, California website. 2018. Available at www.Richmondhealth.org. Accessed June 10, 2018.
3. Maxmen, A. A focus on health to resolve urban ills. *New York Times.* April 19, 2017. Available at https://www.nytimes.com/2017/04/19/opinion/a-focus-on-health-to-resolve-urban-ills.html. Accessed June 10, 2018.
4. Leigh Brown, P. How a forlorn playground became one of America's most innovative public spaces. *Christian Science Monitor.* 2017. Available at https://www.csmonitor.com/World/Making-a-difference/2017/0524/How-a-forlorn-playground-became-one-of-America-s-most-innovative-public-spaces. Accessed June 10, 2018.
5. Health in All Policies strategy, 2013-14. City of Richmond, CA website. Available at http://www.ci.richmond.ca.us/2575/Health-in-All-Policies-HiAP. Accessed June 10, 2018.

36

Case Studies in Urban Health

Nairobi, Kenya

ALEX EZEH AND BLESSING MBERU

1 Urbanization and Health in Nairobi: Introduction and Overview

Africa remains mostly rural, with 43% of its population living in urban areas. However, Africa is the most rapidly urbanizing region in the world and its population is projected to reach 59% urban by 2050.[1] Kenya typifies this pattern of rapid urbanization with Nairobi for years holding the title of one of the most rapidly growing cities in the world. In the last intercensal period, the city's population grew by about 4% per annum.[2] A characteristic consequence of this rate of rapid urbanization in Africa is the inability of governments to expand urban infrastructure to accommodate growth in urban population. For decades, increasing numbers and proportions of the urban population in sub-Saharan Africa (SSA) have lived in informal settlements characterized by limited access to water and sanitation, poor housing conditions, limited employment opportunities, and near absence of the public sector.[3-6] Current estimates suggest that about 56% of the urban population in SSA lives in slums, down from 70% in 1990.[7] While the proportion of urban population living in slums in SSA is declining, the absolute number continues to grow as a result of overall population growth in the region. By 2016, the number of slum dwellers in SSA had doubled from its 1990 figure.[8] Unfortunately, slum populations are not uniquely identified in censuses and national surveys, and current global estimates rely on a definition of households that lack certain basic amenities or that live in houses with defined characteristics.[8,9]

In Nairobi, more than 60% of the population lives in informal settlements.[10] Yet little is known from official statistics on this population. In order to address this gap, the African Population and Health Research Center (APHRC) designed and implemented the Nairobi Cross-Sectional Slums Survey (NCSS) in 2000, which highlighted the plight of slum residents in Nairobi, Kenya, showing their excess mortality and disease burden compared to other subgroups in the country. The survey also identified the limited access to healthcare and family planning services; the debilitating environment that characterizes the physical living conditions in slums; and the inadequate access to water and sanitation, poor housing conditions, poor livelihood opportunities, and the near-absence of public sector services in slum areas.[3] This survey was repeated in 2012 to take stock of changes that had taken place in key well-being indicators among Nairobi slum residents since the 2000 survey. APHRC also initiated in 2003 a prospective, longitudinal study among residents of two slum communities in Nairobi, Korogocho and Viwandani. This platform, the Nairobi Urban Health and Demographic Surveillance System (NUHDSS), has continued to collect data on various aspects of life among the residents of these two slum communities and serves as an effective platform to understand the process of urbanization and urban health in SSA.

In this chapter, we draw on nearly two decades of work by APHRC among slum populations in Nairobi, Kenya, to highlight the unique health challenges of slum populations and how these are changing. We summarize various efforts to improve health in Nairobi's informal settlements since 2000 and their evaluations; we conclude with reflections on strategies that could support evidence-based policy and action in improving health outcomes among the urban poor in Nairobi, Kenya, and across SSA.

2 Highlights from the 2000 and 2012 NCSS

The 2000 NCSS was the first real effort to quantify the magnitude of health deficits for a representative sample of slum settlements in any given city in SSA. The results showed unconscionable levels of poor health outcomes among slum populations, with up to one in four children born in slums in Embakasi division of Nairobi dying before their fifth birthday. It also showed that slums are not the same even within a single city. Health outcomes among slum residents in different divisions of Nairobi varied by as much as a factor of 2.5 for the under-5 mortality rate to a factor of 6.8 for the neonatal mortality rate (see Table 36.1). Compared to national and other subgroups in Kenya, slum residents had the poorest health outcomes.

The poor health outcomes among slum residents observed in the 2000 NCSS led many agencies to swing into action, with the worst-off slums receiving the greatest attention. Twelve years later, the 2012 NCSS data showed remarkable improvements in child health outcomes across all the divisions of Nairobi except the Dagoreti division, which had the best child health outcomes in 2000. Despite child health indicators improving by almost 50% over the 12-year period, inequities across slum areas persisted and even widened. The 2014 Kenya Demographic and Health Survey (KDHS) also showed similar decreases in child mortality across the country. The slum health deficit, however, continued to persist for the under-5 mortality rate. Indeed, compared to national, rural, and all urban areas, Nairobi consistently recorded the poorest neonatal, infant, and under-5mortality rates, which could reflect the poor health outcomes among the majority of Nairobi residents living in slums. The data reiterate intra- and interslum differences, with persistent ethnic differentials (data not shown) highlighting the heterogeneity of urban slums and the importance of disaggregating data on urban health by multiple dimensions of inequities to enable targeted interventions to the most vulnerable groups.

Table 36.1 **Child health indicators from the Nairobi Cross-Sectional Slums Survey (2000 and 2012) and the Kenya Demographic and Health Survey (1998 and 2014) per 1,000 live births**

	Nairobi Cross-Sectional Slums Survey (NCSS) 2000 and Kenya Demographic and Health Survey (KDHS) 1998			Nairobi Cross-Sectional Slums Survey (NCSS) 2012 and Kenya Demographic and Health Survey (KDHS) 2014		
	Neonatal mortality rate	Infant mortality rate	Under-five mortality rate	Neonatal mortality rate	Infant mortality rate	Under-five mortality rate
Divisions in Nairobi						
Central	24.5	68	123.1	16.1	48.6	146.5
Makadara	34.1	86.3	142.7	14.6	32	82.5
Kasarani	19.2	77.4	124.5	8.1	19.9	42.4
Embakasi	111.1	163.6	254.1	8.5	31.5	68.4
Pumwani	16.3	72.6	134.6	4.2	14.3	49.4
Westlands	23.1	103	195.4	27.2	58.5	100.5
Dagoreti	0	35	100.3	26.7	46.7	93
Kibera	35.1	106.2	186.5	9.3	33.2	78.5
NCSS Slum Total	31.3	88.2	136.4	14.4	39.2	79.8
KDHS National	27	70.7	105.2	22	39	52
Nairobi	19.5	41.4	66.1	39	55	72
Urban	20.3	55.4	88.3	26	43	57
Rural	28.4	73.8	108.6	21	40	56

3 Highlights from NUHDSS

Just as the NCSS show large differentials in health status across slums in the same city, differences in rates of progress in improving health outcomes among slum populations, and continuing large health deficits relative to other population subgroups, the NUHDSS provides a unique opportunity to take an in-depth look at the drivers of poor health outcomes in two specific slum communities in Nairobi. Data on causes of death using verbal autopsies from the NUHDSS between 2003 and 2017 show that the burden of disease profile for urban slum communities differs significantly from any known burden of disease profile for SSA populations. In particular, the role of acute respiratory infections as the driver of under-5 mortality; injury deaths as the driver of adult, and especially adult male, mortality; and the overall burden of tuberculosis (TB) are features that are not as evident in other burden of disease studies in SSA.

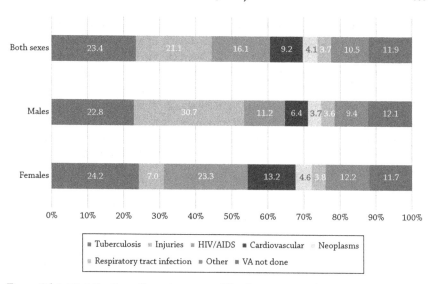

Figure 36.1 **Distribution of top six causes of death among residents 15 years and older, by gender, NUHDSS 2003–2017.**

Figures 36.1 and 36.2 provide an assessment of the main causes of death among adults 15 years and older (Figure 36.1) and among children under 5 years of age (Figure 36.2) using data from the NUHDSS verbal autopsies collected between January 2003 and December 2017 and covering almost 6,300 deaths. For adults, the role of

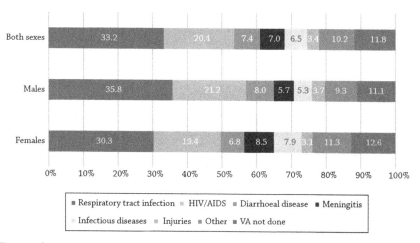

Figure 36.2 **Distribution of top six causes of death among children under 5 by gender, Nairobi Urban Health and Demographic Surveillance System (NUHDSS) 2003–2017.**

injury—especially for adult male mortality, where it accounts for nearly one in three deaths—is notable. Overall, TB is the leading cause of adult deaths, and, combined with HIV, both account for 40% of all adult mortality and about half of the deaths among adult females. The importance of noncommunicable diseases (NCDs) in the slums is also evident. For children, acute respiratory infections account for more than a third of the deaths among children under 5 years of age, and this has been linked to the high levels of both indoor and outdoor pollutions in the slums.[11,12]

The longitudinal nature of the NUHDSS data also permits an assessment of how the health profile of the slum communities has changed over time, providing insights into the temporal and enduring drivers of poor health outcomes among slum populations in a SSA city.

For children under 5 years of age, acute respiratory infection has remained the leading cause of death since 2003, and its significance has continued to increase over time (Figure 36.3). The worrying spike since 2014 is currently being investigated. HIV continues to decline as a major cause of under-5 mortality among children in slum communities. Most other causes have remained relatively stable over the years. For adults 15 and older, injury deaths have continued to increase over time, with major causes identified as assault (54%), road traffic accidents (20%), and exposure to smoke/fire/flame (14%) (Figure 36.4). The spike in injury deaths in 2011 reflects a fire incident in a petroleum pipeline that passed through one of the slum communities and that resulted in hundreds of fire deaths and injuries.[13] The dramatic drop in HIV deaths from 2003 to 2005 coincides with the US President's Emergency Plan for AIDS Relief (PEPFAR) rollout in Kenya in 2003; deaths from HIV has remained relatively stable over time, varying between 10% and 15% of all adult deaths. TB remains the leading cause of all adult deaths between 2003 and 2010. Since 2010, it has continued to vie with injury deaths for the top leading cause position.

4 Efforts to Address Health Challenges of Slum Residents in Nairobi

The consistent provision of evidence on the health deficits borne by slum dwellers in Nairobi has led to many different efforts by various agencies to address health issues among the urban poor. Many of these efforts have focused on child health, including nutrition and breastfeeding interventions, HIV/AIDS, maternal health, and NCDs, among others.[14–19] But other challenges, including injuries (largely from interpersonal violence and road traffic accidents) and indoor and outdoor pollution, have remained largely unaddressed. These interventions have also resulted in noticeable improvements in health outcomes, as is evident from both the NCSS 2012 and NUHDSS data, indicating the massive potential to improve health outcomes in slum communities through properly targeted interventions.

Several studies by researchers at APHRC have documented significant improvements in health outcomes among slum dwellers in Nairobi within relatively short periods. An intervention research program on maternal and child health—the Partnership for Maternal, Newborn and Child Health (PAMANECH) in Korogocho and Viwandani

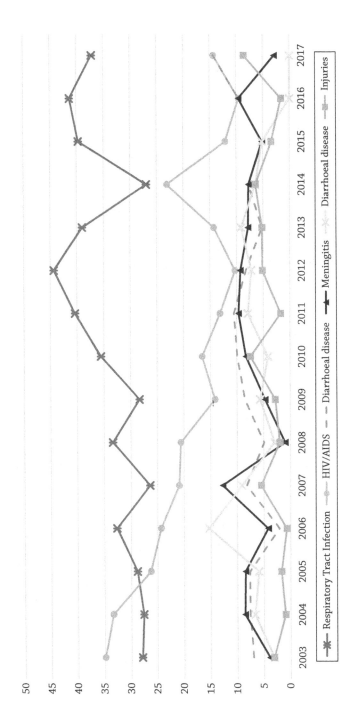

Figure 36.3 **Trends in leading causes of death among children under 5, Nairobi Urban Health and Demographic Surveillance System (NUHDSS) 2003–2017.**

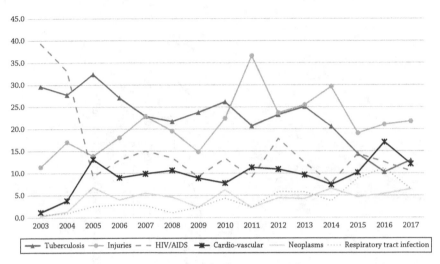

Figure 36.4 **Trends in leading causes of death among residents 15 years and older, Nairobi Urban Health and Demographic Surveillance System (NUHDSS) 2003–2017.**

slums—implemented between 2012 and 2016 increased the capacity of private health facilities in the slums to provide basic emergency obstetric care and significantly reduced home deliveries.[20,21] An intervention to address poor nutritional status among children in the slums focused on personalized home-based counseling by community health workers on exclusive breastfeeding for 6 months. Despite acknowledged design limitations, researchers found a large increase in exclusive breastfeeding from a baseline of 2% to 55%, with only an increase from 2% to 3% over the same period in a parallel observation study on comparable women who gave birth in the surveillance area but were not recruited into this study.[22] A community-based intervention for primary prevention of cardiovascular diseases (CVD) in the slums of Nairobi (SCALE-UP) led to the screening of up to 5,000 slum dwellers aged 35 years or older; the identification of leakages across the continuum of NCD risk reduction; more than 1,000 hypertension diagnoses, referrals, and improved quality of care for hypertension patients; and the identification of the most affordable, feasible, and cost-effective health service delivery package for prevention of cardiovascular disease in the slum settlements.[23] As part of the search for successful interventions and pathways to address the challenge of health inequity between slum and non-slum urban dwellers, Mberu and colleagues identified the specific advantage of slum dwellers over the rest of the country to specific HIV prevention interventions delivered through mobile clinics. The study highlights the complementary roles of mobile outreach services in expanding healthcare access to hard-to-reach but vulnerable groups in informal settlements beyond public facilities and other traditional service delivery models.[24]

5 Conclusion

This chapter summarizes two decades of urban health research in Nairobi, Kenya. It shows the earlier findings of massive health burdens borne by slum residents and how a platform of rigorous research provided the impetus for action to address some of these health burdens and the significant impact achieved by specific interventions in relatively short periods. It also highlights areas of increasing health burden where, as yet, little or no action is being undertaken (such as injuries and indoor and outdoor pollutions). The summary contributes to a nuanced understanding of urban health in Kenya and much of SSA, where rapid rates of urbanization and limited expansion of affordable housing, urban infrastructure, and amenities are forcing increasing numbers of the urban population to live in slum settlements. It underscores the known fact that, even in a single city, slums vary significantly in size, their degree of deprivation, and on the magnitude of health deficits they experience. While significant progress has been made to improve slum health outcomes in Nairobi since 2000, their disadvantage relative to other subgroups in Kenya persists.

As we strive to "make cities and human settlements inclusive, safe, resilient, and sustainable" by "ensuring access to safe and affordable housing, and upgrading slum settlements,"[25] targeted action to improve access to basic services and amenities, including health and education services, must not wait. The heterogeneous nature of slums within a city underscores the need for data at very local levels to support contextualized policy and program interventions. The specific case studies highlighted here responded to clear gaps identified through research in poor urban settings of Nairobi, and they were shown to have worked well in improving health outcomes. They all have elements that can be scalable across other urban poor settings in Kenya and across low- and middle-income countries of the Global South, but they will need to be validated against local evidence in other settings. The PAMANECH service delivery model shows the power of targeted support for public–private partnerships in expanding access to high-quality, accessible, and affordable healthcare among the urban poor. The CVD SCALE-UP intervention demonstrates the potential for improved quality of care for hypertension patients that can be applied beyond the slums of Nairobi, and the study on delivering HIV prevention to the urban poor in Nairobi through mobile clinics suggests the potential promise of nontraditional service delivery models that are convenient and adaptable to specific contexts in bridging service access and utilization deficits among disadvantaged populations.

Building resilient and healthy cities will require sustained investments informed by credible local scientific evidence. The chapter provides informed perspectives on existing and new areas of focus that will be of significant value to policymakers and development partners whose programmatic focus is aimed at improving the well-being of city dwellers, including the urban poor. Generating credible evidence will require close collaboration between scientists, local governments, and urban residents, including slum dwellers. Investment in data systems at local levels should be an important component of the push to address urban challenges, especially in monitoring and evaluation of interventions and in determining what works.

References

1. Department of Economic and Social Affairs. *World urbanization prospects: the 2018 revision, online edition.* New York: United Nations; 2018.
2. Kenya National Bureau of Statistics. *Kenya demographic and health survey 2008–09.* Calverton, MD: Kenya National Bureau of Statistics and ICF Macro; 2010.

3. African Population and Health Research Center. *Population and health dynamics in Nairobi's informal settlements: report of the Nairobi Cross-sectional Slums Survey (NCSS)*. Nairobi, Kenya: African Population and Health Research Center; 2002.

4. Fotso JC, Ezeh A, Oronje R. Provision and use of maternal health services among urban poor women in Kenya: what do we know and what can we do? *J Urban Health*. 2008; 85:428–442.

5. Kyobutungi C, Ziraba AK, Ezeh A, et al. The burden of disease profile of residents of Nairobi's slums: results from a demographic surveillance system. *Popul Health Metr*. 2008; 6:1.

6. UN-Habitat. *The state of African cities 2008: a framework for addressing urban challenges in Africa*. Nairobi, Kenya: UN-Habitat; 2008.

7. UN-Habitat. *Slum almanac 2015/2016 tracking improvement in the lives of slum dwellers*. Nairobi, Kenya: UN-Habitat; 2016.

8. Ezeh A, Oyebode O, Satterthwaite D, et al. The history, geography and sociology of slums and the health problems of people who live in slums. *Lancet*. 2017; 389(10068):547–558.

9. UN-Habitat. *The challenge of the slums. Global report on human settlements*. Nairobi, Kenya: UN-Habitat; 2003.

10. African Population and Health Research Center. *Population and health dynamics in Nairobi's informal settlements*. Nairobi, Kenya: African Population and Health Research Center; 2014.

11. Egondi T, Kyobutungi C, Ng N, et al. Community perceptions of air pollution and related health risks in Nairobi slums. *Int J Environ Res Public Health*. 2013; 10(10):4851–4868.

12. Muindi K, Egondi T, Kimani-Murage E, Rocklov J, Ng N. "We are used to this": a qualitative assessment of the perceptions of and attitudes towards air pollution amongst slum residents in Nairobi. *BMC Public Health*. 2014; 14:226.

13. Mberu BU, Wamukoya M, Oti S, Kyobutungi C. Trends in causes of adult deaths in Nairobi's informal settlements, 2003–2012: results from an urban demographic and health surveillance system. *J Urban Health*. 2015; 92(3):422–445.

14. Kimani-Murage EW, Kyobutungi C, Ezeh AC, et al. Effectiveness of personalised, home-based nutritional counselling on infant feeding practices, morbidity and nutritional outcomes among infants in Nairobi slums: study protocol for a cluster randomised controlled trial. *Trials*. 2013; 14:445.

15. National AIDS Control Council. *Kenya AIDS response progress report 2014. Progress towards zero*. Nairobi, Kenya: National AIDS Control Council; 2014.

16. National AIDS and STI Control Programme. *Kenya AIDS indicator survey 2012: final report*. Nairobi, Kenya: National AIDS and STI Control Programme; 2014.

17. National AIDS and STI Control Programme. *Kenya AIDS epidemic update 2011*. Nairobi, Kenya: National AIDS Control Council and National AIDS/STI Control Programme; 2012.

18. Bakibinga P, Ettarh R, Ziraba AK, et al. The effect of enhanced public–private partnerships on maternal, newborn and child health services and outcomes in Nairobi–Kenya: the PAMANECH quasi-experimental research protocol. *BMJ Open*. 2014; 4(10):e006608. doi:10.1136/bmjopen-2014-006608

19. Oti S, van de Vijver S, Kyobutungi C, et al. A community-based intervention for primary prevention of cardiovascular diseases in the slums of Nairobi: the SCALE UP study protocol for a prospective quasi-experimental community-based trial. *Trials*. 2013; 14 (1):409.

20. Bakibinga P, Ziraba AK, Ettarh R, Kamande E, Egondi T, Kyobutungi C. Use of private and public health facilities for essential maternal and child health services in urban informal settlements: perspectives of women and community health volunteers in Nairobi, Kenya. *Afr Popul Stud*. 2016; 30(3):3113–3123.

21. Osindo J, Bakibinga P, et al. Challenges and opportunities for promoting maternal, newborn, and child health (MNCH) in urban informal settlements: perspectives of community health workers in Nairobi, Kenya. *Afr Popul Stud*. 2016; 30(3):3124–3132.

22. Kimani-Murage EW, Griffiths PL, Wekesah F, et al. Effectiveness of home-based nutritional counselling and support on exclusive breastfeeding in urban poor settings in Nairobi: a cluster randomized controlled trial. *Global Health*. 2017;13:90.

23. van de Vijver S, Oti S, van Charante EM, et al. Cardiovascular prevention model from Kenyan slums to migrants in the Netherlands. *Global Health.* 2015; 11:11.

24. Mberu BU, Elungata P, Kabiru CW, Ezeh AC. Reaching the urban poor with health interventions: the case of HIV testing in Nairobi urban informal settlements, Kenya. *Afr Popul Stud.* 2016; 30(3):3103–3112.

25. United Nations, 2015. Transforming our world: the 2030 Agenda for Sustainable Development; Resolution adopted by the General Assembly on 25 September 2015. Goal 11 and Target 11.1. https://documents-dds-ny.un.org/doc/UNDOC/GEN/N15/291/89/PDF/N1529189.pdf?OpenElement. (Accessed September 18, 2018).

37

Observatory for Urban Health in Belo Horizonte City

An Innovative and Cross-Sectoral Collaboration in Urban Health

WALESKA TEIXEIRA CAIAFFA AND AMÉLIA AUGUSTA DE LIMA FRICHE

1 Background and Conceptual Framework

The Observatory for Urban Health in Belo Horizonte (OSUBH, in Portuguese) is a partnership—in place since 2002—between the Brazilian Federal University of Minas Gerais (UFMG) and the Belo Horizonte Municipality. Created by academics associated with the Epidemiology Research Group at UFMG, registered with the Brazilian National Research Council (GPE-CNPq) and municipal technicians in the Belo Horizonte Health Department, and driven by a common interest in finding ways of bridging the gap between science and public health policies, OSUBH's mission is to build workforce capacity in population health research and to conduct urban-themed studies that can drive planning for improving urban health.[1]

Under a well-defined urban health conceptual framework and throughout its 16 years of existence, OSUBH has been a space for reflection and elaboration of urban health themes.[2-4] Focusing on intra-urban health inequities, OSUBH compiles urban health metrics and scrutinizes social, environmental, and spatial conditions of urban life and related consequences.

In addition, OSUBH is involved in training and mentoring of scholars and undergraduate and graduate students from various fields of knowledge (physicians, nurses, architects, engineers, lawyers, psychologists, speech therapists, statisticians, nutritionists, and physical educators) by including trainees in project realms, in working groups around thematic areas, or around the development of proposals for dissertations and theses on urban health. OSUBH researchers and scholars also engage with health and non-health sectors in a collaboration across sectors to provide an empirical basis for determining the health benefits and co-benefits of urban public policies (Figure 37.1).

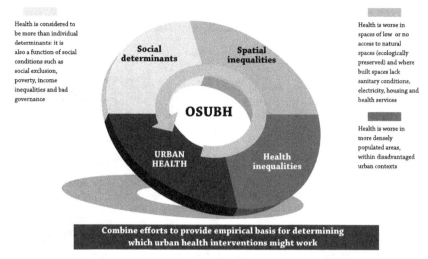

Health is considered to be more than individual determinants: it is also a function of social conditions such as social exclusion, poverty, income inequalities and bad governance

Social determinants

Spatial inequalities

OSUBH

URBAN HEALTH

Health inequalities

Health is worse in spaces of low or no access to natural spaces (ecologically preserved) and where built spaces lack sanitary conditions, electricity, housing and health services

Health is worse in more densely populated areas, within disadvantaged urban contexts

Combine efforts to provide empirical basis for determining which urban health interventions might work

Figure 37.1 **The Observatory for Urban Health in Belo Horizonte team framework.**
OSUBH home-based health survey (BH Health Study) in Belo Horizonte, Southeast Brazil, using a leisure time physical activity (LTPA) levels (≥150 minutes/week), measured by the International Physical Activity Questionnaire (IPAQ) and self-perception of the neighborhoods. Environmental data were assessed through systematic social observation (SSO) on street segments of respondents' residences. Twenty-one neighborhood-level environment variables were reduced to six environment factors using principal component analysis with covariance matrix.

1.1 Core Projects

OSUBH has been developing urban health evaluation models to assist government agencies in their elaboration of public policies in the health sector and beyond. Figure 37.2 shows the ongoing project realms developed by the OSUBH team, including innovative studies on urban health and their different levels of attributes from the individual to the governmental level.

Across these projects, OSUBH observes health outcomes and health behaviors in the urban context, including (1) urban lifestyle (diet and physical activity), (2) neighborhood physical and social environments, (3) comprehensive community interventions in vulnerable urban areas, (4) transport and mobility, (5) health services, and (6) models of participatory governance.[5-27]

1.2 Metrics: Data Management, Analysis, and Sharing Plan

Over the course of its existence, OSUBH has managed and updated a city-wide database of urban indicators for Belo Horizonte, collected through primary or secondary resources such as (1) intra-urban-level data obtained from household surveys for various

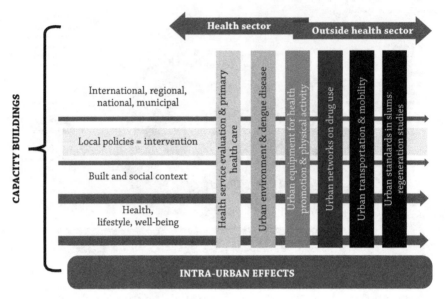

Figure 37.2 **Observatory for Urban Health in Belo Horizonte team projects: from health sector to outside health sector.**

years; (2) intra-urban-level data obtained from Systematic Social Observation that is harmonized with household survey data; (3) intra-urban-level secondary data from vital records; (4) surveillance system and hospitalization data linked to intra-urban indicators of social vulnerability, such as the Health Vulnerability Index, from the entire city; and (5) selected data about pre- and post-public policy interventions linked to intra-urban-level data for core projects.

All this information has been valuable to researchers for the investigation of a myriad of research questions or for linkage or combination with other data resources.

1.3 Partnerships

Locally, OSUBH is engaged in partnership with several sectors of the municipality working together in the health impact evaluation of public policies and providing feedback in several local, national, and international agendas of the city. OSUBH has been actively participating in (1) the Millennium Development Goals (MDG) and the Sustainable Development Goals (SDG) indicators, along with the Municipal Secretary of Planning, Budgets, and Information, through Belo Horizonte's Millennium Observatory; (2) *Projeto Vida no Trânsito*—the Brazilian Road Safety Project with the City Health Department, Transit Department, and the Health Surveillance Secretariat of the Brazilian Ministry of Health (MoH), for whom OSUBH is a collaborative center; (3) *Academias da Saúde* in Belo Horizonte as a model for Brazil, in partnership with the City Health Department and Brazilian MoH; and (4) *Projeto Vila Viva*, together with the Urbanization and Housing Company of Belo Horizonte (URBEL), in partnership with the Oswaldo Cruz Foundation (FIOCRUZ) and the Brazilian MoH. In this chapter, we will briefly present the *Academias da Saúde Project*.

OSUBH also has developed several international partnerships. These include (1) a partnership with the University of Michigan through its Center of Social Epidemiology and Population Health, to undertake collaborative research projects and the training of doctoral and postdoctoral candidates through the CNPq-Science Without Borders Program; (2) with the World Health Organization (WHO) Center for Health Development in Kobe, Japan, and the Pan American Health Organization (PAHO), to undertake joint efforts that have led to the publication of technical reports based on studies of urban health and health observatories; and (3) with the New York Academy of Medicine through participation in the board of the International Society for Urban Health (ISUH) and also through studies on the experience of Belo Horizonte with participatory governance and participative democracy. Also, in 2011, OSUBH chaired the Tenth International Conference on Urban Health (ICUH) in Belo Horizonte, which allowed for the exchange of experiences between a wide network of national and international researchers and practitioners.

More recently, OSUBH scholars were founders of the Urban Health Network for Latin America and the Caribbean (LAC-Urban Health). LAC-Urban Health is a regional learning network focused on exchange and collaboration for research, training, and policy translation; it was founded by academics and representatives from international organizations following a meeting on urban health in September 2015 at the Dornsife School of Public Health in Philadelphia. It includes representatives from Argentina, Brazil, Colombia, and Peru, along with the Economic Commission for Latin America and the Caribbean (ECLAC) and the United Nations University International Institute for Global Health (UNU-IIGH). The most significant collaboration to emerge from LAC-Urban Health is an ongoing 5-year interdisciplinary project named *Salud Urbana en América Latina* (SALURBAL) funded by the Wellcome Trust's *Our Planet, Our Health Initiative*, aimed to investigate how variations in urban environments in cities across Latin America affect population health, social equity, and environmental sustainability.[28]

2 Belo Horizonte City: A Case Study

Belo Horizonte City (BHC), translated as City of the Beautiful Horizon, is about 120 years old, located in southeastern Brazil, and the capital of the State of Minas Gerais. It covers an area of 331 square kilometers and has an estimated population of 2,523,794 in 2017, and a population density of 7,167 inhabitants/km². BHC scores 0.81 (in 2010) on the Human Development Index (HDI) and its gross domestic product (GDP) per capita is US$10.058,73. However, the Gini index of 0.6106 is one of the most unequal among the 26 Brazilian state capitals.[29]

The city has about 460,000 dwellers living in informal settlements characterized by inadequately urbanized spaces with poor habitability conditions and subject to geological risks; this corresponds to 19% of the total residents living in 5% of the city's territory, reaffirming high density and inequalities in the quality of life of its citizens.[29,30]

Founded in 1897 with an urban plan that emphasized a model city both in terms of physical layout and with the goal of becoming disease-free, its population grew by 55% from 1940 until the end of the decade, well exceeding the initial urban plans for the city.[31] Sprawling slums started to appear in the 1960s, reflecting a housing deficit and the population's need to reduce commuting distances. Growing to a million inhabitants in the 1970s, the city struggled to absorb this population influx. From 1991 to 2006, BHC was the fourth most rapidly expanding city among Brazilian cities with more than 100,000 inhabitants.

Although today it ranks as the sixth most populated Brazilian city, continuous and disorderly growth has been aggravated by intense construction of low-income housing developments without basic sanitary infrastructure and services. This construction, especially in proximity to existing middle- and upper-class neighborhoods, exacerbated the contrasts in living conditions.[32]

Like any other large urban center in Brazil, the city has faced multiple challenges— waste accumulation, air pollution, traffic, insufficient housing, and other complex social dynamics. These have led to unfavorable living conditions and increased social problems with consequent significant health implications, mainly associated with an aging population, high rates of chronic diseases, and vector-borne diseases together with other emergent and reemergent diseases. Associated with these conditions is the magnitude of the sprawling city peripheries, especially throughout the metropolitan area (Figure 37.3), with large clusters of vulnerable areas characterized by social deprivation, greater vulnerability to disease and death, and the lack of access to goods and services further deepening health inequities in the region.

With a democratically elected popular government from the end of the 1990s to the early 2000s, the city established the foundation of a process of participatory governance, defined by UN-Habitat as "the sum of the many ways individuals and institutions, public and private, plan and manage the common affairs of the city."[32] Despite current economic and political obstacles, among other challenges, Belo Horizonte City Hall has worked together with other sectors to maintain a participatory budgeting process—an inclusive participatory, transparent, and accountable democratic process for distribution of funds application in public works—and other extensive initiatives designed to improve urban living for vulnerable populations, such as the Vila Viva Project.[33]

The organization of health services has focused primarily on comprehensive care and the interconnection of various public policies for mitigating disease processes.[34]

3 Case Study

Belo Horizonte aimed to increase the physical activity of its residents. The example given here illustrates a community health promotion model of evaluation of the *Academia da Cidade* program experience.

3.1 Background

Physical activity has been considered a priority theme in health promotion, given the epidemiological importance and the social gradients of this behavior in the population.[35,36] With a low overall prevalence of leisure-time physical activity (LTPA) in the city (30.2%), the OSUBH team worked with the City Health Department to design a study aiming to (1) understand physical and social contextual factors (perceived and

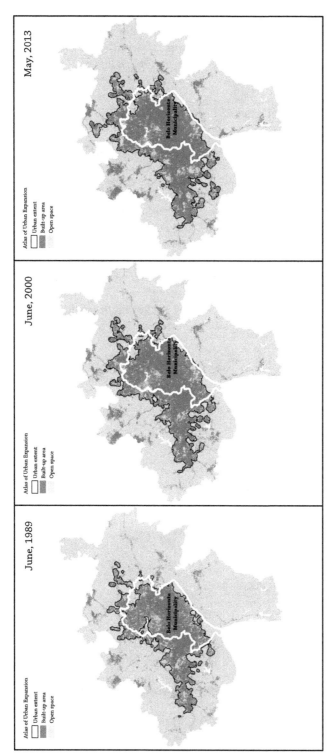

Figure 37.3 **Sprawl of built-up Belo Horizonte and metropolitan area over time.** *Source:* Angel S, Blei A, Parent J, et al. *Atlas of urban expansion—2016 edition, volume 1: areas and densities.* New York: NYU Urban Expansion Program at New York University, UN-Habitat, and the Lincoln Institute of Land Policy. 2016. Elaborated by Yuanyuan Zhao, postdoctoral candidate at University of California Berkeley College of Environmental Design Salurbal Project.

objectively measured) beyond the individual level related to low LTPA prevalence rates in the city; (2) develop an evaluation model to estimate the impact of a city-level agenda aiming at promoting more active lifestyles—the *Academia da Cidade* (AC) program, which was derived from a participatory budgetary process implemented in 2006; and (3) further extend the city model of AC to a national model for evaluation of the scaled-up program, the *Academia de Saúde* (AS), for physical activity interventions in Brazil from the Health Academy Program (Law No. 719/GM/MS of April 7, 2011).[37]

3.2 The *Academia da Cidade* Program

The AC program is a public, city-wide intervention prioritized to areas of high vulnerability to health and planned by the City Health Department of Belo Horizonte since 2005. Between 2007 and 2008, there was an expansion of the program in the city that was incrementally increased by national policy in 2011.[38] It offers universal access as part of the Unified Health System of the city, and it represents a facility built with simple infrastructure for physical activity classes and other health-promoting activities. It is located in deprived urban neighborhoods as part of the urban planning and participatory budgeting process of the city.

The AC program receives people referred by primary healthcare units or by spontaneous demand in centers that operate in up to three shifts per day.[38]

3.3 Research Methods

Briefly, using a specially designed sampling process for this purpose, OSUBH conducted a home-based health survey in Belo Horizonte, named *Saúde em Beagá (2008–9)* (SB) under a conceptual model presented in Figure 37.4.[39]

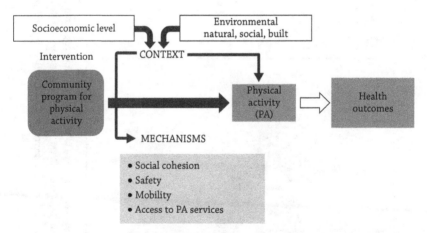

Figure 37.4 **Conceptual model of Community Program for Physical Activity and its effects on health outcomes.** Source: Adapted from Mehdipanah R, Manzano A, Borrell C, et al. Exploring complex causal pathways between urban renewal, health and health inequality using a theory-driven realist approach. *Soc Sci Med.* 2015; 124:266–274.

The survey was a probabilistic sampling design, stratified in three stages (census tracts, household, and one resident of 18 years of age or older).[40] To ensure the representativeness of residents in the vicinity of the AC Program, the probabilities of selecting each census tract were differentiated according to distance to the centers. The census tracts closest to the in-service centers and to centers planned to be built were included in the survey without randomization. Census tracts located within 500 meters and between 500 and 1,000 meters were, respectively, 8 and 4 times more likely to be selected compared to those located at more than 1,000 meters from AC program centers. Individual and environmental data were obtained using instruments designed for assessing subjective perception and objective measurements of the social and physical neighborhood environment. Several domains were included. For subjective perception, services, aesthetics, safety, and social cohesion were some of the measured domains. For the objective assessment under the Systematic Social Observation (SSO) model, indicators of walkability, places for physical activity, aesthetics, physical disorder, safety, and services were collected in a final sample consisting of 1,295 street segments randomly chosen using interviewee residential addresses obtained from the survey and nested in 147 neighborhoods.[41]

3.4 Summary of the Main Results and Further Studies

A total of 4,048 nonuser participants of the program living at different distances from the three AC centers planned to be built and those living near an in-service center were interviewed. The study outcome was LTPA of 150 minutes/week or longer, as measured by the International Physical Activity Questionnaire.

Selected LTPA study data are shown in Table 37.1. Results were assembled to furnish evidence on determinants of increased LTPA in an urban context that go beyond individual characteristics, such as social capital and environmental attributes like safety, walkability, and the public policies associated with increased physical activity.

As member of the MoH physical activity monitoring network, OSUBH is in charge of assessing the program in Belo Horizonte City from 2006 onward, starting even before the first center opened. OSUBH is now expanding this methodology to the entire city in order to apply the evaluation model under the new Academia da Saúde (AS) Program federative bill (Law No. 719/GM/MS of April 7, 2011 2012–2015), with provision for implementation of 2,702 units in 2,186 Brazilian cities.[38-40] As a result of this national law, currently coexists in Belo Horizonte City two typologies of programs: AC and AS. Therefore, following the first large cross-sectional study, *Saúde em Beagá (2008-09)*, which established a baseline to evaluate the impact of the AC program, a new project named "Modes, Lifestyles, and Health: A Study of the Health Academies Program in Brazilian Cities: from Understanding the Program to Effectiveness of the Actions" (MOVE–SE Academias (2014-15) was developed to evaluate the impact of the AC, the AS, and their combination on the city, consolidating the evaluation 6 years after the first study. Up to February 1, 2017, of the 76 existing centers, 57 qualified as similar. A random sample of them is part of the ongoing OSUBH process of evaluation.[37]

Table 37.1 **Selected studies on physical activity in leisure time developed by the Observatory for Urban Health in Belo Horizonte team**

Author and year	Sample size (adults)	Main exposure	Analysis	Main results	Main conclusion
Fernandes et al. (2015)[17]	1,621	Linear distance from households to the Academia da Cidade (AC) categorized in radial buffers: <500; 500–1,000; 1,000–1,500 m and self-perception score rates of the physical environment of non-users of the AC living in these buffers in: the vicinity of an in-service AC (exposed Group I) or in the vicinity of two sites reserved for future installation of centers (non-exposed Groups II and III)	Binary logistic regression using GEE method	Residents living within <500 m of the operating AC gave better ratings to the physical environment when compared to those living in the 1,000 and 1,500 m buffers regardless AC presence. They also reported more physical activity in leisure time (LTPA) (odds ratio [OR] = 1.16), independently of SES	AC may have potential for influencing the surroundings as rated by the population living closer to it and thus providing a strategic alternative for mitigating inequalities in neighborhoods regarding LTPA
Andrade et al. (2015)[15]	3,597	Scales of subjective characteristics (self-perception) of the social and physical neighborhood environment for services, aesthetics, safety, and social cohesion domains	Multilevel logistic regression stratified by socioeconomic status (SES)	LPTA overall prevalence of 30.2%, stratified of 20.2% in low, 25.4% medium, and 40.6% high SES. Higher perception of social cohesion was associated with increased LTPA only among participants of lowest SES (OR = 1.43)	Social cohesion is important for the promotion of LTPA in economically disadvantaged groups, supporting the need to stimulate interventions for enhancing social relationships in this population

Author	N	Measure	Analysis	Results	Conclusion
Andrade et al. (2018)[42]	3,597	Scales of objective characteristics of the physical and social neighborhood environment, through Systematic Social Observation (SSO)** for walkability, places for physical activity, aesthetics, physical disorder, safety, and services domains	Multilevel logistic regression	Individuals living in neighborhoods with higher walkability (OR = 1.20) and safety (OR = 1.18) indicators were more likely to be active during leisure time, even after adjusting for individual variables	Improving built and social environments is an important step for achieving higher levels of LTPA in the population in a middle-income country
Andrade et al. (2018)[16]	1,581	To be an AC non-user living within 1,500-meter radius of an in-service Academia da Cidade (AC) (exposed group) or to be an AC non-user living in two nonoperational AC (nonexposed group)	Binary logistic regression using generalized estimating equation (GEE) and Propensity score	LTPA prevalence was 26.5% in exposed versus 22.7% in nonexposed group. Exposed group was more likely to be active in leisure time (OR = 1.05), especially when living within a short distance (<500 m) of the AC (OR = 1.18)	Community interventions for physical activity in low-SES neighborhood, such as AC, may affect the practice of LTPA among nonusers living near the intervention centers. LTPA chance increased 5% due to exposure and 18% if the exposure was within the 500 m
Rodrigues et al. (2018)[43]	3,667	Scales of subjective characteristics (self-perception) of collective efficacy and social cohesion in the neighborhood.	Poisson regression using GEE	Individuals living in areas with higher level of social cohesion were more likely to be LTPA even after controlling for potentially confounding individual and area-level covariates (PR = 1.56). Collective efficacy was not significantly associated with LTPA	Interventions to strengthen social cohesion in the community may be an avenue for promoting physical activity

4 Opportunities, Challenges, Reflections, and Ways Forward

Over the years, OSUBH is maturing and progressing in terms of mission, data management, and governance according to the proposed framework for the observatories.[4] Since the creation of OSUBH, the world has been evolving and cities and citizens have become central to ensuring a sustainable future resting on economic, environmental, and social sustainability.[44] These aspirations have encouraged intersectoral collaborations that may provide data that are meaningful for local policy and decision-making.

There are, however, also challenges. First, we note the ongoing need for a review of our urban health conceptual framework to make sure it remains adequate to evolving local needs. Second, we continue to have limited primary and secondary data, and we need to ensure reliable data collection to inform our work. Third, we need to ensure novel conceptualizations and methodological tools that capture the system dynamics and complexities of cities, with multidirectional causality, feedback loops, and unintended consequences of interventions. Fourth, a real challenge for OSUBH is establishing legitimacy and sustainability even after 16 years of existence. To address this, OSUBH has expanded its partnership efforts (with governments, academics from distinct areas, international organizations, and civil society) through intense capacity building and networking activities. In addition, OSUBH has been in the knowledge production field, building models for evaluating the determinants of health and disease and the impacts of policies and services on urban health, thus ensuring that it can contribute plausible evidence that can increase the confidence of stakeholders. Fifth, financial sustainability—the basis for the Observatory to continue the production of knowledge for action—remains a challenge. Partnerships, in part, hold here a solution. A concrete example is the partnership between OSUBH and the Fiocruz Foundation in developing a joint study and, possibly, an outline for a network of observatories and recent involvement in the LAC Urban Health Network. The sixth challenge is related to publicizing the knowledge produced to policy, especially among the target populations, by creating strategic and appropriate mechanisms so that all subjects can understand health, equity, and their determinants in urban settings along with the various dimensions of health.

Despite such challenges, OSUBH has been optimistically observing and analyzing the city and health through a broad social determinants of health approach, as well as suggesting means of overcoming the challenges of building cities that focus on the well-being of their inhabitants.

References

1. Dias MA, Friche AA, Oliveira VB, Caiaffa WT. The Belo Horizonte Observatory for Urban Health: its history and current challenges. *Cad Saude Publica.* 2015; 31(S1):277–285.
2. Galea S, Vlahov D. *Handbook of urban health: populations, methods, and practice.* New York: Springer; 2005.
3. Caiaffa WT, Ferreira FR, Ferreira AD, Oliveira CD, Camargos VP, Proietti FA. Urban health: "the city is a strange lady, smiling today, devouring you tomorrow." *Cien Saude Colet.* 2008; 13(6):1785–1796.

4. Caiaffa WT, Friche AA, Dias MA, et al. Developing a conceptual framework of urban health observatories toward integrating research and evidence into urban policy for health and health equity. *J Urban Health*. 2014; 91(1):1–16.

5. Mattos Almeida MC, Caiaffa WT, Assuncao RM, Proietti FA. Spatial vulnerability to dengue in a Brazilian urban area during a 7-year surveillance. *J Urban Health*. 2007; 84(3):334–345.

6. Caiaffa WT, Almeida MC, Oliveira CD, et al. The urban environment from the health perspective: the case of Belo Horizonte, Minas Gerais, Brazil. *Cad Saude Publica*. 2005; 21(3):958–967.

7. Dias CS, Dias MA, Friche AA, et al. Temporal and spatial trends in childhood asthma-related hospitalizations in Belo Horizonte, Minas Gerais, Brazil and their association with social vulnerability. *Int J Environ Res Public Health*. 2016;13(7).

8. Meireles AL, Xavier CC, Andrade ACdS, Friche AAdL, Proietti FA, Caiaffa WT. Self-rated health in urban adults, perceptions of the physical and social environment, and reported comorbidities: The BH Health Study. *Cad Saude Publica*. 2015; 31:120–135.

9. Meireles AL, Xavier CC, de Souza Andrade AC, Proietti FA, Caiaffa WT. Self-rated health among urban adolescents: the roles of age, gender, and their associated factors. *PLoS One*. 2015; 10(7):e0132254. doi:10.1371/journal.pone.0132254

10. Andrade RG, Chaves OC, Costa DA, et al. Overweight in men and women among urban area residents: individual factors and socioeconomic context. *Cad Saude Publica*. 2015; 31(S1):148–158.

11. Caiaffa WT, Bastos FI, Freitas LLd, et al. The contribution of two Brazilian multi-center studies to the assessment of HIV and HCV infection and prevention strategies among injecting drug users: the AjUDE-Brasil I and II Projects. *Cad Saude Publica*. 2006; 22:771–782.

12. Friche AA, Caiaffa WT, Cesar CC, Goulart LM, Almeida MC. Maternal and child health indicators in Belo Horizonte, Minas Gerais State, Brazil, 2001: an analysis of intra-urban differences. *Cad Saude Publica*. 2006; 22(9):1955–1965.

13. Cunha MCM, Caiaffa WT, Oliveira CDL, et al. Fatores associados à infecção pelo vírus do dengue no Município de Belo Horizonte, Estado de Minas Gerais, Brasil: características individuais e diferenças intra-urbanas. *Epidemiol Serv Saude*. 2008; 17(3):217–230.

14. Fernandes AP, Andrade ACS, Ramos CG, et al. Leisure-time physical activity in the vicinity of Academias da Cidade Program in Belo Horizonte, Minas Gerais State, Brazil: the impact of a health promotion program on the community. *Cad Saude Publica*. 2015; 31(S1):195–207.

15. Andrade ACS, Peixoto SV, Friche AA, et al. Social context of neighborhood and socioeconomic status on leisure-time physical activity in a Brazilian urban center: The BH Health Study. *Cad Saude Publica*. 2015; 31(S1):136–147.

16. Andrade ACS, Mingoti SA, Fernandes AP, et al. Neighborhood-based physical activity differences: evaluation of the effect of health promotion program. *PLoS One*. 2018;13(2):e0192115. doi:10.1371/journal.pone.0192115.

17. Fernandes AP, Andrade AC, Ramos CG, et al. Leisure-time physical activity in the vicinity of Academias da Cidade Program in Belo Horizonte, Minas Gerais State, Brazil: the impact of a health promotion program on the community. *Cad Saude Publica*. 2015; 31(S1):195–207.

18. Ramos CGC, Andrade RG, Andrade ACS, et al. Contexto familiar e atividade física de adolescentes: cotejando diferenças. *Rev Bras Epidemiol*. 2017; 20:537–548.

19. Ward J, Friche AA, Caiaffa WT, Proietti FA, Xavier CC, Roux AV. Association of socioeconomic factors with body mass index, obesity, physical activity, and dietary factors in Belo Horizonte, Minas Gerais State, Brazil: the BH Health Study. *Cad Saude Publica*. 2015;31(S1):182–194.

20. Friche AA, Diez-Roux AV, Cesar CC, Xavier CC, Proietti FA, Caiaffa WT. Assessing the psychometric and biometric properties of neighborhood scales in developing countries: Saude em Braga Study, Belo Horizonte, Brazil, 2008–2009. *J Urban Health*. 2013; 90(2):246–261.

21. de Almeida Célio F, Friche AAL, Jennings MZ, et al. Contextual characteristics associated with the perceived neighbourhood scale in a crosssectional study in a large urban centre in Brazil. BMJ Open 2018;8:e021445. doi:10.1136/ bmjopen-2017-021445

22. Bentes AA, César CC, Xavier CC, Caiaffa WT, Proietti FA. Self-rated health and perceived violence in the neighborhood is heterogeneous between young women and men. *BMC Public Health*. 2017; 17(1):967.

23. Friche AA, Dias MA, Reis PB, Dias CS, Caiaffa WT, Project BH-V. Urban upgrading and its impact on health: a "quasi-experimental" mixed-methods study protocol for the BH-Viva Project. *Cad Saude Publica*. 2015;31(S1):51–64.

24. Oliveira DF, Friche AAL, Costa DAS, Mingoti SA, Caiaffa WT. Do speed cameras reduce speeding in urban areas? *Cad Saude Publica*. 2015; 31:208–218.

25. Paixão LMMM, Gontijo ED, Mingoti SA, Costa DAS, Friche AAL, Caiaffa WT. Urban road traffic deaths: data linkage and identification of high-risk population sub-groups. *Cad Saude Publica*. 2015; 31:92–106.

26. Souza RCF, Oliveira VB, Pereira DB, Costa HSM, Caiaffa WT. Viver próximo à saúde em Belo Horizonte. *Cadernos Metrópole*. 2016; 18(36).

27. Caiaffa WT, Nabuco AL, Friche AAL, Proietti FA. Urban health and governance model in Belo Horizonte, Brazil In: Vlahov D, Boufford JI, Perason C, Norris, eds. *Urban health: global perspectives*. 1st ed. San Francisco, CA: Jossey-Bass; 2011:437–452.

28. Diez Roux AV, Slesinski SC, Alazraqui M, et al. A novel international partnership for action-able evidence on urban health in Latin America: LAC-Urban Health and SALURBAL. *Global Challenges*. 2018; 1800013. doi: 10.1002/gch2.201800013

29. Instituto Brasileiro de Geografia e Estatística. Portal de Governo Brasileiro website. Available at https://cidades.ibge.gov.br/brasil/mg/belo-horizonte/panorama. Accessed March 29, 2018.

30. Pereira CVL, Afonso AS, Magalhães MCF. Programa Vila Viva: intervenção em assentamentos precários. Available at http://portalpbh-hm.pbh.gov.br/pbh/ecp/comunidade.do?evento=p ortlet&pIdPlc=ecpTaxonomiaMenuPortal&app=urbel&tax=7901&lang=pt_BR&pg=5580 &taxp=0&&idConteudo=22546&chPlc=22546. Accessed April 29, 2018.

31. Atlas of Human Development in Brazil website. Available at http://www.atlasbrasil.org.br/ 2013/en/. Accessed March 29, 2018.

32. United Nations Human Settlements Programme (UN-Habitat) website. 2012. https://www. un-ngls.org/index.php/engage-with-the-un/un-civil-society-contact-points/144-united-nations-human-settlements-programme-un-habitat. Accessed April 29, 2018.

33. Prefeitura Municipal de Belo Horizonte. Participatory budgeting in Belo Horizonte for fifteen years: 1993–2008. Prefeitura Municipal de Belo Horizonte. Available at http://www.pbh. gov.br/comunicacao/pdfs/publicacoesop/revista_op15anos_ingles.pdf. Accessed on April 29, 2018.

34. Secretaria de Vigilância em Saúde, Ministério da Saúde. *Política Nacional de Promoção da Saúde*. Brasília: Ministério da Saúde; 2006.

35. Malta DC, Castro AM, Gosch CS, Cruz D, Bressan A, Nogueira JD, Morais Neto OL, Temporão JG. A Política Nacional de Promoção da Saúde e a agenda da atividade física no contexto do SUS National. *Epidemiol Serv Saude*. 2009; 18(1):79–86.

36. Althoff T, Sosič R, Hicks JL, King AC, Delp SL, Leskovec J. Large-scale physical activity data reveal worldwide activity inequality. *Nature*. 2017; 547(7663):336–339.

37. Fernandes AP, Andrade ACS, Costa DAS, Dias MAS, Malta DC, Caiaffa, WT. Programa Academias da Saúde e a promoção da atividade física na cidade: a experiência de Belo Horizonte, MG, Brasil. *Cien Saude Colet*. 2017; 22(12), 3903–3914.

38. Brasil. Ministério da Saúde. *Secretaria de Vigilância Sanitária em Saúde. Departamento de Análise de Situação em Saúde. Avaliação de efetividade de programas de educação física no Brasil*. Brasília: Brasil Ministério da Saúde (MS); 2013.

39. Mehdipanah R, Manzano A, Borrell C, et al. Exploring complex causal pathways between urban renewal, health and health inequality using a theory-driven realist approach. *Soc Sci Med*. 2015; 124:266–274.

40. Friche AA, Xavier CC, Proetti F, Caiaffa WC. *Saúde urbana em Belo Horizonte*. Belo Horizonte: UFMG; 2015.

41. Costa D, Mingoti SA, Andrade ACS, Xavier CC, Proietti FA, Caiaffa WT. Indicators of physical and social neighborhood attributes measured by the systematic social observation method. *Cad Saude Publica*. 2017; 33(8):e00026316. doi:10.1590/0102-311X00026316

42. Andrade ACS, Mingoti SA, Costa DAS, Xavier CC, Proietti FA, Caiaffa WT. Built and social environment by systematic social observation and leisure-time physical activity report among Brazilian adults: a population based study. Paper presented at the International Conference on Urban Health, 2018.

43. Rodrigues DE, César CC, Kawachi I, Xavier CC, Caiaffa WT, Proietti FA. The influence of neighborhood social capital on leisure-time physical activity: a population-based study in Brazil. *J Urban Health*. 2018 Jul 30

44. Acuto M, Parnell S, Seto KC. Building a global urban science: the study of cities needs to become more than the sum of its parts. An international expert panel investigates why, and how. *Nature Sustainability*. 2018; 1:2–4.

38

Rapid Urbanization in China

BRIAN J. HALL, TENG IENG LEONG, AND WEN CHEN

1 Urbanization in China

Beginning in 1978, post Maoist era economic reforms set China surging toward modernity. An emphasis on economic expansion—and elevation from poverty—fueled massive migration from rural areas to urban city centers. Mega cities with populations numbering in the tens of millions emerged from small fishing villages and were transformed into centers of commerce, ushering in the birth of modern China. Despite clear advances in economic development, urbanization gave rise to critical public health challenges, as well as with opportunities. In this chapter, we will summarize several key signposts along the journey to rapid urbanization in China and how urbanization has influenced population health in the country.

The urban population of China has grown rapidly from 69.4 million in 1950 to 863.6 million in 2018.[1] China's remarkable urbanization was shaped in three stages.[2] During the era of the planned economy (1949–1978), the pace of urbanization in China was slow. By the end of 1978, the proportion of the urban population was less than 18%. Between 1979 and 2008, rapid urban growth was driven by nationwide economic reform. In this stage, massive internal migration emerged in China, and the population started to concentrate in costal and economic zones. In 2008, 46% of China's population lived in urban areas.[3] After 2008, the general layout of economic development in China shifted to industrial structural transformation, and significant attention was devoted to developing central and western China. The strategy of balanced regional growth pushed urbanization forward. By the end of 2017, the proportion of the urban population in China reached 59%; this figure had been just slightly more than 10% in 1950.[4]

2 Epidemiological Transition and the Burden of Disease

China experienced an epidemiological transition starting in the 1980s.[5] This is illustrated by changes in median death rates due to different diseases.[6] Between 1990 and 2010, there was a 59.5% decrease in communicable, maternal, neonatal, and nutritional diseases but a relatively lower decrease in noncommunicable diseases (18.7%). Notable declines in death rates included tuberculosis (73.0%), diarrheal diseases (93.9%), and sexually transmitted diseases (86.8%). Despite great strides made to reduce syphilis and other sexually transmitted diseases within the general population, a key exception was HIV, which showed a dramatic increase in deaths during this period.[6] Within urban centers, key populations most at risk for HIV include men who have sex with men, injection drug users, college students, and migrants.[7] Emerging and neglected tropical diseases are also important, as was seen in 2002 during the severe acute respiratory syndrome (SARS) outbreak. The urban population in China remains at risk of exposure to emerging diseases (e.g., H7N9 or Avian flu) and to possible infectious disease epidemics due to the high concentrations of people in city centers and the preference for purchasing live poultry, sold in local wet markets in some parts of China.[8] Increases in health literacy may be one key strategy to mitigate these risks.

In line with the epidemiological transition, deaths due to some lifestyle diseases increased, with notable increases of ischemic heart disease (120.3%) and diabetes mellitus (141.6%). Especially relevant to our discussion of urbanization is the increase in deaths due to traffic-related pedestrian injuries, accounting for a 188.9% increase.[6] Aside from these critical challenges in health, China has made incredible advances in population health in the past 30 years. Life expectancy increased by more than 10 years for men and by nearly 15 years for women. The infant mortality rate was reduced from 100.6 per 1,000 to 12.9 per 1,000.[9]

3 Health System Reform

Until the early 1980s, the Chinese health system was state-owned.[10] At that time, this largely functional system was changed, which led to massive defunding of hospitals and privatization, which still affects the Chinese medical landscape.[11,12] For example, market reform led to unintended financial incentives for physicians to provide expensive diagnostic tests and medications. Out-of-pocket consumer costs for medical care also ballooned, and citizens were forced to pay exorbitant fees for care. The use of costly procedures and the overprescription of medication eroded the public's trust in doctors and, in some cases, has been linked to medical violence.[13,14] More recent reforms in 1999 improved the overall quality of health services. Strategies were implemented to provide universal insurance, expand the primary healthcare system, introduce pharmaceutical regulations, and institute public hospital reforms. By 2010, 95% of Chinese had healthcare insurance, and, by 2017, universal coverage was achieved in advance of the 2020 goal.[6] Through strategic reforms, China made enormous strides in improving the health of populations. But the health of one group of Chinese lagged behind—migrants.

4 Migration with Chinese Characteristics

One of the key strategies that helped manage population growth in China comes from an ancient household registration system—the *hukou* system. Essentially, there are rural and urban *hukou*, which grant citizens rights to access healthcare, education, and other benefits. This is largely determined by one's parents' birthplace and is difficult to change.

The unintended consequence of this system was to become a key modifiable social determinant of health.[15] The system accounted for unequal health status between rural-to-urban migrants and locals.[16] Rural-to-urban migrant workers were also targets of discrimination and lived in substandard informal housing.[17,18] Migrants are at higher risk of sexually transmitted infections, partly due to poor sexual health literacy.[19] They are also at risk for other infectious diseases like tuberculosis, particularly among those who are living in densely populated urban areas with poor ventilation.

While the *hukou* system remains a key cause of social inequalities, the Chinese government is making progress to remedy this situation. By 2020, 100 million urban *hukou* will be given to migrant workers granting them rights to access "urban residency privileges." However, the chances of acquiring such urban rights is unequally distributed: for cities with a population of more than 5 million, migrants have to fulfill a tough point system based on applicants' education levels and other criteria. Despite the fact that a majority of migrant workers are working in big cities, the tight control of these high-tier cities implies that the majority of migrant workers will still be unable to access local services and privileges in the near future.

Urbanization increased population movement in China, which complicates caring for the elderly. The substantial improvements in life expectancy and the former "one child policy" contribute to population aging in China. A young couple routinely takes care of at least four elders in China. Currently, China is the largest low-fertility country in the world. The fertility dropped from 3.0 births per woman between 1975 and 1980 to 1.63 births per woman between 2015 and 2020. The young generation, especially migrants, face dilemmas between personal development in modern society and caring for aging parents because of the belief in filial piety deeply rooted in Chinese society.

Urbanization, coupled with increased numbers of older adults, led to increases in foreign import labor. Women from across South East Asia migrate to Hong Kong, Macao, and soon, Mainland China, to provide the "emotional labor" of caring for children and elders in addition to household work.[20] These women now number more than 360,000 in both special administrative regions, an increase of 44% in the past 10 years. Recent studies highlighted their difficulties with social integration, poor access to medical care, and heightened risk for mental and physical health issues.[21] A population representative sample of domestic workers showed that fewer than 25% had health insurance.[22]

5 Mental Health: A Critical Yet Neglected Dimension of Health

Another key area of health affected by urbanization is likely the most hidden and neglected within Chinese societies. Common mental disorders like depression and anxiety are often understudied due to stigma and cultural beliefs.[23,24] The general trust people have for one another has eroded over the years, and this is associated with common mental disorders like depression. This was demonstrated in two recent studies in Macao, China, where social capital emerged as a key correlate of depression among the general population and elders.[25,26]

Climate change and natural disasters are another key area of concern for residents living in urban environments. The Wenchuan Earthquake in Southwest China in 2008 led to catastrophic loss of life due in part to population density. On August 23, 2017, Super Typhoon Hato hit Macao and led to 10 deaths and massive economic losses (US$1.42 billion). In the only mental health study conducted following the disaster, a sample of college students reported more than 5% with posttraumatic stress disorder (PTSD).[27]

With increased urbanization, the cost of land increases, and this has effects on vulnerable members of society. For example, among elders who were placed in public housing, the prevalence of depression was greater than 15%. Population density has also soared. In Macao, the population density in 2016 was estimated at 21,340 people per square kilometer, a 15.5% increase compared to 2011.[28] Developing comprehensive mental health services will be critical for continued development.

6 The Great Bay Area and China's New Frontiers

Rapid urbanization may be most obvious in Guangdong Province. Located in south China, the region, once called the Estuary, then the Pearl River Delta, has now transformed itself again. The Guangdong-Hong Kong-Macao Greater Bay Area links cities in an integrated business, economic, and technological hub. It consists of nine cities and two special administrative regions. As of 2016, the population in this region reached 67 million.[29] The longest bridge in the world was built to connect Macao to Hong Kong and Zhuhai and opened in 2018.

The story of rapid urbanization, epidemiological transition, and the rise of population diversity through migration is a story that can be told in many parts of the world. However, as China looks to expand its economic footprint, utilizing the belt and road initiative, the typical notion that "China is for the Chinese" will be challenged.[30] As diverse populations migrate to China, the health of these populations needs to be considered.[31] Efforts made to address the health of populations, improve social cohesion, and increase the quality of life will undoubtedly offer the world examples that can be generalized elsewhere. The graying of populations, now living in urban centers, will necessitate reimagining care structures and provisions to ensure that elders, so important within Chinese culture, are provided the care they need to live a high quality of life. In the post-SARS and more recently post-Zika context, the health of urban populations in China must include enhanced surveillance and rapid response to infectious diseases and potential epidemics, along with enhanced public health infrastructure to complement economic growth and modernity.

7 Conclusion

By 2050, it is projected that China will have added 255 million urban dwellers, which will account for 10% of the projected growth of the world's urban population between 2018 and 2050.[1] Over the past decade, China embarked on the largest health system reform the world has seen and achieved huge domestic successes. In 2016, China ensured that health had become an explicit national political priority with the approval of the "Healthy China 2030" Planning Outline by the central government. The "Healthy China 2030" plan also indicates the political commitment of China to participate in global health in a way that delivers benefits across the world.

References

1. Department of Economic and Social Affairs. *World urbanization prospects: 2018 revision of world urbanization prospects*. New York: United Nations; 2018.
2. China Mohau-rdo. *The 12th Five-Year Plan*. China Architecture and Building Press; 2011.
3. Bureau of Statistics website. The Bureau of Statistics released the 2008 Statistical Report on National Economic and Social Development. 2009.
4. Statistical Communiqué of the People's Republic of China on the 2017 National Economic and Social Development. National Bureau of Statistics of China website. February 28, 2018. Available at http://www.stats.gov.cn/english/pressrelease/201802/t20180228_1585666. html. Accessed June 10, 2018.
5. Wang YH, Li LM. Evaluation of impact of major causes of death on life expectancy changes in China, 1990-2005. *Biomed Environ Sci*. 2009; 22(5):430–441.
6. Yang G, Wang Y, Zeng Y, et al. Rapid health transition in China, 1990–2010: findings from the Global Burden of Disease Study 2010. *Lancet*. 2013; 381(9882):1987–2015.
7. Yu YQ, Xu JJ, Hu QH, et al. High-risk behaviour and HIV infection risk among non-local men who have sex with men with less than a single year's residence in urban centres: a multicentre cross-sectional study from China. *Sex Transm Infect*. 2018; 94(1):51–54.
8. Tong MX, Hansen A, Hanson-Easey S, et al. Infectious diseases, urbanization and climate change: challenges in future China. *Int J Environ Res Public Health*. 2015; 12(9):11025–11036.
9. Wang H, Dwyer-Lindgren L, Lofgren KT, et al. Age-specific and sex-specific mortality in 187 countries, 1970–2010: a systematic analysis for the Global Burden of Disease Study 2010. *Lancet*. 2012; 380(9859):2071–2094.
10. Blumenthal D, Hsiao W. Privatization and its discontents—the evolving Chinese health care system. *N Engl J Med*. 2005; 353:1165–1170.
11. Ramesh M, Wu X, He AJ. Health governance and healthcare reforms in China. *Health Policy Plan*. 2014; 29(6):663–672.
12. Li L, Chen Q, Powers D. Chinese healthcare reform: a shift toward social development. *Modern China*. 2012; 38(6):630–645.
13. Hall BJ, Xiong P, Chang K, Yin M, Sui XR. Prevalence of medical workplace violence and the shortage of secondary and tertiary interventions among healthcare workers in China. *J Epidemiol Community Health*. 2018; 72(6):516–518.
14. Shan L, Li Y, Ding D, et al. Patient satisfaction with hospital inpatient care: effects of trust, medical insurance and perceived quality of care. *PLoS One*. 2016; 11(10):e0164366. doi:10.1371/journal.pone.0164366
15. Hesketh T, Jun YX, Lu L, Mei WH. Health status and access to health care of migrant workers in China. *Public Health Rep*. 2008; 123(2):189–197.
16. Chen W, Zhang Q, Renzaho AMN, Zhou F, Zhang H, Ling L. Social health insurance coverage and financial protection among rural-to-urban internal migrants in China: evidence from a nationally representative cross-sectional study. *BMJ Glob Health*. 2017;2(4):e000477. doi:10.1136/bmjgh-2017-000477
17. Wang B, Li X, Stanton B, Fang X. The influence of social stigma and discriminatory experience on psychological distress and quality of life among rural-to-urban migrants in China. *Soc Sci Med*. 2010; 71(1):84–92.
18. Huang Y, Tao R. Housing migrants in Chinese cities: current status and policy design. *Environ Plan C: Government and Policy*. 2015; 33(3):640–660.

19. Chen W, Zhou F, Hall BJ, et al. Spatial distribution and cluster analysis of risky sexual behaviours and STDs reported by Chinese adults in Guangzhou, China: a representative population-based study. *Sex Transm Infect.* 2016; 92(4):316–322.
20. Remitio R. 300,000 jobs in China available for Filipino workers. CNN Phillipines website. February 8, 2018. Available at http://cnnphilippines.com/news/2018/01/28/dole-jobs-ofws-china.html. Accessed June 10, 2018.
21. Hall B, Garabiles M, Latkin C. Filipino domestic workers in China: a qualitative needs assessment. Under review.
22. Hall B. Discrimination modifies the effect of cumulative adversities on PTSD symptom severity among Filipino Domestic Workers in China. Presented at International Society of Traumatic Stress Studies, on November 8, 2017, Chicago, IL.
23. Yang LH. Application of mental illness stigma theory to Chinese societies: synthesis and new directions. *Singapore Med J.* 2007; 48(11):977–985.
24. Hall B, Chang K, Chen W, Sou K-L, Latkin C, Yeung A. Exploring the association between depression and shenjing shuairuo in a population representative epidemiological study of Chinese adults in Guangzhou, China. *Transcult Psychiatry.* 2018. doi:10.1177/1363461518778670.
25. Hall BJ, Lam AIF, Wu TL, Hou WK, Latkin C, Galea S. The epidemiology of current depression in Macau, China: towards a plan for mental health action. *Soc Psychiatry Psychiatr Epidemiol.* 2017; 52(10):1227–1235.
26. Wu TL, Hall Bj Fau-Canham SL, Canham Sl Fau-Lam AIF, Lam AI. The association between social capital and depression among Chinese older adults living in public housing. *J Nerv Ment Dis.* 2016; 204(10):764–769.
27. Hall BJ, Xiong Y, Yip PSY, Lao C, Shi W, Sou EKL, Chang K, Wang L, & Lam AIF (in press). The association between disaster exposure and media use on posttraumatic stress disorder following Typhoon Hato in Macao, China. *European Journal of Psychotraumatology.*
28. Statistics and Census Service. Detailed Results of 2016 Macau Population By-Census. 2016. https://www.dsec.gov.mo/getAttachment/e20c6bab-ada4-4f83-9349-e72605674a42/E_ICEN_PUB_2016_Y.aspx
29. Editors. Fast facts of the Guangdong-Hong Kong-Macau Bay Area. *Fung Business Intelligence.* 2017(12).
30. Tang K, Li Z, Li W, Chen L. China's Silk Road and global health. *Lancet.* 2017; 390(10112):2595–2601.
31. Hall BJ, Chen W, Latkin C, Ling L, Tucker JD. Africans in south China face social and health barriers. *Lancet.* 2014; 383(9925):1291–1292.

39

Regional Planning for Health

DAVID SISCOVICK, MANDU SEN, AND CHRIS JONES

1 Introduction

New York City (NYC) is one of the world's largest and most diverse metropolitan areas; it has also been a leader in thinking about how to promote health by improving the physical structures, social conditions, and natural environment around us. NYC has the oldest and largest Department of Public Health and Mental Hygiene (DOHMH), and it is home to multiple world-class academic institutions and healthcare systems. NYC is also the home of an independent, nonprofit, civic institution, the Regional Plan Association (RPA), that has worked to improve the prosperity, sustainability, and quality of life in the NYC metropolitan region for the past 90 years. In this case study, we tell the story of how the RPA reconnected health and equity with planning in the Fourth Regional Plan for Metropolitan New York. We then discuss the strengths and limitations, the lessons learned, and the challenges related to implementation of the Plan. The Fourth Regional Plan was developed over the course of 5 years and released on November 30, 2017. It provides a model for integrating health and equity into planning in large metropolitan regions nationally.

1.1 The New York Metropolitan Region

Large metropolitan regions offer unique opportunities and major challenges for planning. Metropolitan New York includes a tri-state area stretching from New Haven, Connecticut, to Trenton, New Jersey. The region includes urban, suburban, and rural areas; 783 municipalities (one of the municipalities is New York City); and 23 million people, and it accounts for 10% of the US economy. The tri-state region includes common physical, social, and natural environments. The region shares the most extensive transit system in the United States, a lack of affordable and quality housing, and a legacy of residential segregation. Its coastline covers 3,700 miles and wetlands are common across the region.

1.2 The Regional Plan Association

Given that no single government is charged with planning for the tri-state region, the RPA, a nongovernmental organization, has been the de facto regional planning organization for metropolitan New York since the 1920s. RPA is a source of ideas and plans for policymakers across the region. RPA has produced four plans to guide the region's growth: the plans identify major challenges facing the region and propose forward-looking solutions. RPA conducts research, planning, advocacy, and public engagement. Some of the region's most significant public works, economic development, and open space projects have their roots in RPA initiatives.

In the 1920s, the first regional plan for metropolitan NYC addressed the opportunities associated with the increasing use of automobiles; in the 1960s, the second plan addressed the challenge of urban flight to the suburbs; and, in the 1990s, the third plan reimagined the role of transit in the region. The decision by the RPA to launch the most recent regional plan came about in part because of the continued lack of investment in aging infrastructure in the region, the unequal economic recovery following the financial crisis of 2008, and the ravages to the metropolitan NYC region of Superstorm Sandy in 2012. The plans have no formal standing but gain their power from the depth of the research and outreach conducted by RPA. While RPA's plans seek to benefit all residents, especially those who are most vulnerable, the main audience for the plan are decision-makers at all levels of government. In between plans, RPA works as an advocate to implement the recommendations in their plans and promote good planning practice across the region.

With the goal of transforming the region, the Fourth Regional Plan sought evidence-based solutions to four major regional challenges: governance, affordability, transportation, and climate change.[1] It was developed by RPA staff with input from hundreds of residents, public and private sector leaders, and advocates from multiple sectors. It laid out a vision for the region over the next 25 years, and it included specific recommendations and indicated what would be required to implement those recommendations. For the first time in its history, the Plan included health as an explicit focus.[2] Equity was a theme in RPA's third plan in the 1990s, but it was more systematically embedded within the Fourth Plan's analysis and recommendations. Together with prosperity and sustainability, health and equity were identified as intrinsic values that shaped the Plan. How did this expanded focus happen?

2 Social Determinants of Health

The social determinants of health (SDOH), defined by the World Health Organization as "the conditions in which people are born, grow, work, live, age, and the wider set of forces and systems shaping the conditions of daily life," are responsible for health inequalities.[3] There is mounting evidence related to the consequences of the SDOH on physical, mental, and behavioral health. For this reason, the health impact of regional planning needs to be considered across multiple sectors. For this to occur, health professionals need to work with urban planners, policymakers, engineers, architects, and other disciplines; communities need to be actively engaged; and the public and private sectors need to collaborate on the development and implementation of solutions focused on the SDOH.

2.1 The Culture of Health Model

The *culture of health* (COH) model, developed by the Robert Wood Johnson Foundation (RWJF), seeks to address the social determinants of health through multisectoral community-based efforts. It is intended to identify priorities for taking action and driving change. It requires communities, organizations, and individuals to work together to develop scalable solutions and to take targeted actions. Given this commitment, RWJF awarded grant funding to the RPA to integrate health and equity into the Fourth Regional Plan for Metropolitan New York.

3 RPA Technical Advisory Committee on Health

The RPA formed a Technical Advisory Committee on Health to obtain input from outside consultants. The Committee included experts in population health, community engagement, health policy, urban planning, and economic development from the New York Academy of Medicine. The Committee also included experts in social epidemiology, chronic disease epidemiology, environmental health, climate change, and health services research from academic institutions and government agencies from the tri-state region. NYC DOHMH staff were also members of the Technical Advisory Committee.

3.1 The Problem

With the support of the Technical Advisory Committee on Health, RPA drafted a report, *State of the Region's Health*, with a focus on the health needs of the region and their root (upstream) causes. The report highlighted the lack of health equity in the region, due at least in part to poverty; lack of affordable and healthy housing; lack of access to transportation; environmental hazards; and low health literacy. The report identified common conditions related to these root causes, such as asthma, diabetes, obesity, cardiovascular disease, mental and behavioral health, and well-being. It noted the large inequalities in health, for example, across contiguous neighborhoods in NYC, counties in northern New Jersey, and towns in Connecticut.

In response, the RPA adopted the following vision in the Fourth Regional Plan: "Everyone deserves the opportunity to live the healthiest life possible regardless of who they are or where they live." The RPA identified what would be required to reduce the overall burden of suffering in the region while promoting health equity. The RPA conducted hundreds of small meetings, roundtables, and an annual large assembly where input was solicited from various stakeholders. Key informant and stakeholder input complemented the expertise of RPA staff and it was used in the development of white papers related to the core areas of regional planning, such as transportation, housing, displacement due to gentrification, and rising sea levels due to climate change.

RPA staff met with experts in community engagement, evidence-based policy, and governance to address the process of decision-making at the local and regional levels. The RPA systematically listened to community voices across the tri-state region around these and other issues, such as community planning and design, land use and zoning, and affordable and healthy housing. The broad input on these issues is reflected in the recommendations incorporated into the Fourth Regional Plan. There was vigorous debate on plan recommendations, and the inclusion of both community groups and the health advisory committee helped to expand the reach of the recommendations. For example, the housing section included a focus on both affordable and healthy housing, and the RPA embraced civic engagement as core to its governance reforms.

4 Integrating Health into the Fourth Regional Plan

The Fourth Regional Plan adopted four values—prosperity, sustainability, equity, and health—to guide its development. The Plan includes 61 recommendations; their potential impact on the four values was rated high, medium, or low. In the introductory sections, the definition and rationale for the focus on each of the four guiding values were addressed. Of note, the impact of the recommendations on health and equity was considered throughout the Plan. As a result, the Plan sought to make the New York Metropolitan Region "an easier, healthier, and more affordable place to live and work."[1]

4.1 Health Equity

In the New York metropolitan region, residents commonly live in segregated neighborhoods. As a result, low-income residents and people of color are far less likely to have access to the resources needed to live healthy lives. As stated in the Plan, "The Fourth Regional Plan provides a roadmap to address health inequities rooted in the built environment and create a healthier future for all."[1] It argues that planning decisions should not prioritize efficiency over health and well-being. The Plan noted the need to make different investments and policy decisions to improve health outcomes in marginalized communities.

4.2 Infrastructure

The Plan also noted that the long-term neglect of critical infrastructure related to transportation had resulted in both daily inconveniences that impact commute time (and cause related stress) and the potential for major transit disasters/disruptions that would impact the economy of the US Northeast Corridor. The multiple existing governing bodies related to transit in the region, many established more than 50 years ago when the challenges to the region differed, had "failed to make the hard choices necessary to address these most intractable problems."[1,4] Additionally, despite the lessons learned from Superstorm Sandy, the coastal region of the tri-state area was not prepared for the next big storm and rising sea levels.

4.3 Reform Institutions to Incorporate Health into Decision-Making

The Plan suggests institutional reform to incorporate health into decision-making. Regional, state, and local agencies would need to embrace the concept of Health in All Policies (HiAP). To achieve this goal, transit, housing, and other agencies would need to create a new leadership position, a Chief Health Officer (CHO), within their agencies.

The CHO would assure that health effects were considered fully when evaluating various funding priorities of the agency. A newly created Regional Coastal Commission would integrate considerations of health impact into funding decisions that address the consequences of superstorms and rising sea levels. Local planning processes would be more inclusive, predictable, and efficient, and they would include health impact assessments (HIAs), when appropriate, as part of master planning. Data-driven planning would focus, for example, on street redesigns in low-income communities to improve health.

4.4 Rebuild and Expand the Transportation Network to Serve Everyone

The Plan addresses the need for fast and reliable public transportation, such as subway, light rail, and bus service, that works better for all, connects more low-income communities with jobs and other opportunities, and reduces traffic congestion. Six million people ride the subways daily in NYC, and the use of shields (a physical barrier) would reduce exposure to noise, air pollution, heat stress, and risk of serious life-threatening injury. Subway stations would be rebuilt so they are healthier and accessible to families and people with disabilities. Light rail service that is integrated with other transportation options would better connect people across the outer boroughs of NYC (the Bronx, Queens, and Brooklyn) with employment opportunities and reduce commute time. Safe streets and more walkable communities would also be goals of regional transportation initiatives. Reducing near-road exposure to diesel exhaust by burying or decking over highways that have disrupted communities of color has the potential to improve air quality, and it also would increase green space and walkability in low-income communities.

4.5 Create Affordable and Healthy Communities

More jobs, healthy and affordable housing, public spaces, and access to healthy food and services are critical to creating healthy communities, and healthy communities make living a healthier life an easier choice for all. Additionally, local land-use and zoning policies need to be designed to ensure that growth benefits existing residents, including low-income and communities of color, because low-income residents in areas at risk for gentrification need to be protected from displacement. Recommendations in the Plan address each of these issues.

4.6 Meet the Challenge of Climate Change by Creating a Healthier Environment

Extreme heat, flooding, displacement, and loss of property and life are potential consequences of climate change. The Plan suggests that now is the time to take action to mitigate the impact of climate change. Other recommendations focus on the electrical grid, carbon emissions, and energy sources; cleaner air and water, strategies to protect coastal communities from storms and flooding; mitigation of the urban heat island effect; and connecting open spaces in the region.

5 Comment

The New York metropolitan region is characterized by density, diversity, and complexity. Health needs are likely to vary across communities, defined by the SDOH and the life cycle (women of reproductive age, pregnant women, children, adolescents, and young, middle-aged, and older adults). However, health needs share common social determinants. For subsets of the population, the nature and timing of the health impacts of various solutions are likely to differ. If nothing else, the Plan shines a light on the reality that a healthier future for all must address the lack of social and health equity rooted in the physical, social, and natural environments.

The Fourth Regional Plan for Metropolitan New York has articulated a compelling approach that reconnects health and equity with planning. It has identified the problems and recommended solutions for the region that would impact prosperity, sustainability, equity, and health. If realized, it would transform the region. Based on the experience of the Fourth Regional Plan, it is clear that communities want to be engaged in this process. On the other hand, whether reconnecting regional planning with equity and health will increase the likelihood that the aspirational recommendations in the Plan are implemented remains to be determined.

Comparative cost-effectiveness analyses and/or HIAs might help us to understand better the value of different long-term investments and frame health and equity in terms of prosperity and sustainability. Whether these assessments will help to build the broad consensus needed to take action and drive change is unclear. The broader society, both the public and private sectors, will need to value health and equity as it does prosperity and sustainability, given the commitment of capital needed to implement many of the recommendations.

6 Conclusion

The Fourth Regional Plan reconnected regional planning with health and equity. Health and equity were values that were reflected in many of the 61 recommendations included in the 374-page plan. Taken as a whole, the Plan is a blueprint for a better social, physical, and natural environment. If implemented, it has the potential to impact health and equity not only over the next generation but over the next 100 years. For the Plan to be realized, however, regional and local planning, policies, and decisions need to align resources with the four values—prosperity, sustainability, equity, and health—that motivated the recommendations in the Plan. Implementation of the recommendations is now the priority of the RPA. While implementation will present enormous political, economic, and social challenges, the blueprint offered in the RPA Fourth Regional Plan for Metropolitan New York has the potential to impact health and equity in the region and beyond.

Acknowledgments

Dr. Siscovick was a member of the RPA Committee for the Fourth Regional Plan, the Community Planning and Design Committee, and the Technical Advisory Committee on Health. He currently is a member of the RPA Committee on New York. The co-authors are RPA senior staff.

References

1. Regional Plan Association. *The Fourth Regional Plan: making the region work for all of us.* Regional Plan Association website. Published November 30, 2017. Available at http://fourthplan.org/. Accessed April 1, 2018.
2. Regional Plan Association. *The Fourth Regional Plan: health.* Regional Plan Association website. Published November 30, 2017. Available at http://fourthplan.org/values/health. Accessed April 1, 2018.
3. World Health Organization. *Social determinants of health.* World Health Organization website. 2018. Available at www.who.int/social_determinants. Accessed November 2, 2017.
4. Sen M. *State of the region's health: how the New York metropolitan region's urban systems influence health.* Regional Plan Association website. Published July 11, 2016. Updated November 30, 2017. Available at http://fourthplan.org/reports/state-of-the-regions-health. Accessed April 1, 2018.

40

Going Biophilic

Living and Working in Biophilic Buildings

JIE YIN AND JOHN D. SPENGLER

1 Biophilia, Biophilic Design, and Health: Why It Matters

1.1 Nature Contact and Human Health

The rapid trend toward global urbanization, resulting in more than half of the world's population living in cities, is associated with decreased access to natural environments. Additionally, the industrialized world spends up to 90% of its time inside buildings, further distancing people from nature. This urban living is associated with increased stress-related diseases.[1] One factor contributing to this increase may be the routine separation of humans from contact with nature when indoors. Research in recent decades has yielded substantial evidence that exposure to nature is associated with positive impacts on human health and well-being.[2] Specifically, epidemiological studies provided population-level evidence that greater exposure to greenness is associated with reduced absenteeism in schools; improved student academic performance; increased physical activity; improved mental health, brain development, and cognitive function; higher birth weights; and lower mortality rates.[3-7] In addition, experimental studies showed positive effects of contact with nature on stress reduction, improvement of cognition and affect, enhanced immune function, and increased parasympathetic and lower sympathetic nerve activity.[8-11] However, because most of the previous studies were conducted in outdoor spaces, the potential for similar health benefits of incorporating natural elements indoors remains unclear. To address this gap, we review current theories, tools, and research opportunities in this chapter.

1.2 Biophilia: Hypothesis and Theories

Biophilia, defined as "love of life or living systems," was introduced within the context of preserving life and fighting against death by psychoanalyst and social philosopher Erich Fromme in 1964.[12] The concept was later popularized by Harvard biologist

E. O. Wilson in 1984, who suggested that human beings, from an evolutionary biology perspective, have an inherent affinity for the natural world.[13] This biophilia hypothesis has since been supported by two complementary theories: *Stress Recovery Theory* (SRT) and *Attention Restoration Theory* (ART). SRT explored the physiological impacts of contact with nature on stress reduction, indicating that natural elements could activate our parasympathetic nervous system and lead to decreased heart rate, blood pressure, skin conductance, and salivary cortisol levels.[14] These responses could induce relaxation and help to reduce stress and autonomic arousal. ART explained how the experience of nature influences cognition, suggesting that natural environments could invoke involuntary attention in people.[15] This attentional recovery could in turn have restorative effects on the mental fatigue caused by overstimulation from the urban environment and thus improve people's cognitive performance that requires direct attention.

2 Biophilic Design and Well-Being: Evidence and Practice

2.1 Design Attributes and Health Benefits

Stephen Kellert initiated biophilic design to incorporate natural features and systems into indoor environments.[16] To operationalize and promote the adoption of biophilic design, he developed six elements (environmental features, natural shapes and forms, natural patterns and processes, light and space, place-based relationships, evolved human–nature relationships) and 72 attributes of biophilic design.[15] Ryan et al. summarized these attributes into three categories (nature in the space, natural analogues, and nature of the space) and 14 patterns, prioritizing the most prominent nature–health relationships in the built environment and providing a framework to study their health impacts more directly.[17]

Specific aspects of the physiological and psychological benefits of biophilic design elements in buildings have been studied.[18] For example, indoor plants have demonstrated benefits for stress reduction and pain tolerance, as well as producing increased emotional satisfaction and productivity.[19] Viewing nature through a window has also been shown to have beneficial effects in the hospital setting, including reducing recovery times and reliance on pain medication.[20] In addition, having natural views through windows could also increase productivity, decrease sick days, and decrease absenteeism in office settings.[18] Natural light has known benefits for circadian rhythm and sleep quality, and it can boost cognitive attention and memory, which could increase worker productivity.[18] The use of interior wooden materials has been found to have similar biorestorative effects on the autonomic, respiratory, and visual systems and contributes to a decrease in tension and fatigue and an increase of positive emotions and comfort.[21] Last, natural analogues (e.g., a mural of a natural scene) in a patient's room or other healthcare space can help to reduce stress levels and relieve pain.[16] Interestingly, while the health benefits of individual design attributes have been studied, there is limited research examining the impact on health and well-being when multiple design attributes are combined.

2.2 From Green Building to Healthy Building: Role of Biophilia

Green building design has been broadly accepted as an approach to minimize the detrimental impacts to the environment through reductions in both energy and water usage. However, the impact of improved indoor environmental quality on population health in green buildings has only recently been investigated.[22] Evidence from nine foundational environmental elements has demonstrated how buildings affect human health.[23] Previously, most research on the health impact of green building focused on negative factors, including poor indoor air quality, inadequate ventilation, uncomfortable thermal conditions, extensive artificial lighting, mold, dust and pests, and materials made of toxic chemical substances. These factors are commonly associated with various symptoms identified as "sick building syndrome." Biophilic design dovetails with the green building movement to provide specific building design strategies. Inclusion of natural elements indoors are considered positive attributes encompassing views to nature, natural ventilation and daylight, access to green plants and water features, and the use of natural materials and biomorphic forms for indoor elements.

The increasing evidence for health benefits from nature-inspired spaces has given rise to building rating systems like the WELL building standard and Living Building Challenge (LBC), both of which highlight biophilia as an important component of their standards.[24,25] Specifically, the WELL standard examines biophilia qualitatively in terms of nature and pattern incorporation and natural interaction. Moreover, it sets up some quantitative indicators of coverage and accessibility to outdoor greenery, percentage of wall and potted plants in indoor spaces, and water features.[24] LBC requires the design team to have a 1-day exploration of potential biophilic features, as proposed by Kellert, to provide a biophilic framework and plan early in the design process. It also requires that goals be tracked during and after construction to ensure they are met.[16,25]

3 New Approaches to Quantify the Health Impact of Biophilic Indoor Environments

Although the health benefits of biophilic design have been part of the green building conversation, they are not easily quantified in comparison to energy and water consumption. Here, we propose several research approaches to generate more evidence about how biophilic design could affect population health.

3.1 Biophilic Exposure Simulation and Assessment

Modern advancements in virtual reality (VR) technology provide an opportunity to replicate and customize visual environmental exposures through an immersive experience that is more effective than photographs or panoramas.[26] *Eye tracking*, a sensor technology that measures eye positions and movement, has been integrated into VR goggles to measure attention to specific elements in simulated environments. Specific elements within the visual field that hold attention can be identified and, with other sensors of physiologic responses (e.g., electroencephalography, heart rate variability, skin conductance, blood pressure), help to identify positive or negative responses. Doing these experiments with VR offers the advantage of testing many more participants across many standardized visual fields. A pilot study indicated that participants could gain similar acute physiological and cognitive benefits via exposure to virtual biophilic indoor environments as compared to real ones.[27] This suggests that VR might have the potential to reduce stress and improve cognitive function by providing exposures to natural elements in a variety of indoor settings where access to nature may not be possible, as in places where patients are treated for posttraumatic stress disorder (PTSD), pain, and palliative care. However, more evidence is needed to detect differences between virtual exposures versus the real environment since the experience of nature is multisensory.[28] Another challenge to coherent findings is the specification of the biophilic exposure in different indoor settings. To address this issue, a tool has been developed to allow observers to rate indoor environments based on their biophilic qualities.[27] This tool, the Biophilic Interior Design Index (BIDI), was developed using the 14 patterns of biophilic design [17] and centers around a questionnaire asking participants to rate their perceptions of biophilic features such as plants, water, air flow, light, materials, biomorphic patterns, and long-distance view; responses to these questions are used to calculate a space's score.

3.2 Objective Outcome Measures

With increasingly affordable, comfortable, and accurate wearable biomonitoring sensors, researchers will be able improve data collection of objective physiological measurements. Many studies have used noninvasive biomonitoring sensors to measure acute physiological markers including heart rate, heart rate variability, skin conductance level, and blood pressure to estimate nervous system arousal and assess autonomic function and short-term stress responses to stimuli. Electroencephalography (EEG) could objectively measure the potential connection between the biophilic environmental exposure and changes in brain activity in real time. Combining VR and wearable biomonitoring sensors makes it possible to quantify subjects' acute physiological responses to many simulated biophilic-enhanced indoor spaces.[27]

3.3 Longitudinal Study Design

To date, most experimental studies have only tested acute effects of biophilic exposure on health outcomes. Longitudinal cohort studies at the building level, such as the Harvard Global Buildings COGfx study in the United States, the Biophilic Site Offices study in Australia, and the BRE Biophilic Office project in the United Kingdom, are needed to test the chronic health impacts of long-term indoor biophilic exposures.[29]

4 Conclusion

In this chapter, we presented the development of biophilic design and its application in buildings, but more evidence regarding the health benefits of bringing natural elements indoorsis needed. Emerging technologies like VR, eye tracking, and wearable biomonitoring sensors could provide a powerful way for designers and public health professionals to quantify human responses—both physiological and cognitive, short-term and long-term—to biophilic buildings.

Beyond the building level, however, the larger challenge facing us is the threat posed by the egregious losses in our ecosystem. "The extinction of our swimming, trotting, slithering, and flying companions on Earth is a building global disaster on a par with climate change, but one that has a solution," according to E. O. Wilson, who believes that "setting aside half of the Earth's land and half of its oceans would be enough to save 85% of species, which are becoming extinct at a rate between 100 and 1,000 times the rate before humans."[30] We need to address how to change the collective consciousness to truly value nature. Testing for the short-term benefits of being surrounded by plants or having a park view from our office window is a beginning for urban dwellers; now we propose to extend our quest to discover the "biophilic phenotype" and the formative experiences that translate into a reverence for all living species.

References

1. Florian L, Peter K, Leila H, et al. City living and urban upbringing affect neural social stress processing in humans. *Nature.* 2011; 474(7352):498.
2. Frumkin H, Bratman GN, Breslow SJ, et al. Nature contact and human health: a research agenda. *Environ Health Perspect.* 2017; 125(7):75001.
3. MacNaughton P, Eitland E, Kloog I, Schwartz J, Allen J. Impact of particulate matter exposure and surrounding "greenness" on chronic absenteeism in Massachusetts public schools. *Int J Environ Res Public Health.* 2017; 14(2). doi:10.3390/ijerph14020207
4. Wu CD, McNeely E, Cedeno-Laurent JG, et al. Linking student performance in Massachusetts elementary schools with the "greenness" of school surroundings using remote sensing. *PLoS One.* 2014; 9(10):e108548. doi:10.1371/journal.pone.0108548
5. Dadvand P, Pujol J, Macia D, et al. The association between lifelong greenspace exposure and 3-dimensional brain magnetic resonance imaging in Barcelona schoolchildren. *Environ Health Perspect.* 2018; 126(2):027012.
6. James P, Banay RF, Hart JE, Laden F. A review of the health benefits of greenness. *Curr Epidemiol Rep.* 2015; 2(2):131–142.
7. Fong K, Hart J, James P. A review of epidemiologic studies on greenness and health: updated literature through 2017. *Curr Environ Health Rep.* 2018; 5(1):77–87.
8. Berto R. The role of nature in coping with psycho-physiological stress: a literature review on restorativeness. *Behav Sci (Basel).* 2014; 4(4):394–409.
9. Bratman GN, Daily GC, Levy BJ, Gross JJ. The benefits of nature experience: Improved affect and cognition. *Landsc Urban Plan.* 2015; 138:41–50.
10. Ming E. How might contact with nature promote human health? Exploring promising mechanisms and a possible central pathway. *Front Psychol.* 2015; 6:1093.
11. Park B, Tsunetsugu Y, Kasetani T, Kagawa T, Miyazaki Y. The physiological effects of Shinrin-yoku (taking in the forest atmosphere or forest bathing): evidence from field experiments in 24 forests across Japan. *Environ Health Prev Med.* 2010; 15(1):18–26.
12. Formm E. *The heart of man: its genius for good and evil.* New York: Harper & Row; 1964.
13. Wilson EO. *Biophilia.* Cambridge, MA: Harvard University Press; 1984.
14. Ulrich R. Stress recovery during exposure to natural and urban environments. *J Environ Psychol.* 1991; 11:201–230.

15. Kaplan S. The restorative benefits of nature: toward an integrative framework. *J Environ Psychol*. 1995; 15(3):169–182.

16. Kellert SR, Heerwagen J, Mador M, eds. *Biophilic design: the theory, science, and practice of bringing buildings to life*. Hoboken, NJ: John Wiley & Sons; 2008.

17. Ryan C, Browning W, Clancy J, Andrews S, Kallianpurkar N. Biophilic design patterns: emerging nature-based parameters for health and well-being in the built environment. *International Journal of Architectural Research*. 2014; 8(2):62–76.

18. Kaitlyn G, Birgitta G. A review of psychological literature on the health and well-being benefits of biophilic design. *Buildings*. 2015; 5(3):948–963.

19. Bringslimark T, Hartig T, Patil GG. The psychological benefits of indoor plants: A critical review of the experimental literature. *J Environ Psychol*. 2009; 29(4):422–433.

20. Ulrich RS. View through a Window May Influence Recovery from Surgery. *Science*. 1984; 224(4647):420–421.

21. Zhang X, Lian Z, Wu Y. Human physiological responses to wooden indoor environment. *Physiology & Behavior*. 2017; 174:27–34.

22. Allen J, MacNaughton P, Laurent J, Flanigan S, Eitland E, Spengler J. Green buildings and health. *Curr Environ Health Rep*. 2015; 2(3):250–258.

23. Cedeño-Laurent JG, Williams A, Macnaughton P, et al. Building evidence for health: green buildings, current science, and future challenges. *Annu Rev Public Health*. 2018; 39:291–308.

24. The WELL Building Standard: V1 with Q1 2018 addenda. International WELL Building Institute website. 2018. Available at https://www.wellcertified.com/en/resources/well-building-standard-english. Accessed September 15, 2018.

25. International Living Future Institute. *Living Building Challenge 3.0*. Seatte, WA: International Living Future Institute; 2014.

26. Higuera-Trujillo JL, López-Tarruella Maldonado J, Llinares Millán C. Psychological and physiological human responses to simulated and real environments: a comparison between photographs, 360° panoramas, and virtual reality. *Appl Ergon*. 2017; 65:398–409.

27. Yin J, Zhu S, Macnaughton P, Allen JG, Spengler JD. Physiological and cognitive performance of exposure to biophilic indoor environment. *Building and Environment*. 2018; 132:255–262.

28. Kellert SR. *Nature by design: the practice of biophilic design*. New Haven, CT: Yale University Press; 2018.

29. Gray T, Birrell C. Are biophilic-designed site office buildings linked to health benefits and high performing occupants? *Int J Environ Res Public Health*. 2014; 11(12):12204.

30. Powell A. A "moon shot" to protect Earth's species. *The Harvard Gazette*. March 29, 2018. Available at https://news.harvard.edu/gazette/story/2018/03/biologist-e-o-wilson-suggests-moon-shot-conservation-effort/. Accessed May 22, 2018.

THE FUTURE OF CITIES, THE FUTURE OF HEALTH

41

City Health Departments

Leading Urban Public Health Practice

DANIEL KASS, THOMAS MATTE, AND ADAM KARPATI

1 Introduction

The United Nations' New Urban Agenda reenvisioned the nature of urban develop-ment to ensure that "all facets of sustainable development to promote equity, welfare and share prosperity."[1] Elsewhere in this book, authors have made the case for why a multisectoral approach is necessary to address the leading determinants of health and why demographic trends compel a focus on cities. In cities, opportunities exist to influ-ence advances in healthcare, food systems, housing, transport, and the social, physical, and built environments to promote equity, well-being, and health.

The role of government in advancing the welfare of the public has been vari-ously described. In the United States, its role in health promotion is to some extent constrained by liberal economic theory: that government exists to intervene in an imperfect economic market by regulating externalities, promoting public goods, and correcting asymmetric information.[2] But the speed of urban development, the rapidity and distributed nature of decision-making, and the complexity of governance is leading to a call for a shift in the urban governance paradigm.[3,4] For cities to accommodate population increases and ameliorate existing conditions, they must seek greater local authority to act and regulate, decentralize power and revenue control from state and na-tional governments, build stronger relationships among governmental sectors and civil society, and build technical and political capacity.

In this chapter, we address a critical mechanism by which public health as a sector must engage with these changes via local public health governance. We identify challenges and constraints and offer recommendations for going forward.

2 Emerging Challenges and Opportunities for Urban Public Health

Cities can become places that either amplify or reduce the health risks and disparities of city living that accompany economic development and the epidemiologic transition from communicable to noncommunicable diseases (NCDs) as the primary drivers of illness and death. For example, urbanization appears to be playing a role in improving access to improved water sources and reducing risks from waterborne communicable diseases, yet trends in air quality will, without intervention, expose more people to more pollution.[5] As cities grow in size, complexity, and influence, urbanization creates challenges and opportunities for advancing public and planetary health. Three examples are highlighted here to illustrate the impact of cities on health: air pollution, urban planning and transportation approaches to climate action, and social determinants of health.

2.1 Air Pollution

Air pollution causes more than 6 million deaths globally. In many rapidly growing cities in low- and middle-income countries, growing emissions from "modern sources" like motor vehicles and electric power generation are added to pollution from "traditional sources," like the use of coal, charcoal, or wood for cooking or heating, and trash burning. Among cities with pollution monitoring data reported to World Health Organization (WHO), more than 9 in 10 have levels of particulate matter ($PM_{2.5}$; the best indicator of air pollution health risks) that exceed the WHO guidance level.[6]

Reducing air pollution in cities requires national actions to address regional pollution sources, energy policies, and vehicle standards. But cities are key venues for strengthening the health sector response to the global air pollution crisis. Using available evidence, data, and methods analogous to those used in the Global Burden of Disease project, local estimates of air pollution disease burdens can be developed and disseminated to raise awareness to build public support and pressure for clean air measures.

2.2 Built Environment

Regular physical activity, sustained over long periods of time, reduces the risk of a wide range of chronic health conditions, including obesity, diabetes, cardiovascular disease, hypertension, cancer, osteoporosis, depression, and dementia.[7] A large body of evidence indicates that urban form and built environments—products of local governmental decision-making—can promote physical activity as part of routine travel ("active transportation") or for purposeful exercise ("active recreation"). Activity-supporting physical environment features include compact development, housing density, public transit access, mixed land use, and access to open space, all of which are within the purview of local authority.[8]

2.3 Social Determinants

Urbanization has the potential to affect health via influences on social determinants of health. Globally, poverty rates are lower for urban than for rural residents, but while migration to urban slums in some cities is associated with improvements in economic opportunity, in others it increases poverty and its resultant threats to well-being.[9,10]

The global growth of urban sprawl and private vehicle–dependent transportation systems could further exacerbate disparities by hindering access to employment opportunities.[11] Urban-based workforce and development strategies are critical to addressing economic inequalities.

With this context of how cities' characteristics drive population health and illness, we turn our focus to urban public health governance and its potential to influence and shape these features. We use examples primarily from the United States, but the principles are relevant to city governments in both high- and low-resource settings.

3 Features of City Health Departments

City governments were drivers of public health practice in many US states in the nineteenth and early twentieth centuries. Typical functions focused on the control of infectious diseases and provision of clinical and supportive services for vulnerable populations. To the extent that these issues were associated with urban squalor and density, and given the limitations of scientific knowledge, they entailed engaging broadly around sanitation, housing, urban design, safety net systems, and other social/environmental issues relevant at the urban level.[12] However, trends in the late twentieth century drew urban health departments away from these traditional domains of focus. City health departments, though ill-equipped, were faced with adapting to shifts in the drivers of morbidity and mortality toward NCDs and to increased public health emphasis on behavioral determinants of risk. Moreover, emerging specialized disciplines, including transportation planning, air quality management, housing design and maintenance, and water management and security, separated these disciplines from general public health practice.

Contemporary city public health agencies are extremely varied in their size and mandates. In the United States, the National Association of County and City Health Officials conducts periodic surveys of local health departments that document these features.[13] The largest city health departments, which serve cities of more than 1,000,000 people, may employ hundreds to thousands of employees and are engaged in a wide variety of activities including population health promotion, clinical services, emergency response, epidemiology and surveillance, environmental health services, and policy advocacy.[14] Some large city health authorities, such as in Los Angeles, also oversee and manage the city's entire public healthcare system, though most are distinct public health organizations with limited and focused clinical services (e.g., infectious diseases, immunizations, school health, and correctional health). In general, cities' mandates for public health practice align with the essential public health services articulated by the Institute of Medicine or WHO.[15]

In the United States, city health departments are a subset of the broader group of agencies known as "local" health departments (which often correspond to county jurisdictions). All local health departments maintain funding, coordination, and communication relationships with their state counterparts. Depending on their size and degree of local investment, city health departments rely to a greater or lesser degree on their state agencies for guidance, direction, resources, and authority.

Financial resources for city health departments typically flow from their states, which in turn receive funds from national agencies like the US Centers for Disease Control and Prevention (CDC). In some larger cities, the CDC provides funds directly to local government, although the CDC's primary relationship is most often with states, and a minority of the CDC's funding flows directly to cities.[16] The CDC's direct funding to local governments tends to be for infectious disease control, such as for tuberculosis, sexually transmitted diseases (STDs), immunizations, and HIV/AIDS, and for some environmental health issues, such as lead poisoning prevention and vector control. Nationwide resources for NCDs or injury prevention are scarce and rarely extend to all states (the most recent increase in drug overdose mortality is an exception, and federal funds are now flowing to state and local agencies). Resources for mental illnesses, substance-using populations, and developmental delays and disabilities are directed primarily to states. Non-federal—local and state—tax levy funds are provided to health departments primarily around their regulatory enforcement functions, such as food safety and other inspection regimes. As a result, most city health departments suffer from underinvestment in NCD surveillance, data-driven policy formation, and adequate staffing for noncategorically funded initiatives.

4 Impediments and Enablers for City Health Departments to Promote Healthy Cities

City health departments are uniquely able to lead public health actions for the benefit of their residents. A variety of features common to cities position them to embrace this role, especially when framed in contrast to state and national government agencies. City governments are literally closer to the populations they serve, and they are able to identify community-level needs and opportunities for action, including understanding intraurban variability. They have direct engagement with civil society organizations, which are often essential supporters of policy advocacy and program implementation, and city government is best-placed to convene stakeholders and achieve social and political consensus. In US cities, critical functions of government are commonly centralized under chief executive/mayoral authority. This enables, and, with the right leadership, encourages cross-sectoral collaboration and accountability. For example, public health action to reduce fatalities and injuries due to traffic crashes requires interventions and collaborations from the police and the transportation, planning, and health sectors. In many cities in low- and mid-income countries (LMICs), law enforcement is a federal or state function, without city oversight, making such integrated work more challenging. Similarly, public health food policy depends on interactions between the health, education, and retail sectors. In many LMICs, cities do not oversee their school systems, making such alignment difficult. Finally, and perhaps most important, city residents perceive their local government as being responsible and accountable for protecting the public's health. Diffusion of this responsibility across different levels of government is confusing to the public and is inefficient.

There have been calls for nongovernmental entities to assume leadership roles in urban public health practice. For example, the size, resources, and community connections of academic medical centers have been cited as a rationale for their increasing engagement.[17] However, these organizations lack essential qualities that are only possessed by government agencies: an explicit mandate that is not conflicted with fiduciary interests, an inherently population orientation, and the legitimacy to convene a wide range of stakeholders. Academic health centers should play an important role as a partner to government; indeed, public health departments frequently rely on the expertise of academic partners. But government agencies should not cede their authority and leadership to nongovernmental actors.[18]

The sheer complexities of urban governance mean that the potential for city health agencies to maximize their impact is often underrealized. For example, despite unified accountability to a chief executive, city agencies are often balkanized and pursue independent agendas. Also, historical reliance on federal and state funding results in mayors and city legislatures limiting the flow of investment of their cities' always-constrained budgets into public health.

A major impediment to city leadership on public health is the absence of relevant legal authority. As public health practice continues to mature and reengage with the physical and social conditions under which people live, the key levers of public health action are increasingly legislative and regulatory. However, most public health authority rests with states, not cities. One exception is New York City, where, in recent years, its robust health code has been a powerful tool for action around tobacco control, food policy, and chronic disease control.[19] But even this mechanism is limited by historical precedent; for example, mental health and substance use policy is governed at the state level, restricting the city's ability to plan and implement innovative strategies in these domains. State preemption of local authority can also be a major impediment to public health practice.[20] A notable example is alcohol policy. Many states' laws explicitly prohibit localities from establishing laws or rules in most aspects of alcohol policy, including best public health practices such as taxation, regulation of sales, siting of outlets, and marketing restrictions.[21]

5 The Way Forward

For big city health departments to realize their full potential to influence determinants of health that are beyond their traditional regulatory authority and programmatic reach, they must adopt and advance a vision of intergovernmental and intersectoral collaboration.

One approach that has been embraced in the past decade is "Health in All Policies" (HiAP), promoted by a range of public health professional and advocacy organizations.[22,23] HiAP at its core strives to advance public health through assessing and projecting health outcomes and benefits from policy options, often on issues like land-use planning, transportation decisions, economic and employment initiatives, and education. HiAP can be practiced by a variety of stakeholders; here, we are concerned with how local governments and, in particular, local health departments, may prepare themselves to more fully engage in "integrated governance" to promote health and equity.[24]

We have found HiAP to be a valuable framework, but when described as such within the confines of municipal government, it is often met with skepticism and reflexive agency territorialism. The skepticism comes from the implicit premise that all policies *can* be analyzed for their health impacts and the unrealistic expectation that health departments are sufficiently resourced to play this role. The territorialism derives from a belief that the public's well-being is already part and parcel of decision-making processes. A strategy for health departments to overcome such challenges is to apply particular principles and tools of HiAP, such as quantitative health impact assessments (HIAs), with targeted efforts to embed this method in legislation and rules.[25] This has been done, for example, in New York City's Environmental Quality Review Act, which requires a public health assessment of any discretionary governmental action that may have negative public impacts.[26]

Delivering robust HIAs in the service of broad public policy, and thereby demonstrating the value-added activities of health departments, requires sufficient and appropriately trained personnel and an adequate data and analytic infrastructure. Data sharing agreements with transportation, city planning, housing, and environmental agencies help build the institutional relationships and trust to enable cross-sector work. Collaborative problem formulation and methodology selection promote a culture in which findings are less likely to be challenged.

We offer two topical examples of how big city health departments have employed HiAP and HIA to promote health and equity.

5.1 Wage and Economic Equity

Income inequality, independent of other genetic, behavioral, and environmental determinants of health outcomes, is an important driver of disparities in premature mortality.[27] One intersectoral role for urban health departments is to drive economic policies that promote public health. In San Francisco, for example, the Department of Public Health used the department's permitting power to address wage theft from low-income workers in the restaurant industry.[28] The Department sought and acted on referrals from the State Office of Labor Standards to enforce a little utilized requirement in its health code requiring permittees to have complied with all local and state laws. The effort created an ongoing incentive for labor law compliance. A California Bay Area multicounty Health Impact Assessment collaborative that concluded that raising the minimum wage would narrow health disparities and increase the proportion of insured was used to successfully argue for raising the area's minimum wage. Their analysis was data-heavy, bolstering the credibility of its largely directional conclusion that raising the minimum wage would reduce chronic disease incidence and increase survival.[29]

5.2 Air Pollution and Health

Levels of hazardous air pollutants in cities, a leading cause of premature mortality, may be largely locally determined and, by extension, controlled. Urban health departments, generally without authority over air emissions, nonetheless can influence public and policymaker support for air quality improvement. New York City's health department sought and obtained resources under the city's first long-term sustainability plan in 2007 to develop a neighborhood-level air monitoring program to identify local sources and inform local clean air actions beyond those required by national and state regulations.[30] The resulting air monitoring program identified high-sulfur heating oil as an important source of neighborhood air pollution.[31,32] To complement this exposure surveillance initiative, the department developed neighborhood-scale estimates of the health burden from air pollution.[33] This technical capability, developed in the context of interagency convening by a mayoral sustainability office, informed local air pollution control initiatives, including a rapid phase-out of high-sulfur heating oil, which led to a 69% reduction in sulfur dioxide (SO_2) exposure and contributed to an estimated 800 fewer deaths annually through improved air quality.[34]

6 Conclusion

We have outlined the successes of, opportunities for, and constraints on city health departments to realize the ambitious goal of playing an essential leadership role in advancing the health of cities. When a local government's métier is merely a reflection of prevailing attitudes for a limited role in shaping the physical, social, and economic conditions of the city, it will fail to anticipate changing conditions and the public's future needs. Health departments must nurture relationships with civil society to enable nongovernmental actors to advocate for a more expansive role, one that is adequately funded to add value to all aspects of the urban policy sphere.

Academic institutions should do their part to strengthen city health departments by inviting government employees to reflect on their practice, encouraging public service as a career path, fostering collaborations that use and enhance local data, and preparing the multidisciplinary workforce needed to support the New Urban Agenda. Mayors, city legislatures, advocates, community-based organizations, and service providers should promote decentralized and expanded municipal authority to enable locally relevant and timely regulatory and policy interventions. Regional and national governments should embrace local authority and provide cities with technical and financial support, although it has been noted that national and regional-level governments are wary of even disaggregating data to the local level given the potential for local political consequences.[35] And public health leaders should take bold steps to assert the importance of health considerations in decisions made outside the current domain of public health.

References

1. United Nations. *Habitat III revised zero draft of the New Urban Agenda, Quito Declaration on Sustainable Cities and Human Settlements for All.* New York: United Nations; 2016.
2. Pierson J. John Maynard Keynes and the modern political economy. *Soc.* 2012; 49:263.
3. Katz B, Nowak J. *The new localism.* Washington, DC: Brookings Institution Press; 2018.
4. United Nations. *Habitat III Policy Paper: 4—urban governance, capacity and institutional development.* New York: United Nations; 2018.
5. UNICEF. Progress on sanitation and drinking water: 2015 update and MDG assessment. UNICEF website. Available at http://www.unicef.org/publications/index_82419.html. Accessed July 18, 2016.

6. Health Effects Institute. *State of global air 2018. Special report.* Boston, MA: Health Effects Institute; 2018.

7. Reiner M, Niermann C, Jekauc D, Woll A. Long-term health benefits of physical activity—a systematic review of longitudinal studies. *BMC Public Health.* 2013; 13:813.

8. Durand CP, Andalib M, Dunton GF, Wolch J, Pentz MA. A Systematic review of built environment factors related to physical activity and obesity risk: implications for smart growth urban planning. *Obes Rev Off J Int Assoc Study Obes.* 2011; 12(501):e173–e182. doi:10.1111/j.1467-789X.2010.00826.x

9. Ravallion M, Chen S, Sangraula P. New evidence on the urbanization of global poverty. *Popul Dev Rev.* 2007; 33(4):667–701.

10. Ezeh H, Oyebode O, Satterwaite D, Caiaffa W, et al. The history, geography, and sociology of slums and the health problems of people who live in slums. *Lancet.* 2017; 389(10068): 547–558.

11. Ewing R, Hamidi S, Grace JB, Wei YD. Does urban sprawl hold down upward mobility? *Landsc Urban Plan.* 2016; 148:80–88.

12. Institute of Medicine; Board on Health Promotion and Disease Prevention; Committee on Assuring the Health of the Public in the 21st Century. *The future of the public's health in the 21st century.* Washington, DC: National Academies Press; 2003. doi:10.17226/10548

13. National Association of County and City Health Officials. National profile of local health departments. National Association of County and City Health Officials website. Available at http://nacchoprofilestudy.org/reports-publications/. Accessed August 25, 2018.

14. Plough A. Understanding the financing and functions of metropolitan health departments: a key to improved public health response. *J Public Health Manag Pract.* 2004; 10(5):421–427.

15. Centers for Disease Control (CDC). The public health system & the 10 essential public health services. US Centers for Disease Control and Prevention (CDC) website. Available at https://www.cdc.gov/stltpublichealth/publichealthservices/essentialhealthservices.html. Accessed August 25, 2018.

16. Leider JP, Castrucci BC, Hearne S, Russo P. Organizational characteristics of large urban health departments. *J Public Health Manag Pract.* 2015; 21(S1):S14–S19. doi:10.1097/PHH.0000000000000172

17. Washington AE, Coye MJ, Boulware LE. Academic health systems' third curve: population health improvement. *JAMA.* 2016; 315(5):459–460.

18. Goodman A, Karpati A. Roles of academic and public health systems in advancing population health. *JAMA.* 2016; 315(23):2623.

19. Frieden TR, Bassett MT, Thorpe LE, Farley TA. Public health in New York City, 2002-2007: confronting epidemics of the modern era. *Int J Epidemiol.* 2008; 37(5):966–977.

20. Pomeranz JL, Pertschuk M. State preemption: a significant and quiet threat to public health in the United States. *Am J Public Health.* 2017; 107(6):900–902.

21. Mosher JF, Adler SS, Pamukcu AM, Treffers RD. Review of state laws restricting local authority to impose alcohol taxes in the United States. *J Stud Alcohol Drugs.* 2017; 78(2):241–248.

22. Rudolph L, Caplan J, Ben-Moshe K, Dillion L. *Health in all policies: a guide for state and local governments.* Washington, DC: American Public Health Association and Public Health Institute; 2013.

23. National Association of City and County Health Officers. *Health in all policies: experiences from local health departments.* Washington, DC: National Association of City and County Health Officers; 2017.

24. Fafard P. Health in all meets horizontal government. Grenoble, France: First International Conference on Public Policy; 2013.

25. Centers for Disease Control and Prevention (CDC). *Different types of health impact assessments.* US Centers for Disease Control and Prevention (CDC) National Center for Environmental Health website. Available at https://www.cdc.gov/healthyplaces/types_health_assessments.htm. Accessed August 1, 2018.

26. NYC Mayor's Office of Environmental Coordination. *CEQR technical manual.* New York: NYC Mayor's Office of Environmental Coordination; 2014.

27. Lynch J, Smith GD, Harper S, et al. Is income inequality a determinant of population health? Part 1. A systematic review. *Milbank Q.* 2004; 82(1):5–99.

28. HealthEquityGuide. San Francisco leverages health permits to combat wage theft. HealthEquityGuide.org website. Available at https://healthequityguide.org/case-studies/san-francisco-leverages-health-permits-to-combat-wage-theft/#advice. Accessed August 1, 2018.

29. Bay Area Health Inequities Initiative. The minimum wage and health. Bay Area Health Inequities Initiative website. 2014. Available at http://barhii.org/download/publications/barhii_2014_minimum_wage_health.pdf. Accessed August 1, 2018.

30. Climate change. In *PlaNYC: a greater, greener New York.* New York: The City of New York. 2007:130.

31. Matte TD, Ross Z, Kheirbek I, et al. Monitoring intraurban spatial patterns of multiple combustion air pollutants in New York City: design and implementation. *J Expo Sci Environ Epidemiol.* 2013; 23(3):223–231.

32. Clougherty JE, Kheirbek I, Eisl HM, et al. Intra-urban spatial variability in wintertime street-level concentrations of multiple combustion-related air pollutants: the New York City Community Air Survey (NYCCAS). *J Expo Sci Environ Epidemiol.* 2013; 23(3):232–240.

33. New York City Department of Health and Mental Hygiene. *Air pollution and the health of New Yorkers: the impact of fine particles and ozone.* New York: New York City Department of Health and Mental Hygiene; 2011.

34. New York City Department of Health and Mental Hygiene. *New York City trends in air pollution and its health consequences.* New York: New York City Department of Health and Mental Hygiene; 2013.

35. Vlahov D, Agarwal SR, Buckley RM, et al. Roundtable on urban living environmental research (RULER). *J Urban Health.* 2011; 88(5):793–857.

City Leadership for Health, Equity, and Sustainable Development

AGIS D. TSOUROS

1 Introduction

City leaders have the power and the means to make a significant difference in the health and well-being of their people. This chapter will explore and discuss the context, potential, and critical preconditions for city leadership for health in the twenty-first century. Leadership encompasses a variety of qualities, skills, and styles and can be addressed from many perspectives. The focus here will be mainly on four aspects of city leadership: political leadership, leadership for change and innovation, value-based leadership, and capacity for effective leadership and governance for health.

In the past three decades, health has increasingly gained significant political attention and importance at all levels of government. It is widely accepted that health goes hand in hand with social, economic, and sustainable development and that it represents a major issue for global security.[1] The accumulating evidence on the complexity of today's public health challenges and the determinants of health has changed the way health is understood and how it should be dealt with.

Although health was defined as a state of complete physical, mental, and social well-being and not merely the absence of disease or infirmity in the World Health Organization (WHO) Constitution in 1948, only in more recent years has this notion begun to be more explicitly reflected in policies and strategies for health development.

2 Health Is a Political Choice

Dealing effectively with health in the twenty-first century requires actions in a wide range of domains by many actors: political, institutional, multiprofessional, and community. Most of the public health challenges today, such as growing health inequalities, the noncommunicable diseases epidemic, antimicrobial resistance, climate change–related emergencies, and the threat of communicable disease epidemics, are very complex and require action by many sectors and stakeholders globally, nationally, and locally. The rapid urbanization and the changing social landscape with the aging of the population, massive migration, high levels of poverty and unemployment, and growing insecurity also demand awareness and sensitivity to the special needs of these groups.

Even though there are a plethora of country and city strategies inspired by the approaches of modern public health, there is a significant deficit in their implementation for several reasons that will be discussed later. A good example is the strong evidence on equity and the social determinants of health. While the social determinants are much talked about and mentioned in policy documents, we have made relatively limited progress on the social determinants and then only in very few countries.

Today's leaders and professionals need to deal with a complex and changing public health landscape that, it could be argued, is shaped by seven imperatives, reflecting the priorities of twenty-first-century WHO strategies and plans (e.g., Health 2020).[1] These suggested imperatives are (1) putting health and well-being high on the social and political agenda of governments at all levels; (2) upholding the core values of the right to health, universal coverage, equity, and sustainable development; (3) promoting Health in All Policies (HiAP) and accountability for health; (4) addressing the determinants of health through upstream interventions; (5) investing in health promotion, disease prevention, and public health emergency preparedness; (6) promoting community empowerment, people-centered services, community resilience, and health literacy; and (7) strengthening leadership and governance for health.

Therefore, in today's context, striving to protect and promote population health presupposes a capacity to work with complexity, uncertainty, and multiple stakeholders and to apply a wide range of modern public health concepts, as reflected in the preceding seven imperatives. These imperatives require making health a whole-of-government priority. Each one of them represents a key precondition for successfully reaching health development goals and effectively tackling public health challenges, such as the control of noncommunicable diseases.

Given the fact that health and the root causes of ill-health and health inequalities are greatly influenced by the policies and actions of many sectors at all levels of government, the key importance of political leadership is clear. This often implies making tough decisions arguing for community health and well-being. Political leaders must articulate visions of the kind of society they wish to create and the values that underpin their visions.

Health is political because it is unevenly distributed; because many determinants depend on political action; because it is a critical issue of human rights and citizenship; because it is a domain where multiple ideologies and interests are at play; and because the politics of health are often driven by new technological developments, demands from citizens, or new forms of delivery. This is the reason the term "political determinants of health" is increasingly used in the literature.[2]

Ultimately, health is an investment and, above all, a political choice. It is a political choice in embracing the values and adopting the right policies and conditions that create health for all, it is a political choice when investing in upstream strategic interventions that will deliver maximum health impact, and it is a political choice when striving to create the organizational capacity and the resources to support intersectoral work and democratic governance for health and well-being.

The political choice of health is a prominent and integral part of the 2030 United Nations agenda for sustainable development.[3] The Sustainable Development Goals

(SDGs) provide a global framework of political responsibility and accountability, providing powerful political support nationally and locally to those who argue for more inclusive and sustainable economic, social, and environmental policies. Health is explicitly relevant to several SDGs (in particular, Goals 1–6, 10–13, and 16) and implicitly relevant to all 17 of them.

The UN agenda puts strong emphasis on issues critical to health development such as poverty, equity, education, employment, and climate action. Goal 3 on health is positioned as a major contributor to human development, significantly affecting the ability of policies in other sectors to succeed. Worth also noting is that Goal 11 (sustainable cities and communities) focuses on making cities and human settlements inclusive, safe, resilient, and sustainable.

Clearly, the 2030 UN agenda offers political leaders significant added legitimacy and momentum, which could help cities and countries overcome barriers to change and innovation as well as improve health and well-being in the context of sustainable development on a global scale. Across the globe, the implementation of the 17 goals over the next 15 years depends on action at all levels: international, national, regional, and local.

Each country is expected to develop its own policy for SDG implementation at national and local levels. Because of their global political status, the SDGs provide an even more compelling imperative to action than does the science of health determinants. The implementation of the SDGs requires whole-of-government and whole-of-society approaches at all levels of government.

3 The Potential of Local Political Leadership

Leadership for health and health equity takes many forms and involves many actors; for example, international organizations set standards, heads of national or subnational governments prioritize health and well-being, health ministers reach out to ministers in other sectors, parliamentarians express an interest in health, business leaders integrate health considerations in their business models, civil society organizations become increasingly active in disease management and health development, academic institutions provide evidence for the determinants of health and interventions that work, and city governments take on the challenge of HIaP.[4]

Leadership for health and equity in the twenty-first century requires new skills, often using influence rather than direct control, to achieve results. Much of the authority of future health leaders will reside not only in their position in the health system but also in their ability to convince others that health and well-being are highly relevant in all sectors. Leadership will be not only individual but also institutional, collective, community-centered, and collaborative.[5] Such forms of leadership are already in evidence. Groups of stakeholders are coming together to address key health challenges at the global, regional, national, and local levels, such as the global movement on HIV. Similar movements are emerging around noncommunicable diseases, environmental health, and health promotion.

In the complex political world comprised of multiple tiers and numerous sectors of public and stakeholders, local governments have both the power and the mandate to influence the determinants and inequities of health and well-being.

Local governments are well positioned to promote health through policy development, regulations, planning and integrated city development strategies, services and programs, national-local collaborations, and partnership-building across society (community and private stakeholders) as well as advocacy and mediation at all levels. Local leaders can promote the health and well-being of their citizens through their influence in several domains such as health, social services, the environment, education, the economy, housing, security, transportation, sport, urban food production, and emergency infrastructures and services. They can do this through various policies and interventions, including those addressing social exclusion and support, healthy and active living (such as cycle lanes and smoke-free public areas), safety and environmental issues for children and older people, working conditions, preparedness to deal with the consequences of climate change, exposure to hazards and nuisances, healthy urban planning and design (neighborhood planning, removal of architectural barriers, accessibility, and proximity of services), and participatory and inclusive processes for citizens.[6–8]

Intersectoral partnerships and community empowerment initiatives can be implemented more easily at the local level with the active support of local governments. Local leaders acting beyond their formal powers have the potential to make a difference to the health and well-being of local communities by harnessing the combined efforts of a multitude of actors.[5]

Today, municipalities worldwide are evolving as key drivers of health, equity, and sustainable development, providing leadership and innovation and often inspiring and leveraging action nationally and internationally.

4 City Leadership for Health, Equity, and Sustainable Development: What It Takes

In the twenty-first century, local leadership for health and sustainable development means having a vision and a good understanding of the importance of health in sustainable social and economic development, advocating and actively implementing an agenda to address health inequalities and foster sustainable development, possessing the commitment and conviction to forge new partnerships and alliances, promoting accountability for health and sustainability by statutory and nonstatutory local actors, aligning local action with national policy, anticipating and planning for change, and, ultimately, acting as a guardian, facilitator, catalyst, advocate, and defender of the right to maximum health for all residents. All these aspects resonate the imperatives presented earlier in this chapter that shape today's public health landscape and the SDGs.

Effective leadership for health and well-being also requires a strategic approach, supportive institutional arrangements, open platforms for dialogue across society, and alignment and connection with other local, regional, and national actors who are working in complementary areas such as community development, urban regeneration plans, transport and ecological projects, and policy for social support, culture, and education. A strategic approach ultimately delivers better and fairer health outcomes because it focuses on the root causes of ill-health that underpin the twenty-first-century public health imperatives.

Citizens' health and happiness depend to a great extent on politicians' willingness to prioritize choices that address health for all and create cities for all. City leaders' political choices should match their aspirations for protecting and constantly improving the health and well-being of all citizens. This means creating supportive social and physical environments that enable all people to reach their maximum potential for health and well-being.

A systematic and comprehensive approach to leadership for health and sustainable development should cover five main aspects: a value-based vision, broad political support in the city administration and civil society, mechanisms and structures to support change and innovation, an agenda and set of goals to achieve and be accountable for, and mechanisms for listening and dialogue.

Most cities invest in developing mission statements, strategies, and development plans for the future. This is an important starting point for committed leaders. Signing a declaration about health is not enough. Cities must develop visions that embrace and integrate health, equity, and sustainable development. It must be made clear that the city values health and well-being and that it considers health closely linked to social and economic development.

It is important to secure the widest possible support from the members of the City Council (executive and cross-party) and stakeholders from different sectors, including the corporate and voluntary ones. Effective intersectoral leadership starts with openness and opportunities to develop a common understanding and articulate common visions. When reaching out to other sectors, it is important not only to ask "what you can do for health" but also "what health can do for you?" The SDG agenda, which is in fact highly relevant to the local level, will never be fully implemented if it becomes fragmented into "sectoral pieces."

An effective way to engage a wide range of partners in health, equity, and sustainable development is to commonly define goals for the city that will be implemented through joint action, joint planning, and shared accountability. This would be an appropriate approach to develop goals addressing the social determinants of health and the SDG agendas.[9]

Most of today's global agendas call for action across sectors and with a strong engagement of individuals and communities, and this is one of the reasons they often remain unimplemented. An important aspect of leadership is to create horizontal structures and processes to manage change and encourage innovation. Intersectoral collaboration requires political steering, consensus building, coordination, and incentives for joint work.

Putting health high on the social and political agenda of cities should mean thinking about health and integrating health considerations in all cities activities.[10] Box 42.1 proposes an agenda for mayors and city leaders committed to health, equity, and sustainable development, which translates the imperatives just outlined into actionable recommendations.

In this context, it is important to mention Healthy Cities, which was launched by the WHO as a value-based political project that offered cities globally legitimacy as well as a framework and a platform for working with different sectors and society as a

---

Box 42.1 **An Agenda for Local Leaders Committed to Health, Equity, and Sustainable Development**

Recognize that health is a fundamental human right and that every human being is entitled to the enjoyment of the highest attainable standard of health.

Strive to make health and well-being core values in city vision statements, policies, and strategies.

Promote health and equity in all local policies and in alignment with the SDG agenda.[11–13]

Address inequalities through the social determinants and gender perspectives.[14]

Create public spaces that support healthy and active living.

Provide universal coverage to health and social services and community support.[15]

Invest in health promotion and health literacy programs.[16]

Invest in giving children a healthy start in life and support socially vulnerable and disadvantaged groups such as migrants, urban poor, and unemployed.

Strengthen population-based disease prevention programs with an emphasis on obesity, smoking, unhealthy nutrition, and physical activity.

Promote healthy urban planning and design.

Invest in green, clean, child-friendly, and age-friendly environments.

Support community empowerment and community-based initiatives and promote social inclusion and community resilience.

Strengthen local capacity to deal with public health emergencies and effects of climate change.

---

whole for health development.[17] The concept of Healthy Cities caught the interest of city politicians, professionals, and public health activists around the world and spread very quickly, becoming a vibrant and thriving global movement.

Healthy Cities places strong emphasis on strategic thinking, the development of city health profiles, and city health development plans that draw on the contributions of different sectors. In addition, Healthy Cities prioritizes the creation of platforms for dialogue with civil society and public stakeholders and stresses the importance of connecting and developing synergies and alliances with other local development agendas, such as community development strategies.[18]

Experience with the European Healthy Cities movement has shown that the most successful cities were those that invested time in partnerships, those that created platforms for dialogue and listened to their citizens' concerns and expectations, those that invested in creating consensus, those that invested in creating ownership and opportunities for community empowerment, and those that invested in capacity-building to support change, creativity, and openness to new ideas.[19,20] National legislation that gives municipalities a strong mandate for health promotion, as is the case in Finland, can significantly strengthen the hand of local leaders.

Last, it is important to mention the emerging fields of health diplomacy and city diplomacy.[21,22] City leaders increasingly strive to become active, vocal, and influential in international fora as well as through (formal and informal) multilateral and bilateral forms of cooperation for peace, health, security, and sustainable development.

5 Conclusion

This chapter provided key arguments for the importance of dynamic local political leadership for health, equity, and sustainable development and discussed what it takes to be successful. It also stressed the unique position of cities to affect the determinants of health and to be conveners and brokers of civil society interests and expectations.

It was emphasized that political support is indispensable in pursuing a modern public health agenda, which requires a shift in the way health is understood and valued as well as institutional capacity to facilitate change and innovation. Health is a value-based political choice.

Prioritizing health must be an explicit political choice. Multisectoral governance is essential for policy coherence, synergy, and coordination across different sectors and provides a basis for accountability and transparency. To advance health requires increasing the capacity of leaders to transcend boundaries, work collaboratively, and transform their communities.[23] Last, strengthening leadership for health also requires a focus on ensuring an ecosystem that enables participation from diverse actors, nurtures debates, and provides space and mechanisms to explore, embrace, and adapt new ideas. The value of creating more platforms where diverse sets of actors regularly engage in mutually respectful discussions of local and global health challenges and plan for concerted action to address them cannot be overstated.

References

1. World Health Organization. *Health 2020: the European policy for health and well-being.* Copenhagen, Denmark: World Health Organization; 2013.
2. Mackenbach JP. Political determinants of health. *Eur J Public Health.* 2014; 24(1):2.
3. United Nations. Sustainable Development Goals. Sustainable Development Knowledge Platform website. 2015. Available at https://sustainabledevelopment.un.org/?menu=1300. Accessed May 10, 2018.
4. Tsouros AD. *City leadership for health and sustainable development–critical issues for successful Healthy Cities projects.* Kuwait City, Kuwait: Global Healthy Cities; 2017.
5. Kickbusch I, Gleicher D. *Governance for health in the 21st century.* Copenhagen, Denmark: World Health Organization. 2014.
6. Edwards P, Tsouros A. *A healthy city is an active city: a physical activity planning guide.* Copenhagen, Denmark: World Health Organization; 2008.
7. Barton H, Thompson S, Burgess S, Grant M, eds. *The Routledge handbook of planning for health and well-being, shaping a sustainable and healthy future.* New York: Routledge; 2015.
8. Barton H, Tsourou C. *Healthy urban planning.* New York: Routledge; 2001.

9. World Health Organization. *Addressing the social determinants of health: the urban dimension and the role of local government.* Copenhagen, Denmark: World Health Organization; 2012.

10. Healthy Cities Mayors Forum. *Shanghai Consensus on Healthy Cities 2016.* Geneva, Switzerland: World Health Organization; 2016.

11. Barton H. *City of well-being: a radical guide to planning.* New York: Routledge; 2016.

12. de Leeuw E, Tsouros A, Dyakova M, Green G. *Promoting health and equity—evidence for local policy and practice.* Copenhagen, Denmark: World Health Organization; 2014.

13. Pan-American Health Organization. *The Santiago Declaration. Mayors Pre-Forum, Road to Shanghai 2016.* July 25–26, 2016. Santiago, Chile: Pan-American Health Organization; 2016.

14. World Health Organization. *Healthy cities tackle the social determinants of inequities in health: a framework for action.* Copenhagen, Denmark: World Health Organization; 2012.

15. World Health Organization. Health financing. What is universal coverage? World Health Organization website. Available at http://www.who.int/health_financing/universal_coverage_definition/en/. Accessed May 10, 2018.

16. Kickbusch I, Pelican J, Apfel F, Tsouros A. *Health literacy: the solid facts.* Copenhagen, Denmark: World Health Organization; 2013.

17. de Leeuw E, Simos J, eds. *Healthy cities: the theory, policy, and practice of value-based urban planning.* New York: Springer; 2017.

18. Tsouros AD. City leadership for health and well-being: back to future. *J Urban Health.* 2013; 90(S): 4–13.

19. Tsouros AD. Twenty-seven years of the WHO European Healthy Cities movement: a sustainable movement for change and innovation at the local level. *Health Promo Int.* 2015; 30(S1): i3–i7.

20. Green G, Tsouros AD. *City leadership for health.* Copenhagen, Denmark: World Health Organization; 2008.

21. World Health Organization. *Health 2020: foreign policy and health.* Copenhagen, Denmark: World Health Organization Regional; 2015.

22. Acuto M, Morissette M, Tsouros A. City diplomacy: towards more strategic networking? Learning with WHO Healthy Cities. *Global Policy.* 2017; 8(1). doi:10.1111/1758-5899.12382

23. World Health Organization. *Open mindsets: participatory leadership for health.* Geneva, Switzerland: World Health Organization. 2016.

43

Teaching Urban Health

NICHOLAS FREUDENBERG

1 Introduction

Creating healthier, more equitable, and sustainable cities requires an urban health workforce with the knowledge, skills, and capacity needed to achieve those goals. This chapter examines what schools, universities, health departments, and policymakers can do to prepare that workforce.

If the urban health workforce is broadly defined as all those whose work contributes to healthier cities and healthier urban populations, then it includes a wide cross-section of employment professional and paraprofessional categories. Those who have significant health-related responsibilities include clinicians of many disciplines, public health professionals, nutritionists, administrators, sanitarians, and community health workers. These workers are the focus of this chapter, and some of their job categories are listed in Box 43.1. Many other professionals contribute to urban health more indirectly: architects, engineers, educators, police officers, social service providers, transportation and urban planners, and others. These workers also play a vital role in promoting health and preventing disease in cities, and their professional preparation requires the development of skills that will enable them to take on these roles, especially an ability to communicate and work effectively with those working in the healthcare and public health sectors.

On the one hand, health professionals practicing in urban settings need the same basic skills as those working in rural or suburban settings. For example, clinicians need to be able to prevent, diagnose, and treat common communicable and noncommunicable conditions. Public health professionals need to master the three core public health functions of assessment, policy development, and assurance, and managers must know how to budget, plan, supervise, and secure needed resources.[1]

On the other hand, the defining characteristics of cities—population density and diversity, high levels of inequality, dense social networks, exposure to urban physical and social environments, and a complex array of formal and informal health and social services—create distinct patterns of heath and disease and unique opportunities for intervention.[2,3] These characteristics of urban settings require health professionals working in cities to master an additional set of competencies, some of which are proposed in Box 43.2.

Box 43.1 **Health Professionals Involved in Promoting Health and Preventing and Treating Disease in Cities**

Physicians in all specialty areas

Nurses

Allied health practitioners

Social workers

Psychologists

Health educators

Nutritionists and dietitians

Community health workers

Home healthcare workers

Patient navigators

Healthcare administrators

Sanitarians and other environmental health specialists

Epidemiologists

Biostatisticians

Health planners

Policy analysts and advocates

No single guide can prescribe how each training program can best integrate the discipline-specific professional competencies identified by each professional organization with the urban health competencies in Box 43.2.[4–7] Given that the urban health workforce includes people with extensive relevant life experience but limited formal education (e.g., community health workers) and those with advanced graduate training, the level of mastery and the priority of the proposed competencies required for professional practice for each category will differ.

By considering the organizational models and pedagogical strategies described in this chapter, academic institutions and faculty preparing urban health professionals can tailor their professional preparation to build on their institutional assets. Their goals are to prepare their graduates for the specific settings in which they work and the populations they serve. Despite the differences in professional responsibilities, what urban health professionals share is a set of principles, values, and strategies that have emerged from more than a century of practice. This "practice-based evidence" constitutes the foundation for interdisciplinary professional education in urban health.[8]

2 Content of Urban Health Professional Education

The discipline of urban health emerged from medicine, nursing, social work, urban planning, social sciences, and public health.[9] In the past decade or so, several scholars

---

Box 43.2 **Selected Competencies for Urban Health Professionals**

1. Apply theories and frameworks from urban social sciences to identifying social and other determinants of health and developing solutions to major urban health problems.
2. Use epidemiological methods to characterize patterns of health and disease and inequalities in health in urban populations and subpopulations.
3. Employ ecological models to identify appropriate solutions to the health problems of cities at the individual, family, community, municipal, regional, national, and global levels.
4. Engage various constituencies including policymakers, community residents and leaders, civil society organizations, social movements, and public agencies in identifying and reducing health problems facing cities.
5. Identify opportunities for intersectoral action to promote the health and prevent or reduce threats to the well-being of urban populations.
6. Participate in formal and informal governance processes that are used to address urban health and social problems.
7. Communicate effectively with professionals from other disciplines and sectors involved in improving the health of urban populations.
8. Develop policies and programs that contribute to promoting the health of urban populations and reducing urban heath inequalities.
9. Promote and support leaders who can advance urban health, especially those from groups often excluded from democratic decisions.
10. Analyze critically one's own contributions to improvements in urban health and modify practice based on feedback and evaluation.

---

have summarized this intellectual history, highlighting its roots in industrialization, urbanization, globalization, and the social conflicts of the nineteenth and twentieth centuries.[10–13] In recent years, academics from several fields have created or developed bodies of knowledge that constitute a framework for contemporary theory, research, and practice in urban health. To achieve the competencies listed in Box 43.2, urban health professionals must become familiar with these evolving domains of knowledge.

First, urban social scientists, including sociologists, psychologists, geographers, political scientists, historians, economists, demographers, and anthropologists, seek to understand how cities and city living influence individuals, communities, and society and how these actors in turn shape cities.[14–16] As health researchers focus their attention on the social determinants of health and disease, deepening our knowledge of the pathways by which urban social characteristics, structure, migration flows, and patterns of interaction influence behavior, health, and social hierarchies becomes an essential task for developing strategies to improve the health of people living in cities.[17]

A second emerging body of knowledge maps the ways that human biology responds to changing physical and social environments. Research on the microbiome, the roles of the immune and neuroendocrine systems in health and disease and the growing understanding of epigenetics and environment–gene interactions and other biological pathways are illuminating some of the distinct ways that urban settings get "under the skin" to influence human health.[18-21] The most effective public health interventions will be firmly grounded in both urban environments and human biology and in our scientific understanding of how urban exposures influence patterns of health and disease.

A third body of scholarship, systems sciences, aims to uncover the behavior of complex systems.[22] Cities, the essence of complex systems, illustrate how various systems interact to shape health.[23,24] By investigating how various systems influence the macrosocial determinants of the health of urban populations, researchers can illuminate opportunities for interventions to, for example, reduce child obesity or mitigate the impact of climate change on cities.[25]

A key task for urban health professionals is to communicate effectively with the diverse constituencies that contribute to improved health. Moving from one-way to interactive communication is especially important and may require transforming established practices. Health communications researchers have contributed new insights into "framing" health and health policy messages, garnering attention in crowded urban communications environments, and using new communications technologies.[26-29] Teaching urban health professionals how to apply these insights will enable them to more fully engage those actors who can contribute to healthier cities.

New methodologies also provide urban health practitioners and researchers with tools to improve the health of the populations they serve. Implementation science studies methods to promote the adoption and integration of evidence-based practices, interventions, and policies into routine healthcare and public health settings.[30] Public health informatics describes the application of informatics to public health. It assists urban health professionals to create and use interoperable information systems for public health functions such as biosurveillance, outbreak management, electronic laboratory reporting, and prevention.[31] Geospatial sciences enable public health researchers to analyze geographic variations in health and disease. In urban health, geospatial methods are used to assess the impact of, for example, toxic exposures, food environments, and infectious disease outbreaks.[32-34]

The study of cities and of population health are each dynamic, evolving domains of knowledge. Interdisciplinary professionals must be able to synthesize and apply the theories, models, and evidence developing at the intersection of these domains to improve the health of cities and their residents. Preparing their students to translate these bodies of knowledge into practice constitutes the main challenge facing educators of urban health professionals.

3 Teaching Approaches

Universities and other educational institutions have employed a variety of approaches to familiarize their students with these bodies of knowledge and assist them with developing the competencies needed to apply them in practice. Learning opportunities range from single lectures to full courses, certificates, degree programs, or specialized field placements. Each approach has distinct advantages and disadvantages.

Single lectures on various dimensions of urban health are usually easier to implement and institutionalize than more comprehensive approaches. The low burden on teaching time may make it easier to expose all students in a given discipline, rather than the few who choose a specialized elective in urban health. These lectures can be tailored to the unique needs of learners' academic levels and disciplines. By adding lectures on urban health to several courses required of, say, family medicine practitioners, it may be possible to provide a somewhat systematic introduction to urban health principles. The incremental costs of this approach are low. Its disadvantages are its potentially superficial coverage, the lack of opportunity to learn with other disciplines, and the limited opportunities to practice the application of new knowledge.

Full courses on urban health provide the opportunity to develop and apply some of the competencies listed in Box 43.2, exchange ideas with classmates from other disciplines, and practice skills in the classroom or in the community. Required courses ensure that all students in a program learn the material but may necessitate additional resources and faculty expertise.

Elective courses offer interested students the opportunity to develop expertise in urban health but limit exposure to those who elect to take them.

Certificates in urban health usually require three or four courses and can either be a component of a degree program or a stand-alone academic experience. Some urban health programs are interdisciplinary, ensuring that students get exposure to courses and faculty from more than one discipline. Some professional organizations, such as Unite for Sight, a global health nongovernmental organization, and Southern Africa HIV and AIDS Regional Exchange (SHARE) also offer online or classroom-based certificates in urban health.[35,36]

Degree programs in urban health grant degrees in the field of urban health. For example, Northeastern University in Boston offers a Master of Public Health Program in Urban Health, and Charles Drew University in Los Angeles provides a Bachelor of Science in Urban Community Health Sciences.[37,38] These programs enable in-depth study of urban health although they require more dedicated resources than the previous approaches.

Within schools and programs in public health, medicine, health sciences, or urban professions, urban health courses and certificates may be located in departments or institutes of global health, community health, community medicine, social and behavioral health, or elsewhere.

Universities have used a variety of organizational approaches to develop urban health teaching, research, and services. These include departments, centers or institutes, offices for community engagement or public health practice, cross-cutting initiatives, or special programs. These organizational approaches offer varying opportunities for interdisciplinary teaching, experiential learning, and engagement with urban health research. Advantages and disadvantages of these approaches have been discussed elsewhere.[39]

4 Pedagogical Strategies

Just as academic institutions use different organizational approaches to provide courses on urban health, they also employ a variety of pedagogical strategies to help students master competencies.

Experiential learning immerses students in the real-life situations they can expect to encounter in professional practice. By critical analysis and reflection on these experiences, students cultivate new awareness and knowledge. Developed by David Kolb, who defined learning as "the process whereby knowledge is created through the transformation of experience," experiential learning provides urban health students with the opportunity to participate in and reflect on efforts to bring about improvements in the health of cities and their residents.[40] This emphasis on critical analysis and reflexivity distinguishes experiential learning from traditional internships and service work.

Community-engaged pedagogy seeks to bring together students and faculty with community leaders and residents to deepen shared understanding of community health problems and solutions. It is based on a deep respect for the prior knowledge and experiences that community partners bring to the conversation.[41]

Team learning, whether in classrooms or practice settings, offers students from various disciplines (e.g., medicine, public health, nursing) or life experiences an opportunity to exchange viewpoints, develop skills in communicating across boundaries, and produce reports based on collective deliberations.[42] Each of these competencies is a vital component of urban health practice.

Case study teaching enables students to critically analyze specific examples of urban health problems and interventions and to consider the relevance and applicability of this practice-based evidence. Several recent texts provide instructors and students with relevant urban health cases.[43–45]

Each of these pedagogical strategies provide opportunities to engage students in grappling with core values of urban health: a commitment to equity; a willingness to confront manifestations of racism, sexism, homophobia and other forms of stigma inside and outside the workplace; respect for differing cultures; and a capacity to listen and learn from others. By making consideration of these values an explicit part of pedagogy, urban health training programs can ensure that their graduates are prepared for ethical practice.

5 Recruitment, Pipelines, and Career Pathways

All urban health training programs need to develop strategies for recruiting students, launching them on successful career paths, and preparing graduates for lifelong continuing education. An important priority in these tasks is to ensure that the urban health workforce includes people from populations that may lack access to professional education and be underrepresented in the current workforce. A wealth of experience is available to guide these efforts.

Pipeline programs establish relationships between urban health academic programs and other organizations that have experience and capacity in reaching desired population groups. Some schools of public health have begun teaching epidemiology in high schools to interest young people in careers in public health and to mentor them for successful entry into the field, a potentially promising path for recruiting urban low-income students into public health.[46,47] Other baccalaureate and graduate programs have established articulation agreements, say, between an associate degree in community health or human service and a bachelor's degree program in public health. These agreements specify which courses will be accepted toward the higher degree, thus enabling students to avoid repeating several courses. Another approach, the result of a decade-long partnership between community health workers organizations and colleges, developed a college degree program for community health workers, enabling them to gain formal academic credentials to continue and advance in their field.[48]

At the University of Illinois Chicago, the Urban Health Program seeks to recruit, retain, and graduate underrepresented racial/ethnic minority students, specifically African Americans, Latinos, and Native Americans, in the health professions, and to expand educational opportunities for these populations at the pre-college (K–12), undergraduate, graduate, and professional levels.[49] By creating a single office to coordinate these tasks across various health professions, the university develops a capacity and the relationships needed to prepare urban health professionals across the educational and disciplinary spectrum. This is perhaps a more efficient approach than expecting each department to develop this capacity on its own.

6 Conclusion

Academic programs that are preparing the urban health workforce needed for the coming decades face a variety of challenges. The workforce includes professionals and paraprofessionals from a variety of disciplines, each with its own standards, professional organizations, and skills. While the International Society of Urban Health has been advancing the field of urban health since 2002, it does not yet have the status or reach of more established professional groups.[50] The interdisciplinary field of urban health has progressed significantly in the past two decades, but it does not yet have widely accepted theories or models, internationally recognized leaders, or well-recognized training programs. Urban health scholars have explored the similarities and differences among cities in high-, middle-, and low-income countries, yet consensus is lacking on the common and differing competencies needed by urban health professionals practicing in these different settings.[51,52]

These challenges complicate the task of preparing the urban health workforce but also provide opportunities for innovation that more established professions may lack. Over the past two decades, urban health professionals have accumulated a wealth of experience and field tested a variety of approaches to educating the workforce that will be needed. The task now is to synthesize and formalize that experience into a body of knowledge that can help to prepare the next generation of professionals who will create healthier, more equitable cities.

References

1. Institute of Medicine. *The future of public health*. Washington, DC: National Academies Press; 1988.
2. Freudenberg N, Galea S, Vlahov D, eds. *Cities and the health of the public*. Nashville, TN: Vanderbilt University Press; 2006.

3. Rydin Y, Bleahu A, Davies M, et al. Shaping cities for health: complexity and the planning of urban environments in the 21st century. *Lancet.* 2012; 379(9831):2079.

4. The Council on Linkages Between Academia and Public Health Practice. *Core competencies for public health professionals.* Washington, DC: The Council on Linkages Between Academia and Public Health Practice; 2014.

5. Kudless MW, White JH. Competencies and roles of community mental health nurses. *J Psychosoc Nurs Ment Health Serv.* 2007; 45(5):36–44.

6. Wiggins N, Borbon A. Core roles and competencies of community health advisors. In Rosenthal EL, ed. *The national community health advisor study: weaving the future.* Tucson: University of Arizona Press; 1998: 11–17.

7. International Hospital Federation. *Leadership competencies for healthcare services managers.* Bernex, Switzerland: International Hospital Federation; 2015.

8. Green LW. Public health asks of systems science: to advance our evidence-based practice, can you help us get more practice-based evidence? *Am J Public Health.* 2006; 96(3):406–409.

9. Vlahov D, Galea S. Urban health: a new discipline. *Lancet* 2003; 362: 1091–1092.

10. Schell LM, Ulijaszek SJ, eds. *Urbanism, health and human biology in industrialised countries.* Cambridge: Cambridge University Press; 1999.

11. Vlahov D, Gibble E, Freudenberg N, Galea S. Cities and health: history, approaches, and key questions. *Acad Med.* 2004; 79(12):1133–1138.

12. Sheard S, Power H. *Body and city: histories of urban public health.* London: Routledge; 2010.

13. Siri JG, Capon AG. Urban health: history, definitions and approaches. In: Iossifova D, Doll C, Gasparatos A, ed. *Defining the urban: interdisciplinary and professional perspectives.* London, UK: Routledge; 2018:175–186.

14. Gottdiener M, Hutchison R, Ryan MT. *The new urban sociology.* 5th ed. New York: Routledge; 2018.

15. Marsella AJ, Wandersman A, Cantor DW. Psychology and urban initiatives: professional and scientific opportunities and challenges. *Am Psychol.* 1998; 53(6):621.

16. Gmelch G, Kuppinger P. *Urban life: readings in the anthropology of the city.* Long Grove, IL: Waveland Press, Inc; 2010.

17. Marmot M, Wilkinson R, editors. *Social determinants of health.* Oxford: Oxford University Press; 2005.

18. Hertzman C, Boyce T. How experience gets under the skin to create gradients in developmental health. *Annu Rev Public Health.* 2010; 31:329–347.

19. Stamper CE, Hoisington AJ, Gomez OM, et al. The microbiome of the built environment and human behavior: implications for emotional health and well-being in postmodern western societies. *Int Rev Neurobiol.* 2016; 131: 289–323.

20. Low FM, Gluckman PD, Hanson MA. Developmental plasticity, epigenetics and human health. *Evol Biol.* 2012; 39(4):650–665.

21. Schug TT, Blawas AM, Gray K, Heindel JJ, Lawler CP. Elucidating the links between endocrine disruptors and neurodevelopment. *Endocrinology.* 2015; 156(6):1941–1951.

22. Trochim WM, Cabrera DA, Milstein B, et al. Practical challenges of systems thinking and modeling in public health. *Am J Public Health.* 2006; 96:538.

23. Carey G, Malbon E, Carey N, Joyce A, Crammond B, Carey A. Systems science and systems thinking for public health: a systematic review of the field. *BMJ Open.* 2015; 5(12). doi:10.1136/bmjopen-2015-009002

24. Ramaswami A, Russell AG, Culligan PJ, Sharma KR, Kumar E. Meta-principles for developing smart, sustainable, and healthy cities. *Science.* 2016; 352(6288):940–943.

25. Fink DS, Keyes KM, Cerdá M. Systems science and the social determinants of population health. In El-Sayed AM, Galea S, eds. *Systems science and population health.* New York: Oxford University Press; 2017: 139–149.

26. Koon AD, Hawkins B, Mayhew SH. Framing and the health policy process: a scoping review. *Health Policy Plan.* 2016; 31(6):801–816.

27. Randolph W, Viswanath K. Lessons learned from public health mass media campaigns: marketing health in a crowded media world. *Annu Rev Public Health*. 2004; 25:419–437.
28. Grajales III FJ, Sheps S, Ho K, Novak-Lauscher H, Eysenbach G. Social media: a review and tutorial of applications in medicine and health care. *J Med Internet Res*. 2014;16(2):e1–e13.\
29. Best P, Manktelow R, Taylor B. Online communication, social media and adolescent wellbeing: a systematic narrative review. *Child Youth Serv Rev*. 2014; 41:27–36.
30. Chaudoir SR, Dugan AG, Barr CH. Measuring factors affecting implementation of health innovations: a systematic review of structural, organizational, provider, patient, and innovation level measures. *Implement Sci*. 2013; 8(1):22.
31. Joshi A, Thorpe L, Waldron L. *Population health informatics*. Burlington, MA: Jones & Bartlett Learning; 2017.
32. Maantay JA, McLafferty S, eds. *Geospatial analysis of environmental health*. New York: Springer; 2011.
33. Wilkins EL, Morris MA, Radley D, Griffiths C. Using geographic information systems to measure retail food environments: discussion of methodological considerations and a proposed reporting checklist (Geo-FERN). *Health Place*. 2017; 44:110–117.
34. Young AF. Zika outbreak in 2016: understanding Brazilian social inequalities through urban spatial analysis and their consequences to health. *MOJ Eco Environ Sci*. 2017; 2(4):00032.
35. Unite for Sight. Certificate in urban health website. Available at http://www.uniteforsight.org/global-health-university/urban-health-certificate. Accessed May 15, 2018.
36. Southern Africa HIV and AIDS Regional Exchange website. Available at https://www.hivsharespace.net/about. Accessed May 15, 2018.
37. Northeastern University. Master of public health program in urban health. Northeastern University website. Available at https://bouve.northeastern.edu/health-sciences/programs/master-public-health/. Accessed May 15, 2018.
38. Charles Drew University. Bachelor of science in urban community health sciences. Charles Drew University website. Available at https://www.cdrewu.edu/cosh/UCHS. Accessed May 15, 2018.
39. Freudenberg N, Klitzman S. Teaching urban health. In Galea S, Vlahov D, eds. *Handbook of urban health: populations, methods, and practice*. New York: Springer; 2005: 521–538.
40. Kolb DA. *Experiential learning: experience as the source of learning and development*. 2nd ed. Upper Saddle River, NJ: Pearson Education; 2014: 41.
41. Rubin CL, Martinez LS, Chu J, et al. Community-engaged pedagogy: a strengths-based approach to involving diverse stakeholders in research partnerships. *Prog Community Health Partnersh*. 2012; 6(4):481.
42. Reimschisel T, Herring AL, Huang J, Minor TJ. A systematic review of the published literature on team-based learning in health professions education. *Med Teach*. 2017; 39(12):1227–1237.
43. Tanner M. *Urban health in developing countries: progress and prospects*. London: Routledge; 1995.
44. Vlahov D, Boufford JI, Pearson CE, Norris L, eds. *Urban health: global perspectives*. San Francisco, CA: John Wiley & Sons; 2011.
45. Novick L, Morrow C, Novick C, eds. *JPHMP'S 21 public health case studies on policy & administration*. Lippincott Williams & Wilkins; 2017.
46. D'Agostino E. Public health education: teaching epidemiology in high school classrooms. *Am J Public Health*. 2018; 108(3):324–328.
47. St. George DM, Chukhina M, Kaelin MA. Training teachers to teach epidemiology in middle and high schools. *Int Q Community Health Educ*. 2017; 38(1):65–69.
48. Love MB, Legion V, Shim JK, Tsai C, Quijano V, Davis C. CHWs get credit: a 10-year history of the first college-credit certificate for community health workers in the United States. *Health Promot Pract*. 2004; 5(4):418–428.
49. University of Illinois. Urban health program. University of Illinois at Chicago website. Available at http://publichealth.uic.edu/diversity-and-inclusion/urban-health-program. Accessed May 15, 2018.

50. International Society of Urban Health website. Available at https://nyam.org/isuh/about/. Accessed May 15, 2018.

51. Harpham T. Urban health in developing countries: what do we know and where do we go? *Health Place.* 2009;15(1):107–116.

52. Giles-Corti B, Vernez-Moudon A, Reis R, et al. City planning and population health: a global challenge. *Lancet.* 2016; 388(10062):2912–2924.

44

Urban Health

Looking to the Future

DAVID VLAHOV, CATHERINE K. ETTMAN, AND SANDRO GALEA

1 The Evolving Perspective of Urban Health

This book builds on, and hopefully advances, the arc of our thinking in urban health. The term "urban health" has undergone an evolution, from its initial narrow focus on morbidity and mortality among minorities in cities of high-income countries to a wider view of population health and social well-being in a global network of complex and interconnected urban settings. "Urban" is a now observed as a determinant of health, along with the mega trends of demography, globalization, climate change, and inequity shaping the city, and with the city's physical, social, and resource environments influencing population health. This book reports on advances in conceptual clarity and methodological refinement to inspire expansion of the knowledge base and translation of knowledge into policy and action.

2 From Isolated Cities to Complex Interconnected Networks

In 1990, McCord and Freeman created a stir when they reported a shorter life expectancy for black men in Harlem, a low-income city area within the prosperity of New York City, than for men in Bangladesh, one of the lowest income countries in the world.[1] Approaches to address these findings in the United States ran the gamut; some viewed the results as an indication of inadequate access to quality healthcare, while others considered the findings a reflection of environmentally determined forces.[2-4] Our view is that health goes beyond (but includes) healthcare. Therefore, a focus on healthcare as the core driver of health is incomplete, as is a focus on certain parts of cities. Low-income city areas, formerly called "inner cities," are part of larger jurisdictions where boundaries blur and influences blend—for better or worse. Over the past decade, this perspective has evolved and has driven research and informed policies. The framework presented in Chapter 2 builds on this perspective and serves as a guide to organize what urban health has accomplished and the questions that remain.

The classic McCord and Freeman study sharpens our thinking about equity. The physical, social, and resource environments in cities are distributed by class and geography, resulting in health disparities that are compounded and sustained by inequities in programs and policies. A simple example involves dedicated bike lanes that are designed to encourage active transportation but can heighten disparities if not built to be available to all in a way that encourages similar results. Deeper areas of inequities are seen in housing in the United States, with historic "redlining," whereby the Federal Housing Administration (FHA), which was established in 1934, subsidized builders of subdivisions for whites with the requirement that none of the homes be sold to African Americans; the FHA furthered segregation efforts by refusing to insure mortgages in and near African American neighborhoods. The Fair Housing Act of 1968 legally reversed discrimination, but what has occurred in subsequent policies and programs ("urban renewal," HOPE VI) has not erased inequity. These impacts extend well beyond housing to education, food environments, local business and jobs, and public transportation. A foundational premise informing this book is a call to move us toward cities that are fair and sustainable for all residents.

The McCord and Freeman article also agitates for a global perspective. Their comparison was framed as "worse than Bangladesh" (referencing the country and not its largest city, Dhaka) in their intent to emphasize appalling outcomes for blacks in the United States. In doing so, they aimed to shine a narrow shaft of light on disparities within New York City as a zone of privilege, but they did not cast a wider beam on similar if not worse inequities within and across other cities in the world. Our thinking has evolved considerably since then, helping us see a broader world of interurban comparisons, both within and across high- and low-income countries.

This overlap is seen in all aspects of health and how cities relate to health. Despite the Global North being already strongly urbanized and the Global South in various stages of urbanizing, simple divisions of high infectious versus chronic disease burdens do not wholly apply, as diseases like HIV, that, through advanced treatment is becoming a chronic condition rather than a fatal disease, are compounded by epidemiologic transitions to an increasing prevalence of chronic diseases.[5] Likewise, cities in both the Global North and South continue to grow radially, with encroachments on natural areas that have implications for zoonoses, decreased biodiversity of ecological systems that threatens sustainability, less arable land that has consequences for food sufficiency, and more and in many cases prohibitive expenses for sprawling infrastructure. All of this and more has global implications and affects the health of urban populations.

3 Mega Trends for the Twenty-First Century

Global mega trends for the twenty-first century affect the health of urban populations.[6] These trends include demographic changes such as population aging and patterns of migration to urban settings, globalization in finance but also in dissemination of infectious diseases, climate change with rising temperatures and sea levels, and inequalities with widening gaps in income and resources. These trends arise from, operate in, and directly affect cities and population health.

Urbanization is tied directly to demography as a twenty-first-century mega trend. In the Global South, urbanization includes migration to cities as places where residents seek to generate wealth in the formal or informal economies because cities, due to their population size and density, produce the proximity and associations needed to develop relations and markets and, due to their diversity, allow individuals to specialize their talents and levels of skills. This migration becomes more pronounced under either the pull for opportunity or the push from such forces as drought or conflict, causing population size to grow faster than the resources needed to serve and sustain the population. In the Global North, the picture of migration tends to focus more on international migrants, although the pattern of "white flight" from cities to suburbs and exurbs has shaped cities in high-income countries for decades. A substantial amount of this type of migration has now reversed, with the gentrification of increasingly desirable urban areas.

By way of example, Chapter 37 provides a detailed case study of Belo Horizonte in Brazil, describing how urbanization resulted in the creation and growth of slums that had an impact on the physical, social, and resource environments that affect population health. Founded in 1897, Belo Horizonte was built on a radial design for 200,000 people. The population grew by 55% in the 1940s, exceeding the initial urban plans for the city. In the 1960s, slums started to appear, reflecting a housing deficit, and, in the 1970s, the population grew to 1 million residents, and the city struggled to absorb this influx. The city has seen continued expansion of its periphery as its population has grown to its current 2.3 million people. Intense construction of low-income housing without basic infrastructure and resources in proximity to middle- and upper-class neighborhoods made the contrast between rich and poor more obvious. The city experiences challenges with sanitation, air pollution, transportation, and inadequate housing, all of which have significant health implications associated with an aging population and high rates of vector-borne diseases, as well as with the increasing prevalence of chronic diseases. The city has taken on these challenges with innovative strategies, as discussed in Chapter 37.

Globalization is a process by which businesses and organizations operate and develop influence on an international scale. These businesses tend to congregate and concentrate wealth in few select cities (e.g., New York, London, Tokyo). Having a limited number of cities as centers of business and wealth has consequences for unequal distribution of resources between cities in different countries, but also within a country, with unequal distribution of resources between urban and rural areas and between areas within a city. Globalization can take other forms as well, in that cities often represent travel hubs that potentiate the global transmission of disease (e.g., the severe acute respiratory syndrome [SARS] epidemic transmission from Hong Kong to Toronto).

Climate change refers to the shift in worldwide and regional weather phenomenon associated with increasing temperatures and adverse weather patterns. These changes have been stimulated by increased levels of atmospheric carbon dioxide and other pollutants. As noted in Chapter 13, cities are generators of pollutants and heat through such activities as combustion of fossil fuels for transportation, industry, and domestic heating and cooling. They also are heat islands that trap heat and maintain higher temperatures than surrounding areas because dark building materials in three-dimensional structures store and radiate heat between buildings and ground surfaces. And, because concrete surfaces are mostly impervious and do not retain water, urban areas are also less vegetated, thus reducing the evaporation and transpiration from vegetation that would otherwise cool urban areas. The increase in temperatures in urban heat islands exacerbates the effect of heat waves and results in adverse health outcomes, especially in the elderly. Another consequence of the urban heat island on global warming is its effect on increasing both ocean evaporation into the atmosphere and the amount of water vapor the atmosphere can hold. High levels of water vapor in the atmosphere can, in turn, create conditions more favorable for heavier precipitation in the form of intense rain and snow. New York City experienced two "once in a century" events—Hurricane Irene and Superstorm Sandy—back to back in 2011 and 2012, respectively, which some have attributed to global warming. The concentration of people and urban infrastructure, and for many cities, their proximity to coastlines and rivers, makes cities susceptible to adverse weather events and rising sea levels. Thus, human decisions about development of urban structures contribute to climate change and are vulnerable to its effects.

The fourth mega trend is *inequality*, which can be first measured at the broadest level. National geographic data reported to multilateral agencies (e.g., the World Health Organization [WHO]) are separated only on "urban" and "rural" categories. When these data showed that health outcomes were worse in rural than in urban areas, it influenced and prioritized bilateral and multilateral agency funding to rural areas. In the past two decades, more attention has focused on disaggregating data within urban areas.

While aggregate data show better health outcomes on average for residents in urban than rural areas, the picture changes when the data are disaggregated.[7] The case example, discussed in Chapter 36, of Nairobi, Kenya, depicts differences between national, urban, slums, and rural in reports published in 2000 and 2014, where the health outcomes in slums were worse than in rural areas.[8] Similar patterns are observed elsewhere. Disease rates in the United States in 1997 were lower on average in metropolitan than nonmetropolitan areas, which are the most common reporting schemes. When those data from the United States were disaggregated, however, rates of disease or adverse health outcomes tended to be worse in metropolitan statistical area (MSA) central cities than in MSA non-central cities or in non-MSA adjacent areas, but data also showed that the non-MSA non-adjacent (rural) and MSA central city areas were similar.[9] The pattern is changing with the "Great Inversion," where the wealthy are returning to cities and the less affluent are moving out.[10]

Inequity, or the lack of fairness, produces and perpetuates health inequalities. In disaggregated urban enclaves of the United States, prior policy on financing for housing affected the opportunity for quality living conditions (e.g., housing, food, education environments, public safety) to support health and potential. For some cities in Africa and Southeast Asia, local and national governments were resource-constrained to absorb rapid unplanned growth; in these cities, slums were bulldozed to discourage people from settling there, but they quickly cropped up again. In Brazil and Mexico, enlightened policies to promote health equity have emerged and are being piloted or tested in other countries.

4 Effects of Physical, Built, Social, and Resource Environments on Population Health Within Cities

The four mega trends discussed here shape the local physical, built, social, and resource environments that in turn influence population health. As noted in earlier chapters and distilled here, the *physical environment* includes the heat island effect and air and noise pollution, which have adverse effects, and also nature, with evidence documenting its salubrious effects. The *built environment* includes the infrastructure that has developed around the car culture and is influenced by the movement toward active transportation in the Global North and the shortage and inadequacy of housing, water, sanitation, and transportation moving toward slum upgrades in the Global South. The *social environment* includes the degrees of social capital and trust that play out in how people engage with each other and with the built environment. "Build it and they will come" applies when it is seen as safe to do so. The *resource environment* includes essential amenities such as healthcare, public health, social services, housing, education, foodscapes, commerce, and investment that can support population health.

Newer methods and approaches are providing us with perspectives that better inform our understanding of health in cities. Earlier thinking in urban health about how these discrete environments affect behavior that in turn influences health has now been enriched with complex systems analyses, epigenetics, and sensory studies. Intersecting and interacting environments each play with or against each other to affect behavior. Systems analyses using conceptual and statistical modeling techniques can assist us in clarifying the role and weight of simultaneous influences and suggest strategies on where and when to intervene. Active transportation, the food environment, safe streets, and social trust all must be considered to encourage healthy behavior. How manipulation of one affects the others can be obscure, and unintended consequences can result. Complex systems analysis provides a strategy to shape thinking on optimal design.

The earlier thinking on how the environment affects behavior in ways that affect health is incomplete in another way. Environmental exposures, such as exposure to chemical compounds, physical and psychological stress, trauma, diet, physical exercise, and many other factors, affect the way genes (DNA sequences) are ultimately expressed into a protein. A growing body of evidence on epigenetics has shown an association between exposures to environmental changes early in life and the origin of late-onset disease, including metabolic, immune, cardiovascular, and behaviorally complex disorders. In this way, the environment "gets under the skin." The disturbing aspect of this is that the effects can be transmitted to the next generation. The reassuring aspect is that epigenetic patterns change throughout the lifespan, that effects at one time may be reversible later.

Measuring how people process experiences has advanced with the continuing development of sensor technologies. In Chapter 40, on biophilic buildings, using virtual reality to create exposures that are simultaneously tracked with sensors for physiologic response was presented as a way to test environments visually. While more work is needed to create stimuli for other senses and better measures to track physiologic responses, the integration of technology to measure experience and advance knowledge is making strides.

5 The Role of Good Urban Governance and the Future of Cities

Addressing the health of people in urban settings is a complex undertaking. Creating and sustaining healthy cities takes more than programs and policies. Program funding may limit who is covered, for how long, and with what level of fidelity, and this may stir up resentments because there will be losers as well as winners. Policies are only as good as their level of design, implementation, and enforcement.

In this volume, the approach to population health in urban settings has centered on the concept of good urban governance. The WHO EURO Healthy Cities program was explicit from the outset in emphasizing that having a healthy city is a political process. Mayors have led collaborations across local government agencies to embrace Health in All Policies (HiAP), and they engage stakeholders to include civil society, commercial interests, and academia. The Urban Health Observatory in Belo Horizonte provides an example of such collaboration. The goal is to develop a collective mindset with expectation that cities, however complex, can create solutions for population health. Organizations such as WHO EURO and CityHealth provide recognition to cities that can meet certain standards.

The challenges to moving to become a healthier city can be daunting. In some countries, mayors and local governments are more ceremonial than functional, and policy is formed at the federal level. Even in countries with decentralized governments, local health departments have their hands full. When competing interests between local government agencies complicates decision-making and resource allocation, intersectoral collaboration can be challenging. When local policy is constrained by state and federal laws and regulations that were not nuanced to city circumstances, creating change or working around policies can be frustrating. Getting agreement, much less consensus, among a diverse set of constituents is demanding.

We suggest that academia can play an important role in providing expert research that is viewed as impartial and that, through engagement in communities, can empower citizens for health. Academia is vital to the process of training community health workers, health department staff, community organizers, and the next generation of transdisciplinary researchers. Beyond workforce development, expert teachers can influence and inspire a populace to embrace its role in making healthy cities.

The future of population health in cities is one of possibilities. While the imagery of mega cities is generally one of clamorous activity and visualizing them to be healthy is a formidable task of the imagination, it is one with enormous potential and possibility. Working to produce healthy cities through an understanding of the drivers of urban health will require vision, commitment, collaboration, development, and persistence. Given that cities are by far our modal form of existence, we consider this effort well worth making. We hope that this book is a step in that direction.

References

1. McCord C, Freeman H. Excess mortality in Harlem. *N Engl J Med*. 1990; 322:173–177.
2. Andrulis DP. Community, service, and policy strategies to improve healthcare access in the changing urban environment. *Am J Public Health*. 2000; 90(6):858–862.

3. Guerra FA, Crockett SA. Overcoming the hurdles to providing urban healthcare in the 21st century. *Acad Med.* 2004; 79(12):1148–1153.

4. Geronimus AT. To mitigate, resist, or undo: addressing structural influences on the health of urban populations. *Am J Public Health.* 2000; 90(6):867–872.

5. Bygbjerg IC. Double burden of noncommunicable and infectious diseases in developing countries. *Science.* 2012; 337:1499–1501.

6. Vlahov D, Ivey Bufford JI, Pearson CE, Norris L, eds. *Urban health: global perspectives.* San Francisco, CA: John Wiley & Sons; 2010.

7. Vlahov D, Agarwal SR, Buckley RM, et al. Roundtable on urban living environmental research (RULER). *J Urban Health.* 2011; 88(5):793–857.

8. Mberu BU, Haregu TN, Kyobutungi C, Ezeh AC. Health and health-related indicators in slum, rural, and urban communities: a comparative analysis. *Glob Health Action.* 2016. doi:10.3402/gha.v9.33163

9. Jonas BS, Wilson RW. *Negative mood and urban versus rural residence: residence: using proximity of metropolitan statistical area as an alternative measure of residence. Advance data from vital and health statistics. No. 281.* Hyattsville, MD: National Center for Health Statistics; 1997.

10. Ehrenhalt A. *The great inversion and the future of the American city.* New York: Vintage House; 2013.

INDEX

Page numbers followed by *b*, *f*, and *t* refer to boxes, figures, and tables, respectively.